Health Systems in Low- and Middle-Income Countries

D1555486

Health Systems in Low- and Middle-Income Countries

An economic and policy perspective

Edited by

Richard D. Smith
Professor of Health System Economics;
Head, Faculty of Public Health and Policy,
London School of Hygiene and Tropical Medicine, UK

Kara Hanson
Reader in Health System Economics;
Head, Department of Global Health and Development,
Faculty of Public Health and Policy,
London School of Hygiene and Tropical Medicine, UK

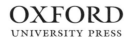

OXFORD
UNIVERSITY PRESS

OXFORD
UNIVERSITY PRESS

Great Clarendon Street, Oxford ox2 6DP

Oxford University Press is a department of the University of Oxford.
It furthers the University's objective of excellence in research, scholarship,
and education by publishing worldwide in

Oxford New York

Auckland Cape Town Dar es Salaam Hong Kong Karachi
Kuala Lumpur Madrid Melbourne Mexico City Nairobi
New Delhi Shanghai Taipei Toronto

With offices in

Argentina Austria Brazil Chile Czech Republic France Greece
Guatemala Hungary Italy Japan Poland Portugal Singapore
South Korea Switzerland Thailand Turkey Ukraine Vietnam

Oxford is a registered trade mark of Oxford University Press
in the UK and in certain other countries

Published in the United States
by Oxford University Press Inc., New York

© Oxford University Press 2012

British Library Cataloguing in Publication Data
Data available

Library of Congress Cataloging in Publication Data
Health systems in low- and middle-income countries : an economic and policy
perspective/edited by Richard D. Smith, Kara Hanson.
      p. ; cm.
  Includes bibliographical references.
  ISBN 978–0–19–956676–1
  I. Smith, Richard, 1968-II. Hanson, Kara.
  [DNLM: 1. Delivery of Health Care—economics. 2. Health Policy—economics.
  3. Health Care Sector—economics. 4. Internationalism. 5. World Health. WA 530.1]
  LC-classification not assigned
  338.4'73621—dc23
                                                                    2011030643

Typeset in Minion by Cenveo, Bangalore, India
Printed and bound by
CPI Group (UK) Ltd, Croydon, CR0 4YY

ISBN 978–0–19–956676–1

10 9 8 7 6 5 4 3 2 1

Foreword

Strong health systems are fundamental to improving the health of the world's population—rich and poor. They are also an important part of the social and economic fabric of a country and, indeed, the globe. There has been increasing recognition of their importance, and efforts to synergize activities to contribute to strengthening of health systems worldwide in recent years. However, many questions remain. What is meant by the term 'health system'? What are the major elements that contribute to a strong health system? What are the threats and opportunities facing health systems? How are events beyond the domestic health sector dealt with, by whom, and with what result?

Looking through a political-economy lens, the contributions within this book help us to construct a better understanding of health systems and an agenda that will advance the health of those in low- and middle-income countries. Combining an analysis of the economic factors which drive many of the challenges and opportunities facing population health and the delivery of healthcare, with the recognition of the political realities within which health and health systems sit, this book helps to lay the foundation for identifying how health activities may be better produced and financed.

Improved health outcomes for the poor and disadvantaged cannot be reached without a clear understanding of the part played by the various elements of the 'health system'. In today's globalized world, this means shared agendas across countries, new and different partnerships, and new funding mechanisms. It also means developing new ways of conceptualizing and thinking about how to address current and future health challenges. This book, with its in-depth, rigorous analysis of the political-economy of health systems, takes us along a key new path—a path that is essential to follow to meet our common goal: better health for all.

Anne Mills CBE MA DHSA PhD FMedSci
Professor of Health Economics and Policy
Vice Director
London School of Hygiene and Tropical Medicine
London, UK

Preface

Strengthening of health systems is firmly on the global health and development agenda. There is a growing acceptance that the improvement of population health can only be achieved if there is an adequate level of physical, human, and financial resources available to deliver services. There have been substantial movements away from investment only in 'vertical' programmes—activities solely focused on the delivery of one programme or addressing a single disease area—with recognition of the waste and inefficiencies this develops. There has thus been increasing emphasis on 'horizontal' programmes, where areas of need are addressed that are of importance for multiple vertical programmes, such as availability of physical infrastructure for storage and delivery of vaccination, and a skilled workforce. Most recently there has been recognition that 'competition' between the vertical and horizontal approaches itself is undesirable, as both are required to maximize attempts to improve global health; this has led to advocacy for a 'diagonal approach'.

This expanding research and policy space devoted to the discussion of health systems and their place in the improvement of global health has, however, often been characterized by opacity in the use of terminology and in the analysis of critical features, following the typical intellectual schism between disciplinary areas. Two of the most important of these, economics and political science and policy analysis, especially have been in operation largely independently. This confusion over the object of study—the health system—and the isolation of the method of study ultimately constrains the development of health system analysis and development.

This has raised more questions than answers, including, for example: What are the elements of a health system? What are the unique features that characterize a system? How does the health system relate to the health sector? Can health systems be compared? And so forth.

With questions such as these in mind, this volume provides the first analysis from a political-economy perspective focused upon low- and middle-income countries, recognizing the current global context within which these systems operate and the dynamics of this context. Although there are a number of volumes—books, substantial reports, and other papers—which discuss and compare the health systems of high-income countries, there is no similar comprehensive coverage of the health systems of low- and middle-income countries. Those publications also often consider health systems from a health service or health policy perspective, rather than an economic perspective. Those that consider the economic issues often do so from a very technical foundation of seeking to assess the economic impact of a specific intervention for instance. Thus, this volume brings a very distinctive economic perspective, but thoroughly grounded within the political and policy context within which the health system operates. Finally, another unique feature of this volume is that it does not focus inward on the workings of a specific domestic health sector—as so often is the case with health system analysis—but locates national health systems as being defined within the broader sectoral and international context.

The work is written from a non-technical perspective, and is suitable for a wide range of readers, including policy makers, advisers, researchers, consultants, practitioners and students in domestic and international public health, economics, and development, in both developed and developing countries.

As outlined in Chapter 1, the conceptualization of health systems taken in this volume is comprehensive and inclusive, and contains not just elements related to healthcare delivery (the typical components of health system analysis), but the wider geographical, sectoral, and temporal contextual factors that affect health and healthcare. The structure of the volume reflects this emphasis by being structured into four sections. Section 1 sets the foundation for the remainder of the chapters by outlining how a health system may be conceptualized and understood from a political-economy perspective, and focuses on the core institutions and institutional relationships that have shaped contemporary health system analysis. Having established the health sector in the wider health system setting, and considered the historical development of health systems analysis, Section 2 then focuses on the more traditional core areas of the domestic health sector, but from a political-economy perspective and with acknowledgement of this wider context beyond the domestic health sector. Section 3 then broadens out the scope again to consider the international and cross-sectoral influences on healthcare and population health, including international trade, international aid, wider social determinants of health, and global changes. Section 4 concludes by considering next steps for health system strengthening and analysis.

The first section of the volume outlines the conceptual and historical background of health systems. The first chapter outlines the breadth of what may be seen to constitute a system of influences upon health, within which healthcare sits as one element or as one subsystem amongst many. This provides the context for the remainder of the volume, arguing that health sector strengthening (which is what most advocacy is concerned with, such as human resources, physical infrastructure, or access to medicines) is one element within the wider goal of improving global health. In this respect there needs to be greater consideration of non-health sector aspects that relate to health, and how these link (including with the health sector) to form the wider 'health' system. The second chapter focuses upon outlining the historical progression concerning the thinking around health systems, and critically the nature of the relationships between key institutions at a health sector level, but within the context of this wider understanding of the health system as being 'beyond' healthcare. This leads in to the second section, which focuses upon the more traditional issues related to healthcare, but from this wider context and the political economy perspective.

Chapter 3, on measuring and evaluating performance, considers the purpose and legitimacy of the comparison and evaluation of health systems. This is a controversial area, but has seen growing popularity, itself with political dimensions. The evolution of comparative approaches is provided, and critiqued in terms of legitimacy and appropriateness given the range of wider contextual factors influencing population health and healthcare delivery outlined elsewhere in this volume.

Chapter 4, on revenue collection and pooling arrangements in health sector financing, uses as its starting point the World Health Assembly resolution calling for healthcare financing systems to provide universal coverage and financial protection for citizens. It focuses on two of the key functions of a healthcare financing system, namely revenue collection and pooling of funds. Revenue collection concerns the sources of funds, contribution structures, and the means by which they are collected, while fund pooling addresses the need to spread the risk of incurring unexpected healthcare costs over as broad a population group as possible. In terms of revenue collection, this chapter reviews the equity, sustainability and feasibility of alternative financing mechanisms (e.g. donor and tax funding, a range of health insurance mechanisms, and out-of-pocket payments) and highlights key lessons from recent research in low- and middle-income countries on these mechanisms. It also highlights the importance of carefully considering who the most appropriate revenue collection organization may be in different political contexts. The main focus of the section on fund pooling is on alternative strategies for reducing fragmentation in healthcare financing in order to maximize both income and risk cross-subsidies in the overall healthcare financing system. Such cross-subsidies are critical to achieving universal coverage and adequate financial protection.

Chapter 5 focuses on supply-side innovations in delivering health services, and their impact. Inadequate and inequitable coverage of effective health services is a common problem in low-and middle-income settings, and is a major barrier to meeting global health targets. In the public sector these problems can be traced to a combination of managerial, financial and incentive-related factors. Private providers are sometimes seen as offering greater responsiveness to patients, but may suffer from problems of low technical quality and financial accessibility. A variety of supply-side approaches have been taken to improving the performance of public and private healthcare providers. These include creating autonomous public agencies to deliver services; 'pay for performance' initiatives linked to the delivery of specific services, and a range of models for working with private healthcare providers, such as contracting and franchising. This chapter develops a classification of service delivery innovations, and reviews the recent evidence regarding their effectiveness.

Chapter 6 then turns attention to one of the two foundations for healthcare in the modern age: human resources for health. Healthcare, as a service sector, relies fundamentally on health professionals for the delivery of health services. The human resource situation in any country is the outcome of the processes in its domestic labour market and the balance between the domestic labour market and the international labour market. The negative effects of migration on source countries' health sectors has been the focus of much attention in recent years, with globalization implicated as a key factor influencing health worker migration. However, other important factors are at play, such as management practices and issues of scope-of-work and task shifting. International codes of practice encouraging ethical recruitment strategies on the part of high income countries are largely seen to be ineffective in stemming the flow of health workers from the poorest countries. The case studies presented in this chapter, from Ghana and Kenya, demonstrate the complexity of factors influencing labour market dynamics. They identify a range of actions that can be taken by source and destination country governments to address both the number of health workers and their distribution within the country.

Chapter 7 considers the other foundation of health systems, that of pharmaceuticals. Pharmaceuticals have become a mainstay of health systems, both as treatment and prevention. Pharmaceuticals comprise a significant element of healthcare expenditure, and in many public systems represent a major interaction with the private sector. They also typify the developed–developing country technological divide. Yet access to medicines, their affordability, and the impact on health expenditure are key issues facing all countries. This chapter takes a broad look at current issues facing low- and middle-income countries with respect to pharmaceutical financing, development, provision, distribution, and the policy situation facing many health systems, especially with respect to access to essential medicines.

The volume then moves on to the next section, Section 3, which focuses upon aspects related to health within the wider context, both geographically and sectorally. Chapter 8 begins this section by considering the impact of international trade on the finance and provision of national health services. Domestic health systems are increasingly the subject of interest for trade policy. Trade in health goods (especially pharmaceuticals), services (e-health, such as remote diagnostics), patients (so-called 'health tourism'), professionals (migration of healthcare workers), capital (foreign investment in health-related infrastructure, such as hospitals), and ideas (health-related intellectual property) is expanding rapidly. Many (especially middle-income) countries are positioning themselves to be leaders in one or more aspects of such trade, such as India for e-health and Thailand and Malaysia for health tourism; many through bi-lateral or regional trade agreements. Moreover, many multilateral trade agreements under the auspices of the World Trade Organization (especially GATS, TRIPS, and SPS) have implications directly or indirectly for domestic health systems. However, negotiation on these issues is predominantly undertaken by trade officials rather than health officials. This chapter reviews developments in these areas, including an overview of key trade agreements affecting health systems, current patterns of trade and major players, important demand and supply side factors influencing this trade, and policies and processes that domestic health systems may consider in response to this, illustrated by country examples and case-studies.

Chapter 9 moves on to look in detail at the impact that increases in external financing are having on health sectors and systems. Domestic health system funding is increasingly influenced by the global context and in low-income countries by global initiatives to support the financing of the health sector. This chapter outlines the global trends in development assistance to health systems in recent years, assesses the current debate on aid effectiveness and describes developments in the international finance architecture. Finally, it examines the implication of the increased attention on aid effectiveness for health systems development in the future.

Chapter 10 brings in the wider social determinants of health, building upon the concept of a health system being more than a health 'care' system by looking at work on non-health sector influences on health. The chapter reviews the broader 'social determinants of health' work, founded on work by the World Health Organization Commission on the Social Determinants of Health. This also establishes some 'boundaries' for the evaluation of health system influences, by demonstrating the relative role played by the health system viz other determinants of disease and health and linkages between health and other governance structures.

Chapter 11 takes this further through considering the wider global influences upon health. Domestic health systems are increasingly impacted upon by wider global developments. These include aspects related to environmental changes (food and water security, natural disaster, energy supplies), economic development and stability (including funding for public health services), and the general expansion in economic liberalization and international trade, the movement of people and animals and animal products (linked with, for instance, zoonotic disease), and technological change. Such developments have implications, for example, for country demographics (growing and ageing populations), demands upon the health system (from changing demographics, economic prosperity) and the supply of healthcare (public financing of health systems, provision of new technologies), communicable disease (e.g. pandemic flu) and non-communicable disease (e.g. diabetes, coronary heart disease), and trade in harmful and hazardous products (such as toxic waste firearms and weapons, and alcohol/fast food). They also involve political, diplomatic, and governance structures outside the health field. This chapter outlines the range and extent of the major external global influences upon the domestic health system, how health systems have, or may, respond to these at the domestic and global level, including country case-studies. The chapter is future looking, considering the major challenges to health systems from external influences in the coming decades, and how health systems may seek to minimize the risks and maximize the opportunities that these present, and the challenges to existing institutional structures that this will create.

The final section, Section 4, consists of a single concluding chapter to review the future of the health system strengthening movement. This chapter draws from the previous substantive chapters in the book, taking the framework from Chapter 1 as the starting point, and summarizes the major points from these chapters through specifying the key risks and opportunities that currently face health systems and will be of import in the coming decades. A specific element that comes through is the need for increased capacity in the 'missing pillar' of negotiation and diplomacy skills for health sector interaction with wider sectors that comprise the health system; increasingly at an international level.

The analysis of how the factors that affect health are linked as a system or set of systems is fundamental to the advancement of global health programmes. Challenges faced in the delivery of health services, as well as wider non-health service influences on the determinants of health, are increasingly interlinked. Critical in the strengthening of health systems is therefore to see the health sector as one element—or sub-system—within the wider geographical, temporal, and sectoral system(s) that impacts on health. Understanding the economic and political forces that drive these systems provides a framework to focus on the challenges faced, and possible solutions to, collective action concerning health system development at the global level.

This volume will assist greatly in progressing the debate concerning the analysis of health system strengthening in low- and middle-income countries. However, the contribution of this volume needs to be built upon and developed to secure novel and sustainable funding and provision of health for the benefit of all. We hope that readers will feel prompted to engage in that debate, and look forward to the next step.

Richard D. Smith
Kara Hanson
Oxford, August 2010

Contents

Section 4 **The future of health systems**

List of contributors

Lucy Gilson is Professor of Health Policy and Systems at the London School of Hygiene and Tropical Medicine, UK, and at the University of Cape Town, South Africa. Her research interests currently focus on governance and decision-making within the health sector, and how to strengthen health system leadership and management. She is also responsible for teaching in this area in South Africa and the UK.

Kara Hanson is Reader in Health System Economics and Head of the Department of Global Health and Development at the London School of Hygiene and Tropical Medicine. Her research has examined the financing and organization of health services in a wide range of low- and middle-income settings, particularly in sub-Saharan Africa. She is especially interested in the role of the private sector and its health system interactions, and in the delivery of malaria interventions.

Joseph Kutzin was at the time of writing Head of the WHO/EURO Barcelona Office for Health Systems Strengthening, where he led a team providing guidance and capacity strengthening on health financing policy and policy analysis. He is a health economist with over 25 years' experience in health financing policy and health system reform, working in Africa, Asia, the Caribbean, and Europe. He has published numerous conceptual and empirical articles as well as co authored and edited books on health financing in Europe as well as in low- and middle-income countries elsewhere. His current position is Coordinator, Health Financing Policy, WHO Headquarters in Geneva.

Rene Loewenson is Director of Training and Research Support Centre and a founder and cluster lead in the Regional network for Equity in health in east and southern Africa (EQUINET). She has worked in academic, trade union and civil society institutions at national and international level, chaired national statutory and global bodies on health, and co-ordinated and implemented national and international research programmes on different aspects of equity in health, social dimensions of health systems, and health and employment. She was strategic advisor to WHO's Commission on the Social Determinants of Health.

Melisa Martínez-Álvarez is a research degree student at the London School of Hygiene and Tropical Medicine. As part of her PhD work she is studying aid effectiveness in Tanzania. Her research interests include health systems, infectious disease, and health economics.

Di McIntyre is Professor of Health Economics at the University of Cape Town and is the South African Research Chair in Health and Wealth. Her key research interests include healthcare financing, health system equity, public–private mix issues, and health service access. She has served on many policy committees, currently serving on the Ministerial Advisory Committee on National Health Insurance. She has also contributed to health economics capacity strengthening in Africa through the health economics Masters programme, the only such program in Anglophone Africa, and through establishing the Health Economics and Policy Network.

Martin McKee is Professor of European Public Health at the London School of Hygiene and Tropical Medicine where he co-directs of the European Centre on Health of Societies in Transition (ECOHOST), a WHO Collaborating Centre. He is also research director of the European Observatory on Health Systems and Policies. He has published over 530 academic papers and 35 books and his contributions to European health policy have been recognized by, among others, election to the UK Academy of Medical Sciences, the Romanian Academy of Medical Sciences, and the US Institute of Medicine, by the award of honorary doctorates from Hungary, The Netherlands, and Sweden and visiting professorships at the London School of Economics, the Universities of Zagreb and Belgrade, and Taipei Medical University, the 2003 Andrija Stampar medal for contributions to European public health and in 2005 was made a Commander of the Order of the British Empire (CBE).

Barbara McPake is a health economist specializing in health policy and health systems research. She has 24 years' experience in these areas based in three UK university departments. She is currently Director, Institute for International Health and Development and Professor of International Health at Queen Margaret University, Edinburgh. She is one of two Research Directors of 'REBUILD', a UK Department for International Development funded Research Programme Consortium on health systems development focusing on post-conflict contexts (from 2011), and formerly (2001–6) Programme Director, Health Systems Development Knowledge Programme. She has extensive research degree supervision and other postgraduate teaching experience and extensive international experience in health systems research and policy analysis including advising United Nations agencies and low- and middle-income country governments.

Ellen Nolte is Director of the Health and Healthcare Policy programme at RAND Europe. She is also honorary Senior Lecturer at the London School of Hygiene. Her research interests are in international healthcare comparisons, performance assessment, and population health analyses.

Richard D. Smith is Professor of Health System Economics and Head of the Faculty of Public Health and Policy at the London School of Hygiene and Tropical Medicine. His research interests and experience range across many facets of health economics, most recently focusing on globalization and the macro-economics of health and health systems. He has also taught widely, and, together with Prof. Kelley Lee at the School, has recently launched a Distance Learning MSc in Global Health Policy.

Anna Vassall is a health economist at the London School of Hygiene and Tropical Medicine. She has significant experience supporting the implementation of health sector development projects in low- and middle-income countries. Current research interests include aid effectiveness, the measurement of development assistance to health and the economics of tuberculosis and HIV.

Prashant Yadav is a Senior Research Fellow and Director of the Healthcare Research Initiative at the William Davidson Institute at the University of Michigan. He also is a faculty member at the Ross School of Business and the School of Public Health at the University of Michigan. Prashant's research explores the functioning of pharmaceutical supply chains using a combination of empirical, analytical and qualitative approaches. He is the author of many scientific publications and his work has also been featured in prominent print and broadcast media. Before academia, Prashant worked for many years in the area of pharmaceutical strategy, analytics, and supply chain consulting.

Section 1

The 'health system'

Chapter 1

What is a 'health system'?

Richard D. Smith and Kara Hanson

1.1 Introduction

There has been a rapid increase in the prominence of 'health systems' in global health discourse. This can be seen, for example, in the creation of new funding streams aimed at health systems strengthening within disease-oriented programmes, such as those of the Global Fund to fight AIDS, Tuberculosis and Malaria (GFATM) and the GAVI Alliance, the activities of the International Health Partnership Plus (IHP+) which seeks to support countries to design and implement national health plans, and the working group report of the recent Task Force on Innovative International Financing for Health Systems [1].[1]

This increasing attention may be attributed to several influences. These include: concerns about system-level support required to deliver on disease-specific targets and the unintended consequences resulting from disease-specific programmes, such as fragmented service delivery systems [2]; the resurgent emphasis of WHO on primary healthcare and its emphasis on service integration [3]; difficulties experienced in some settings in making progress towards the health-related Millennium Developments Goals (MDGs) and more generally in achieving and sustaining improvements in population health [4]; and the Paris Declaration focus on harmonization and aid effectiveness as a means to limit the fragmenting effects of donor funding [5]. The result of these, and

---

[1] The international landscape is populated by a large number of global health initiatives. The Global Fund to Fight AIDS, Tuberculosis and Malaria was created in 2002 to raise resources to dramatically expand activities against these three diseases (see http://www. theglobalfund.org). The Global Alliance for Vaccines and Immunization (GAVI) was launched at the World Economic Forum in 2000 to improve vaccination coverage and accelerate access to new vaccines such as Hib and rotavirus, and evolved into the GAVI Alliance (http://www.gavialliance.org). Recognizing that immunization services require strong health system foundations, GAVI created a new funding stream for health system strengthening activities in 2005. The International Health Partnership Plus (IHP+) is a group of developing country and donor partners committed to improving health and health services by improving aid effectiveness following the Paris and Accra principles. It was launched in 2007 (http://www.internationalhealthpartnership.net).

no doubt other, various initiatives and insights has been a return to what has been termed the 'horizontal' approach to health; looking at the basic needs for the provision of health services across a range of specific disease areas [6,7]; and alongside this, efforts to 'strengthen' health systems to better meet these population health needs.

Given this increase in interest and emphasis on 'health system strengthening', it may seem surprising that there is no operational consensus or definition of what is meant by it. Rather, there are a number of different (one might say competing) approaches, generally advocated and supported by different agencies [8]. For instance, the World Health Organization (WHO) identifies six health system 'building blocks' (service delivery, workforce, information, technology, finance, governance), but it is not clear how they fit together to build a 'system'. Indeed, WHO suggests that perhaps they are formulated differently in different settings, as health systems are seen as 'highly context-specific' [9]. The World Bank approach, in contrast, is to focus upon those areas where it perceives its comparative advantage to lie—health financing, development of public–private partnerships, public sector reform, and macro-economics [10]. However, there remains, as with WHO, no clear explication of the health system they are seeking to affect and how their initiatives fit within and influence it. These represent just two approaches; there are more, as outlined later in this chapter.

We therefore face a paradox: for all this growth in interest and discussion around 'health system strengthening', there remains no clear and universal understanding of the object of such strengthening measures, nor what the implications of it are; rather, we now confront 'a proliferation of models, strategies, and approaches' to health system strengthening [11]. This raises important questions. For instance, how are we to evaluate initiatives which aim to strengthen health systems? What do we understand about factors that contribute to a strong health system? Where do the challenges that threaten health systems come from? Can we compare the relative strength or performance of different health systems? There are, of course, many more such questions.

Critical to these discussions of health system strengthening is, of course, what one understands by a health system; and within this, what is meant by health and what is meant by system. This may sound quite a simple definitional exercise, but is actually a question loaded with values, norms, and, from our perspective, aspects relating to the political-economy. In providing a context for the remainder of this volume, this chapter therefore considers the broad characteristics that may define a 'health system' and the political-economic approach to the analysis and evaluation of health system strengthening.

In this volume, we consider the health *sector* to be made up of the set of actors and activities that are primarily aimed at improving/preserving health status, at individual or population level. In contrast, the health *system* encompasses the broader range of activities that influence health. Our central message is that a clearer understanding of these broader influences, together with the complex set of interactions and linkages among them, are critical for improving population health in a world in which both sectoral and international boundaries have become increasingly permeable. The purpose of this chapter is therefore to elaborate upon, and justify, the deliberately broader approach that is taken in this volume. Before this, however, we begin by providing a brief history of the development of 'health system' thinking to provide the context.

1.2 The development of 'health systems' thinking

The history of health systems thinking is best seen as a tension between a strategy of investment in general health-related activities, supporting a comprehensive package of services, versus one of focusing on the requirements of a narrower range of services and interventions to address specific diseases.

Prior to the 1960s, the focus of the international health community's actions in low- and middle-income countries was on implementing disease programmes, such as malaria eradication programmes. Such programmes would later become termed 'vertical' programmes as they coordinated the finance, production, and delivery of healthcare only in so far as they affected the specific disease/intervention of interest. Through the 1960s, doubts began to surface concerning the nature of the impact of these programmes, and it was recognized that interventions, programmes, and policies focused upon disease-specific interventions, such as polio, tuberculosis, and malaria, relied upon a foundation of basic health service capacity within the context of their execution, in terms of physical infrastructure, human, and financial resources. Thus, a movement to advocate for investment beyond disease-focused, time-limited, service delivery contracts emerged. A seminal publication appeared in 1969 which suggested that health was not best served through sustaining such parallel, independent, programmes [12]. This was followed by others in the 1970s [13]. During this time the terminology of vertical and horizontal approaches developed, referring essentially to the extent to which programme management was integrated into general health sector management, rather than kept separate, and the extent to which health workers had one function as opposed to many functions [14]. In essence, vertical programmes (also known as categorical programmes) had their own financing, management structures, and staff. In contrast, horizontal programmes delivered a number of services through the general health service structure [15]. The 1978 Alma Ata Declaration of

'Health for all by the year 2000' marked the culmination of this thinking, emphasizing the role of integrated delivery of a comprehensive set of preventive, promotive, and rehabilitative health services, together with the participation of communities and greater inter-sectoral collaboration for health.

However, the idea of comprehensive, integrated care was soon supplanted by 'selective primary healthcare' which argued that in the context of scarce resources, greater health gains would be secured through a focus on high priority diseases and a limited package of cost-effective interventions, such as growth monitoring, oral rehydration therapy, breastfeeding, immunization, family planning, and food supplementation [16]. In many cases these disease-specific programmes adopted vertical systems of management, and they continued to attract donor funding throughout the 1980s.

What we might now recognize as 'health system reform' efforts first began towards the end of the 1980s with a number of World Bank publications, including *Health Financing in Developing Countries: An agenda for reform*, which proposed a greater role for user financing and market-based mechanisms in healthcare, and followed with the 1993 World Development Report, *Investing in Health* [17]. These reports, and the broader 'health sector reform' movement of the 1990s drew heavily on the proposals for sharpening incentives and market-oriented approaches, echoing the New Public Management reforms being adopted in some OECD (Organisation for Economic Cooperation and Development) countries (see Chapter 5).

Partly in response to a need for a more explicit evaluative framework for these and other health system reforms, the 2000 World Health Report proposed a definition of a health system ('all the organizations, people, and actions whose primary purpose is to promote, restore or maintain health') and developed a framework for evaluating health system performance, based on the three criteria of health achievement, fairness in financing, and responsiveness [18]. This health system framework was subsequently elaborated in the 2007 WHO report, *Everybody's Business: Strengthening Health Systems to Improve Health Outcomes* [9].

However, even while these analytical developments were taking place, the pendulum had already begun to shift again: the creation in 2000 of the GAVI Alliance, focusing on childhood immunization, and GFATM in 2002, marked a renewed emphasis on disease-specific programmes and a dramatic expansion in funding, particularly for HIV/AIDS. In some countries these increased funding levels for disease-specific programmes began to swamp the health sector, placing particular strain on human resources. For instance, in some high burden countries, funding for HIV/AIDS exceeded 150% of government health budgets [1]. In response to this, both GAVI (in 2005) and GFATM (from 2007) began to entertain proposals for support to health system strengthening, and the IHP+ was created to help countries develop comprehensive health sector plans. This combining of the explicit focus, targets, and goals of disease-specific programmes with the investments in general health sector strengthening needed to deliver these goals, came to be known as the 'diagonal approach'; a 'strategy in which we use explicit intervention priorities to drive the required improvements into the health system, dealing with such generic issues as human resource development, financing, facility planning, drug supply, rational prescription, and quality assurance' [19].

During these last two decades a variety of frameworks for health systems emerged; a fuller analysis of which is provided in Chapter 2. Two of the three broad approaches to conceptualizing health systems in the 1990s remained very focused upon healthcare service finance and delivery [20,21]. The third allowed the inclusion of other sectors which may affect health [22]. Two of the frameworks also highlight the relational nature of components within their definitions of a health system [21,22]. During the last decade, the most influential framework was that proposed by the WHO in its 2007 report, *Everybody's Business: Strengthening Health Systems to Improve Health Outcomes* [9]. This specified six 'building blocks', representing basic functions that a health system must carry out effectively if it is to achieve its goals. These building blocks, outlined earlier, have been used elsewhere to structure thinking, analysis and advocacy for health system support.

So, where are we now with thinking around health systems? Over the last 20 to 30 years the discourse around health systems has been characterized by two broad developments. The first is the gradual appreciation of the broader range of influences, beyond health services themselves, which affect health. The second is the movement beyond a structural or 'inventory' approach, cataloguing core elements of a health system, towards a 'relational' approach, which recognizes the relationships and linkages between such elements. Nonetheless, despite these important developments in thinking, these ideas have yet to be fully reflected in the analytical frameworks used to describe and understand health systems, nor are these ideas firmly integrated into health policy making. A third area, where there has been much less intellectual progress, is in recognizing the importance of influences originating outside of national boundaries.

Perhaps to move forward we need first to step back. The term 'health system' is, obviously, composed of two words—health and system—which both have specific connotations within different audiences and settings. In exploring what a health system is, it is therefore important to take each in turn and consider what is meant by it, which is what the next two sections turn attention to.

1.3 **Health 'system' or health 'sector'?**

Is the focus of health system activity on the health of the population, or more narrowly on the contribution that healthcare can make to it? Most health system research appears to have focused primarily on health *care* (including preventive and promotive care as well as curative care). Yet, adopting WHO's wider perspective on health as 'a state of complete physical, mental and social well-being and not merely the absence of disease or infirmity', suggests that a wider range of influences could legitimately be subject to health system research. These would encompass, for instance, aspects related to diet, employment, and friendships. In this sense, would actors, institutions, and resources that have the primary intent of improving *those* elements also count as belonging to a health system? This is a critical concern when specifying the boundaries for analysis of health systems.

Although the WHO definition of health is often seen more as an aspirational goal than an operational definition, it is important to consider what the object of analysis is, and in this case it *is* health of some description (very few would be concerned to strengthen a health system that did not have a meaningful impact upon health). The debate then concerns the aspects of health that are of relevance, and especially with respect to the elements that may influence it. For instance, Figure 1.1 provides a simple illustration of this possible breadth.

In the centre—the core concern—is individual health, which may be defined narrowly, such as cholesterol level, more widely such as a measure of overall mental or physical health, or even more broadly, including aspects of social well-being. Immediately outside of this we might think of the relationship of

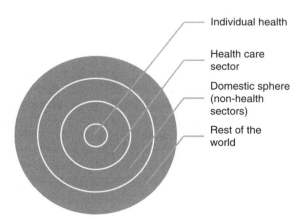

Fig. 1.1 Ever-increasing circles of relationship to health.

health to the health sector—those actors, institutions, and resources whose primary intent is to improve population health. However, beyond this there are factors related to the rest of what we have termed the domestic circumstance—the range of environmental, social, and economic factors that can impact upon health and upon the healthcare sector, and hence encircles them both. For instance, a financial crisis, such as that which occurred in 2008/9, can affect job security, employment, and government incomes. These will directly impact households, and thus indirectly their health (in a narrow or broad sense). But they will also impact on the affordability of health service provision, for instance through their effects on work-related entitlements to health insurance. The final ripple concerns aspects outside of the domestic sphere, which we have termed the 'rest of the world'. These are factors beyond the country of concern that will impact upon health directly and indirectly, and upon health and non-health sectors. For instance, an outbreak of pandemic influenza may affect individual health directly as it travels between countries. Natural disasters may increase the price of specific food items, affecting health indirectly. Currency appreciation elsewhere may make pharmaceuticals more expensive for the domestic health sector. Reduced demand for meat products in another country may reduce the agricultural sector and create health impacts associated with unemployment and urban migration.

We would suggest that a health system thus should be concerned with all the factors that may, directly or indirectly, impact upon population health; taking the WHO definition of health as the starting point. The implication of this is presented, in a simplified form, in Figure 1.2 (a more comprehensive exposition is provided elsewhere [24].

The lower half of the figure represents the individual country under consideration (the domestic sphere), and the upper half the 'rest of the world'. Taking the domestic sphere first, at the foot of the figure health looms large as the core concern for those from the health profession. Around this are the core categories of factors that together have been shown to influence health status. Thus, we have risk factors, representing genetic predisposition to disease, environmental influences on health, infectious disease, and other factors; the household economy, representing factors associated with human capital and the investment in health by individuals/households; the health sector, representing the impact of goods and services consumed principally to improve health status; and the national economy, representing the meta-influences of government structures and general economic well-being (see Chapter 2 for more on the importance of institutional structures and influences). The range of interlinkages between these factors is also illustrated. Those concerned with the health sector as a health system would thus focus on one small part of this

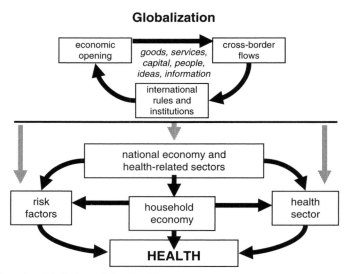

Fig. 1.2 A simplified view of the 'health' system.

jigsaw—the linkages between the health sector and health (as illustrated in the first ripple in Figure 1.1). However, as Chapter 10 demonstrates, the broader 'social determinants of health' are widely acknowledged to be significant, if not perhaps more significant, than the health sector in improving population health.

In the upper half of Figure 1.2, the influences of factors outside the national context, which we refer to in Figure 1.1 as the 'rest of the world', are illustrated, where the main linkages to the domestic context are highlighted. For example, there are a wide variety of international influences which operate directly upon risk factors for health, including: an increased exposure to infectious disease through the rapid cross-border transmission of communicable diseases; increased marketing of unhealthy products and behaviours; and increased environmental degradation as a result of increased industrialization. International linkages will also affect health through influences upon the national economy. There is an extensive literature concerning the relationship between health and wealth, and to the extent that trade influences economic growth, and the distribution of positive and negative aspects of this growth will also influence health (e.g. changes in consumption of various goods beneficial or detrimental to health). Finally, trade will affect health through the direct provision and distribution of health-related goods, services, and people, such as access to pharmaceutical products, health-related knowledge and technology (for example, new genomic developments), and the movement of patients and professionals. These aspects are considered in more detail in Chapters 7 and 8. Also of note in the upper half of Figure 1.2 is the importance of international structures for governance, both of health and elsewhere, which are discussed especially in Chapter 12. Despite comments, some quoted earlier, that health system strengthening should be encompassing and incorporate these broader factors and relationships, these voices are the minority. The majority of work around health systems, and their strengthening, continues to focus on the narrow centre of Figure 1.1, or just the bottom right-hand corner of Figure 1.2, on aspects related to the domestic health sector.

In this respect one interesting development has been the proposals for methods to assess the impact of disease-specific (vertical) initiatives on country health sectors [25]. Such methods have been termed 'health system impact assessments' (HSIAs), and focus upon the six health systems building blocks identified by the WHO. However, we can contrast the focus of these proposed HSIAs, as considering the effect of initiatives on these six elements of healthcare, with that of an alternative tool—health-impact assessments—whose use has been suggested as an approach to anticipating the health effects of proposals from sectors *outside* health [26,27]. We would suggest that in order to provide a useful analytical framework, the focus of HSIAs should be extended to encompass the interactions that run in both directions between the health sector and other sectors. Thus, for example, the provision of medicines within a health sector is affected by the price of these medicines. This is a function of national exchange rates, negotiation with the supplier/industry, levels of import tariffs if the medicines (as most are) are imported, and the result of negotiations concerning intellectual property rights and patents. These factors are explored in more detail in Chapter 7. These broad international influences lie outside the remit, control, or often sphere of interest, of the health sector. Similarly, international policies regarding trade in services, such as medical tourism, will have an effect on relative wages in the public and private healthcare sectors, with downstream impacts on the availability of nurses to work in rural areas. This is explored in more detail in Chapter 8. It is also the case that the healthcare sector has influences on other sectors that affect health. For instance, policies on whether to pay community health workers will influence local labour markets, and potentially the availability of casual labour for agricultural work during seasonal labour demand peaks.

To summarize our concern here is with the nature of the breadth of meaning in the term 'health system': whether it is applied to the broad set of elements that directly or indirectly affect health status, or the narrower set of components that comprise a typical health sector. We have suggested that most of the discussion on health systems, as indicated in Section 2, has maintained a steady tension between these two, with 'health system', 'health sector', and 'healthcare' all used fairly interchangeably. However, we would argue that a broader perspective is needed in order to allow for the possibility that these cross-sectoral effects and interactions may be substantial and may even swamp their 'primary' effects. This is not to suggest that a focus on the health sector is any less legitimate or appropriate than a focus on the wider influences on health, but that they are very different propositions in terms of the analysis and policy implications of the discussion around strengthening the health 'system'. For instance, if this encompasses more than the health sector, then it could be that efforts for strengthening to improve population health are focused more on diet and nutrition, and hence the agricultural or food retail sectors, than the health sector itself.

We would therefore suggest that it is more accurate to distinguish discussion concerning the health sector—those actors, institutions, and resources that undertake actions with the *primary intent* to improve population health— from those concerning the health system—which encompasses wider non-health sector determinants of health, and in turn, their influences upon the health sector.

1.4 The importance of the 'system'

The second crucial element in exploring health system strengthening is what is meant by system. The definition of the health system commonly used, as comprising 'organizations, people and actions whose primary intent is to promote, restore or maintain health', does not encompass well the dynamics that may be present in the linkages between elements within and beyond the health sector. There is a focus upon the elements that are seen to comprise a health system, rather than the relationships between these elements. Although there is acknowledgement that 'A health system, like any other system, is a set of interconnected parts that must function together to be effective' [9, p.4], this remains narrow in its focus upon the health sector and also does not stress the importance of the form and dynamics of these relationships. The focus remains, as Chapter 2 elaborates, a static analysis of components rather than a dynamic analysis of their interaction.

We may characterize a system as having a number of properties. Perhaps the most important are that:

- A 'system' refers to a set of elements, individuals, or organizations, connected together to form a whole and that itself possesses properties distinct from those of its component parts [29].

- Systems are nested within other systems, so change in one subsystem affects other subsystems, making it difficult to determine the boundaries of a system.

- Systems are necessarily complex and adaptive: 'a collection of individual agents with freedom to act in ways that are not always totally predictable, and whose actions are interconnected so that one agent's actions changes the context for other agents' [30, p.625].

- Multiple direct and indirect feedback loops between agents not only mean that agents influence other agents, but also that their own actions are fed back to them and this, in turn, affects the way they behave in the future. The past influences current behaviour, providing a basis for learning [31].

- Agents also belong to several systems at the same time, and membership of such systems changes over time as agents move in and out of them. So change is constant in systems.

In terms of relationships and linkages with respect to health systems, Figure 1.2 demonstrates this with the bi-directional flows between elements. Here, the solid black arrows indicate those core relationships between elements at the global or national level, many of which have been the subject of other literature and are the topic of other chapters in this volume (e.g. Chapters 4 and 5). The shaded black arrows indicate the three core forms of linkages between the global and domestic levels—between the two outer circles of Figure 1.1. For instance, global interactions are associated with changes in risk factors for disease. These will include both communicable diseases, as people and goods which are associated with such diseases (e.g. poultry and bird flu, cows and bovine spongiform encephalopathy (BSE)) cross borders, and non-communicable diseases, as changes in the patterns of food consumption, for instance, are influenced by changes in income and industry advertising (see Chapter 11). Second, as indicated earlier, global economic interaction will impact upon the domestic economy through changes in income and the distribution of that income, as well as influencing the levels of tax receipts and form of tax receipts (e.g. reduced import taxes). This will influence the household economy and also the abilities of government to be engaged in public finance and/or provision of healthcare (see Chapters 4 and 5). Finally, the health sector itself is engaged in relationships beyond the domestic borders, with trade in health-related goods and services, such as pharmaceuticals and associated technologies, healthcare workers, patients, and so forth (see Chapters 6, 7, and 8). Clearly the import and export of these will generate a variety of risks and opportunities for the health sector directly, and thus impact upon the breadth and depth of healthcare provision. Linkages and relationships are therefore critical for health systems *and* health sectors.

A critical feature of a system is that its behaviour is non-linear and unpredictable, which reflects the cultural context of policy implementation [30,32,33].

To date, the largely reductionist thinking associated with the development of health system strengthening has generate a mostly mechanical organizational and implementation model, where there is linear causality, and predictable, replicable, and knowable links between component parts, such that a focus on the components is sufficient. For instance, the 'control knob' perspective suggests linear relationships and predictable responses between health system components [34]. In contrast, a focus on the system as a whole, and the complexity associated with that, demands new thinking skills that acknowledge the complex interactions among system elements, and an ability to respond to them; these differences are highlighted in Table 1.1.

This systems approach, given the emphasis on dynamics, learning, and adaptation, also stresses the temporal context which much health systems literature does not. Elements within a system are constantly evolving their position and evaluating their relationships with others within the system. This starts from the individual level, where patients learn from their interaction with healthcare providers which influences their next consultations. It applies at the local healthcare level, where, for example, the prospect of introduction of performance targets might reduce health worker effort in order that targets

Table 1.1 Systems thinking as an approach

Usual approach	Systems thinking approach
Static thinking:	Dynamic thinking:
Focusing on particular events	*Framing a problem in terms of patterns of behaviour over time*
Systems-as-effect thinking:	System-as-cause thinking:
Viewing behaviour generated by a system as driven by external forces	*Placing responsibility for a behaviour on internal actors who manage the policies and 'plumbing' of the system*
Tree-by-tree thinking:	Forest thinking:
Believing that really knowing something means focussing on the details	*Believing that to know something requires understanding the context of relationships*
Factors thinking:	Operational thinking:
Listing factors that influence or correlate with some result	*Concentrating on causality and understanding how a behaviour is generated*
Straight-line thinking:	Loop thinking:
Viewing causality as running in one direction, ignoring (either deliberately or not) the interdependence and interaction between and among causes	*Viewing causality as an on-going process, not a one time event, with effect feeding back to influence the causes and the causes affecting each other*

Source: Reproduced from [32] with permission from the World Health Organisation.

are 'easy' to achieve in the first period, and leading to a cycle of suboptimal service delivery. It applies at the domestic level, where a decision to issue a compulsory licence leads to a medicine being withdrawn from the market in retaliation. It applies at the global level, where decisions by a wealthy country to eat more fish increases the price of fish causing less to be consumed in a poor country, who now export more, and with that extra income buy more processed food which contributes to increased levels of obesity. An emphasis on the dynamics of a system highlights the need for continual monitoring of the status of such relationships and likely impacts of actions on other parts of the system and the consequences of those, in order that the next moves can be forecast and evaluated.

In sum, our concern here is with the relationships between the various components of the health system (or the health sector as a subsystem)—their nature and how these evolve adaptively over time. We have suggested that most of the discussion on health systems, as indicated in Section 2 earlier, has focused upon elements and not the linkages and relationships between them. In doing so, this misses the fundamental importance of health system strengthening as also building capacity for those within the health professions in understanding, managing, and engaging in these relationships. The health system, or the health sector as a subsystem, requires an up-skilling in negotiation skills, at the local, domestic, and global levels. A particular gap when considering health system strengthening (or health sector strengthening more specifically) is the capacity to engage with those outside of the health sector in an effective manner. This is important at both the domestic and international levels. This is explored in more detail in Chapter 12.

1.5 The need for a political-economy approach to health systems

The prime purpose of delineating and understanding what is meant by a health system is to be in a position to provide analysis of the workings of that system, how it reacts to external shocks, and how the structure of the system itself performs in order to evaluate changes made to it. Equally critical, therefore, is the evaluative paradigm used in such analysis. As with the understanding attributed to 'health' and 'systems', the evaluative paradigm utilized in health system analysis may similarly vary in breadth, as well as in form. As highlighted elsewhere, the requirements imposed in evaluation of a complex and multifaceted system, such as described in Section 2, requires methodology that is similarly complex and multifaceted [32,35]. This has three main implications for the analysis of health systems, and health sectors as subsystems.

First, the context is critical. There is a trend towards attempting to classify or develop typologies of health sectors, grouping those that appear to have a similar structure. The (explicit or implicit) purpose of this is to indicate what the effects of changes to that structure and organization are likely to be across a range of different settings, but each with similar health sector structures. It also allows evaluation of different forms of health sector structure. However, as Figure 1.2 outlined, the complexity in the links between various aspects influencing health, and more narrowly the health sector, and the bi-directional nature of these linkages, means that such attempts to provide a typology may be fraught with problems. At worst, such evaluations may be wholly misleading as the context within which the aspects of the health system or health sector sits is critical to how it functions. At the most basic level, the structure of any health sector (and health system) will be the result of a political process, and will be influenced by the level of economic development and the structure of the economy in general; at its most crude, between a largely socialist, publicly regulated political-economy or a liberal, largely unregulated, private industry focused economy. This is explored in more detail in Chapters 3 and 7.

Second, following from the point above concerning context, the boundaries of the 'system' being evaluated will be related to the question posed, and it may be appropriate to set different boundaries for different questions. For instance, when considering the system-wide effects of a pay-for-performance scheme, it may be necessary to look beyond the influences on the health sector (e.g. looking at the interactions between health financing and health workers) to the effects on the local economy arising from changed patterns or levels of health worker remuneration, or the effects on local accountability structures of a specific form of performance monitoring. So whether it will be possible to limit evaluations of such schemes to the health system building blocks, or necessary to look more outside the health sector to local economic and governance structures, will depend both on the nature of the question and on the evaluator's prior expectations about the magnitude of such second-level effects.

Third, the political nature of health is critical. Much of the traditional evaluative approach, building upon methods designed around technology assessment and even wider public health measures, is undertaken within a broadly 'apolitical', mechanistic, context [35]. However, health and healthcare is a highly politicized area within all countries; from the design of the health sector, to policies that determine the broader social determinants of health, aspects related to the health system and health sector are predominantly political decisions and the result of a political process. To the extent that much policy development, and especially health reforms in recent years, is driven by economic and financial factors, then the political-economy nature of health systems is a core factor in analysis.

1.6 Implications for strengthening health systems

Efforts to strengthen health systems must start with an appropriate understanding of the object of their efforts. In this chapter we have argued that what constitutes a health system is broader than healthcare, and needs to encompass the wide variety of other influences on health. However, it is accepted that a more narrow definition may be appropriate for specific questions, and thus a health sector focus may be suitable. Moreover, health systems are concerned not only with the component parts (wherever the boundaries are set) but also with the relationships among the parts, the feedback loops that link them, and the process of learning and adaptation over time. This systems thinking requires new tools and models. Finally, health systems are explicitly political: this is because they are subject to political decision-making (e.g. about resource allocation, laws and regulations concerning entitlements, regulation, etc.). But the political nature of health systems is also reflected in the need to recognize the distribution of power and authority within the health sector, e.g. between patients, health workers, and their managers; between sectors such as health and the other sectors that influence health; and between nations and global level actors and institutions. Health system analysis thus needs to go beyond a narrow technocratic approach, and must recognize the contested nature of health and health policy if it is to contribute actionable new insights for improving population health.

References

1 Task Force on Innovative International Financing for Health Systems (2009). *Constraints to scaling up and costs: Working Group 1 Report.* Available at: http://www.internationalhealthpartnership.net//CMS_files/documents/working_group_1_-_report_EN.pdf.

2 Naimoli JF (2008). Global health partnerships in practice: taking stock of the GAVI alliance's new investment in health system strengthening. *International Journal of Health Planning and Management,* **21**, 1–23.

3 Chan M (2008). Return to Alma Ata. *Lancet,* **372**, 865–6.

4 World Health Organization (2005). *Health and the Millennium Development Goals.* WHO, Geneva.

5 OECD (2005). *The Paris Declaration on Aid Effectiveness and the Accra Agenda for Action.* OECD, Paris. Available at: http://www.oecd.org/dataoecd/30/63/43911948.pdf.

6 Unger JP, De Paepe P, Green A (2003). A code of best practice for disease control programmes to avoid damaging health care services in developing countries. *International Journal of Health Planning and Management,* **18**(suppl 1), 27–39.

7 Biesma RG, Brugha R, Harmer A, Walsh A, Spicer N, Walt G (2009). The effects of global health initiatives on country health systems: a review of the evidence from HIV/AIDS control. *Health Policy and Planning*, **24**, 239–52.

8 Mills A, Rasheed F, Tollman S (2006). Strengthening health systems. In Jamison DT, Breman JG, Measham AR, *et al.* (eds) *Disease control priorities in developing countries*, 2nd edn, pp.87–102. Oxford University Press and the World Bank, New York.

9 World Health Organization (2007). *Everybody's Business: Strengthening health systems to improve health outcomes. WHO's framework for action*. WHO, Geneva.

10 World Bank (2007). *Healthy Development: the World Bank strategy for health, nutrition and population results*. World Bank, Washington, DC.

11 Reich MR, Takemi K (2009). G8 and strengthening of health systems: follow-up to the Toyako summit. *Lancet*, **373**, 508–15.

12 Bryant J (1969). *Health and the developing world*. Cornell University Press, Ithaca, NY.

13 Newell KW (1975). *Health by the People*. World Health Organization, Geneva.

14 Gonzalez CL (1965). *Mass Campaigns and General Health Services*. World Health Organization, Geneva.

15 Mills A (2005). Mass campaigns versus general health services: What have we learnt in 40 years about vertical versus horizontal approaches. *Bulletin of the World Health Organization*, **83**, 315–16.

16 Walsh J, Warren K (1979). Selective primary health care: an interim strategy for disease control in developing countries. *New England Journal of Medicine*, **301**, 967–74.

17 World Bank (1993). *World Development Report: Investing in Health*. The World Bank, Washington, DC.

18 WHO (2000). *World Health Report 2000: Health Systems: Improving Performance*. WHO, Geneva.

19 Frenk J (2006). *Bridging the Divide: Comprehensive Reform to Improve Health in Mexico*. Lecture for WHO Commission on Social Determinants of Health, Nairobi, June 29, 2006. Available at: http://www.who.int/social_determinants/resources/frenk.pdf.

20 Roemer MI (1991). *National health systems of the world. Volume 1: The countries*. Oxford University Press, Oxford.

21 World Health Organization (1993). *Evaluation of recent changes in the financing of health services* (WHO Technical Report No. 829). WHO, Geneva.

22 Frenk J (1994). Dimensions of health system reform. *Health Policy*, **27**, 19–34.

23 Frenk J (2010). The Global Health System: strengthening national health systems as the next step for global progress. *PLoS Medicine*, **7**(1), 1–3.

24 Woodward D, Drager N, Beaglehole R, Lipson D (2001). Globalization and health: a framework for analysis and action. *Bulletin of the World Health Organization*, **79**, 875–81.

25 World Health Organization Maximizing Positive Synergies Collaborative Group (2009). An assessment of interactions between global health initiatives and country health systems. *Lancet*, **373**, 2137–69.

26 Swanson RC, Mosley H, Sanders D, *et al.* (2009). Call for global health-systems impact assessments. *Lancet*, **374**, 433–5.

27 Cole BL, Shimkhada R, Fielding JE, Kominski G, Morgenstern H (2005). Methodologies for realizing the potential of health impact assessment. *American Journal of Preventive Medicine*, **28**, 382–9.

28 Moon S, Szlezak NA, Michaud CM, *et al*. (2010). The global health system: lessons for a stronger institutional framework. *PLoS Medicine*, **7**(1), 1.

29 Atun R, Menabde N (2008). Health systems and systems thinking. In Coker R, Atun R, McKee M. (eds) *Health systems and the challenge of communicable diseases: experiences from Europe and Latin America* (European Observatory on Health Systems and Policies Series), pp.121–40. Open University Press, Maidenhead.

30 Plsek PE, Greenhalgh T (2001). The challenge of complexity in health care. *British Medical Journal*, **323**, 625–8.

31 Hudson J (2007). Learns lesson from policy experience. In Bochel H and Duncan S (eds) *Making policy in theory and practice*, pp.191–210. The Policy Press, Bristol.

32 de Savigny D, Adam T (eds) (2009). *Systems thinking for health systems strengthening*. Alliance for Health Policy and Systems Research, WHO, Geneva.

33 Kernick D (2004). An introduction to complexity theory. In Kernick D (ed) *Complexity and health care organisation*, pp.23–38. Radcliffe Medical Press, Oxford.

34 Roberts M, Hsiao W (2008). *Getting health reform right: A guide to improving performance and equity*. Oxford University Press, New York.

35 Smith RD, Petticrew M (2010). Public health evaluation in the 21st century: time to see the wood as well as the trees. *Journal of Public Health*, **32**, 2–7.

Chapter 2

Health systems and institutions

Lucy Gilson

2.1 **Introduction**

As outlined in Chapter 1, richer understanding of the dynamics of health sectors is necessary in thinking through how to strengthen the health system and enable performance improvements in health sectors [1,2]. To support such understanding, this chapter adopts an institutional lens in considering both the nature of health systems and ways of strengthening them.

Building on Chapter 1, five widely known health system conceptual frameworks are reviewed first. The review highlights the different types of agents, organizations, and organizational arrangements that are embedded within each framework, and seeks to identify the nature of relationships among actors, and the institutions each identifies or implies as underpinning these relationships. Second, recent thinking on health system governance—a central, but less considered, function of every health system that is particularly relevant to health system strengthening—is presented. Third, three complementary bodies of theory (organizational and policy implementation theory, and systems thinking) that draw on institutional perspectives in considering organizational functioning and change, are briefly presented and applied in critique of the health system frameworks. The critique highlights the dominance of a mechanical perspective of organizational functioning within existing frameworks, and a primarily command and control approach to health system strengthening. Finally, two alternative approaches to supporting change within health systems, both of which acknowledge complexity and seek institutional change, are introduced: soft systems methodology and strengthening trust-based relationships.

The concept of an institution is central to this discussion. Where organizations are the social settings within which activities take place, institutions are the rules, laws, norms, and customs that shape behaviour in those settings, generating patterned or shared behaviour over time among groups of actors involved in specified relationships with each other [3]. It has been argued that such institutions have three main components: the regulative pillar of rules that constrain and regulate behaviour (commonly understood to include economic incentives); the normative pillar of norms and values that confer both responsibilities that constrain social behaviour, and rights that enable social action; and the cultural-cognitive pillar of shared routines, conceptions, and frames through which meaning is made [4]. Although institutions are fairly stable social structures they can and do change over time because there is a two-way process of influence: individual preferences and values are both shaped by, and shape, institutions [3].

2.2 Conceptualizing health 'systems'

Five conceptual frameworks are discussed here, allowing examination of different and changing understandings of the nature of a health system, thus complementing Chapter 1. In order of chronological development, these are: Roemer's 1991 outline framework [5]; the World Health Organization's (WHO') 1993 healthcare financing framework [6]; Frenk's 1995 relational framework [7]; WHO's 2007 version of the building block framework [1]; and Roberts et al.'s 2008 'control knobs' framework [8].

2.2.1 A focus on healthcare or on health?

Of these five frameworks, three focus squarely on healthcare and health services [5–6,8]. Only two encompass activities relevant to promoting, restoring, or maintaining health (but see also [9], discussed in Chapter 10). The Frenk framework [7], for example, includes other sectors and their production of services with health effects. It also gives the population, through community participation, a role in and influence over healthcare organizations, as well as recognizing its role in providing people, money, and data for the overall system. The broader focus of the WHO building block (WHO BB) framework [1] is more hidden. However, it describes the health *information* system as encompassing the collection and use of information on 'health determinants, health systems performance and health status', and notes that leadership/governance includes concern for the health-promoting actions of other government sectors.

2.2.2 An inventory or relational approach?

Both the WHO BB framework [1] and Roemer [5] appear to adopt an inventory approach [7] to understanding a health system: that is, they identify a set of core functions but do not specify the health system actors engaged in these functions nor the relationships among them. Figure 2.1, thus, gives no sense of the interactions among health system building blocks, nor how they impact on performance outcomes. Similarly, although Figure 2.2 signals interactions among a set of five health system functions that result in service delivery,

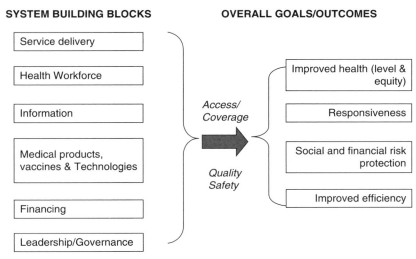

Fig. 2.1 WHO BB [1] framework.
Source: Reproduced from [1] with permission of the World Health Organization.

it does not clarify their basis or nature: 'These types of approaches are helpful for describing health systems… However, the categorizations are less helpful for understanding how well health systems perform. This would require more detailed subcategories and greater elaboration of the relationships within each category but particularly between categories' [10, pp.514–15].

Nonetheless, the report presenting the WHO BB framework notes that 'A health system, like any other system, is a set of inter-connected parts that must function together to be effective. Changes in one area have repercussions

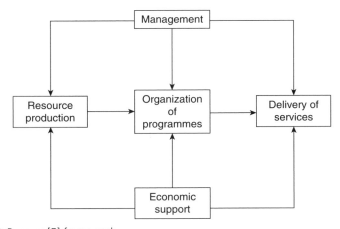

Fig. 2.2 Roemer [5] framework.
Source: Reproduced from [5] by permission of Oxford University Press.

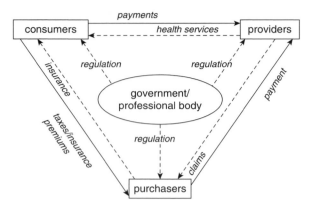

Fig. 2.3 WHO HCF [6] framework.
Source: Reproduced from [6] with permission of the World Health Organization.

elsewhere. Improvements in one area cannot be achieved without contributions from the others. Interaction between building blocks is essential for achieving better health outcomes' [1, p.4]. This relational nature of health systems is more clearly represented in the next two frameworks discussed.

Four functions required in any health system (regulation, financing, resource allocation and service provision) are identified in the WHO healthcare financing (HCF) framework [6] (Figure 2.3), as well as four agents and the relationships among them that underpin the functions. Although not discussed in any detail, the figure also highlights the key institutions that shape these relationships: regulatory authority (based on rules and involving sanctions or economic incentives); payments by patients/population (economic incentives); and provider claims on financing agents (underpinned by rules) (Box 2.1). In a further specification of the framework, government's regulatory role is noted to include structuring the system in line with social consensus on the ethical principles (e.g. ability to pay or social rights) on which it is founded [10].

A more complex set of dynamics among elements of the health system, and between them and the external environment, are represented in Frenk's framework [7] (Figure 2.4).

In illuminating this complexity, the framework highlights, first, the various roles played by the state (the collective mediator), noting that 'there are many public agencies that are not part of the health system per se, but that constitute a key element of its organizational environment. This is the case of the legislative and judicial branches of government, as well as the executive officers dealing with public budgets, taxation and law enforcement. We may conclude, therefore, that the state occupies multiple positions in the health system and its environment' [7, p.27]. Figure 2.4 shows that the state exercises control over health sector agents (here, healthcare providers and resource generators),

Box 2.1 Health system relationships and their institutional bases [6]

- *Government/professional body and providers*: regulatory authority used to secure, e.g. available and good quality service provision to patients.

- *Government/professional body and financing agents*: regulatory authority used to, e.g. contain costs for patients (controlling pricing and reimbursement levels).

- *Patients and providers*: financial payments exchanged for service provision.

- *Population and financing agents*: financial payments exchanged for insurance coverage.

- *Providers and financing agents:* claims (based on service provision to clients) exchanged for resource allocation (using funds raised from the population).

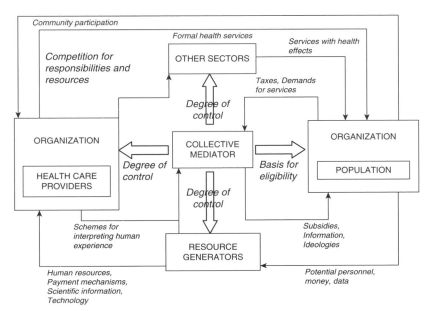

Fig. 2.4 Frenk [7] framework.
Source: Reprinted from [7] with permission from Elsevier.

through some combination of financing, regulation and direct delivery of services (in effect, ownership). However, it also exercises control over other sectors (recognizing variations among systems in the degree to which broader health promoting functions rest in other sectors) and explicitly acts as the mediator between patients and providers. Finally, the state's relationship to the population involves, on the one hand, offering the subsidies, information, and ideologies that shape population interactions with the health sector and, on the other hand, is based on the basic eligibility principles on which the health sector is founded (which vary between countries from purchasing power, to poverty, to the socially perceived priorities accorded particular population groups, to citizenship). The relationship between the state and the population is thus itself influenced by the prevailing sociocultural norms or consensus that is embedded in these principles.

Indeed, the second layer of complexity embedded in Figure 2.4 is its recognition of both the layers of exchange embedded within health system relationships and the range of institutions underpinning them. Considering the relationship between the population and healthcare providers, Figure 2.4 indicates that the provision of taxes and demand for services is exchanged for service delivery. However, the figure also shows that the population not only receives services from providers, but also participates in decision-making *with* healthcare providers, or *about* them. The nature of these exchanges suggest that the underpinning institutions are likely to comprise economic incentives, the rules of decision-making and the norms and values demonstrated by each actor through the experience of decision-making. Healthcare providers, for example, not only deliver care to the population, but also offer frameworks for interpreting human experience to patients. Frenk [9, p.27] explains these as 'alternatives to magical and religious explanations [presumably of health and illness] that can be used to legitimize modernizing ideologies and to exercise control over the population (for example, in such cases as infectious diseases and mental disorders)'. Providers, thus, offer new frames of understanding, new norms, to shape health seeking behaviour and legitimize healthcare interventions. Finally, as members of the population and individual providers belong to various organizations at the same time, these organizations (the interests of which may themselves conflict) also influence their members' interactions with other actors.

2.2.3 Descriptive, analytical, or predictive?

The four frameworks so far presented either describe health system components [1,5], or support analysis of their functions and operations [6,7]. The framework of Roberts et al. [8], illustrated in Figure 2.5, goes further, seeking

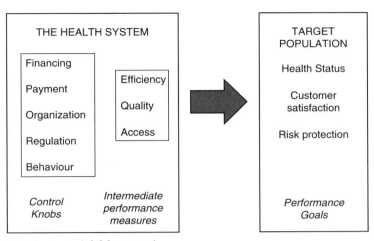

Fig. 2.5 Roberts et al. [8] framework.
Source: Reproduced from [8] by permission of Oxford University Press, Inc.

to answer the question, 'what factors influence how well the functions perform in a system?' [2, p.9].

Focused only on healthcare, this framework identifies five 'control knobs' that can be adjusted by government action to influence the relationships among health system elements. Although several of these knobs resemble the functions of other frameworks, they are seen here as 'power mechanisms' through which actors adjust the health system and generate measurable changes in system outcomes [2]. As Table 2.1 illustrates, they do this by adjusting the institutional drivers of the behaviour of health system agents.

Table 2.1 The institutional drivers underpinning the control knobs framework

Control knob	Influences
Financing	Who pays and who benefits from health care, as well as generating funding for the system as a whole;
Payment	The ways in which money is transferred to health care providers, creating financial incentives influencing how they behave;
Regulation	The use of state coercion to control the behaviour of other actors within the system;
Organization	The incentives for the organization; and the incentives, authority, skills and attitudes of both managers and workers; and
Behaviour	Information provision and marketing, incentives and coercion shaping how patients and providers act in relation to health and health care (addressing treatment seeking behaviours, health professional behaviours, and patient compliance, lifestyle and prevention behaviours).

The health system strengthening interventions highlighted by this framework include those discussed in the health reform debates of the 1990s [10,11], such as financing, resource allocation, regulatory and service delivery reforms. Possible organizational reforms include changing: the mix of organizations or division of tasks among them, through, for example, privatization; the interactions among health sector agents and their relationship with the rest of the system, through strategies that change incentives such as competition or contracting out; or what happens inside healthcare organizations through decentralization, total quality management, and other types of management strengthening or corporatization. Reforms focused on the behaviour knob, meanwhile, include quality improvement programmes targeting provider behaviour and social marketing programmes targeting patient behaviour. In broad terms, this knob acknowledges the importance of provider–patient and state–patient relationships in overall health sector and system performance.

However, Roberts et al. [8] emphasize that achieving performance and equity improvements also demands paying careful attention to six steps in the reform process:

1 Clarifying goals and related policies, prioritizing among the range of performance outcomes through ethical reflection, as well as political and technical analysis of feasibility.

2 Carrying out an honest diagnosis of current problems, to identify where action is required.

3 Developing a plan that can be realistically expected to work in a specific national context; recognizing also that the process of plan development will itself influence its acceptability to key actors and interest groups.

4 Embracing politics: health sector change affects interest groups differently and is subject to broader contextual changes, so all reform processes require active political management.

5 Focusing on implementation, as health sector actors often resist change, either from self-interest or anxiety, and it is always necessary to keep an eye on results and outcomes.

6 Learning from mistakes—even successful reform generates new problems.

2.2.4 Recognizing international influences?

None of these five frameworks consider international influences. Yet, as discussed in more detail in other chapters (especially Chapters 8–11), international factors directly impact on national health systems, through trade in goods, services, and people, and related international agreements, bio-technological advances, and through levels of, and approaches to, channelling, financial and technical support. They also indirectly impact on the causes of disease, to which health systems must respond, and, by influencing the wider economic situation, on national health funding levels. Finally, international factors have influenced the institutional underpinnings of health sectors: for example, the market-oriented health sector reforms promoted by international agencies have implications for the eligibility principles (or social contract) of some national health sectors [12]. Future conceptualization of health systems must, therefore, recognize that national health systems are open systems that interact with their external environment, including international factors (for example, by adopting the systems thinking approaches discussed later).

2.3 **Governance and governance reforms**

Although not well reflected in Figure 2.1, the function of governance is sometimes portrayed in the WHO BB framework as the central point around which the other building blocks turn (reflecting the collective mediator of Frenk [7], Figure 2.4). Synonymous with the notion of stewardship, it involves the protection of the public interest or 'the careful and responsible management of the well-being of the population' [13, p.2]. More specifically, governance involves guiding the whole health sector through six subfunctions that emphasize both some areas of health sector reform and the need to pay attention to the reform process (Table 2.2).

However, an explicit focus on governance also offers new insights about health system relationships and the actions required to strengthen them. The dominant institutions underpinning these relationships are not economic incentives and regulatory rules. Instead they are the rules, norms and values that confer responsibilities and rights. These 'can be both formal, embodied in institutions (e.g. democratic elections, parliaments, courts, sectoral ministries), and informal, reflected in behavioural patterns (e.g. trust, reciprocity, civic-mindedness)' [14, p.3]. Power is also recognized as a dimension of relationships, with the state and providers seen to be generally more powerful than citizens. The focus on governance, thus, clearly highlights the normative institutional pillar of any health system.

From this perspective, health governance is about putting in place effective rules that 'condition the extent to which the various actors involved fulfil their roles and responsibilities, and interact with each other, to achieve public purposes' [14, p.3]. When these interactions operate well they ensure:

1 Some level of accountability of key actors to the beneficiaries and broader public;

Table 2.2 Leadership and governance sub-functions [1]

Subfunction	Tasks
Policy guidance	Formulating sector strategies and also specific technical policies
	Defining goals, directions, and spending priorities across services
	Identifying the roles of public, private, and voluntary actors and the role of civil society
Intelligence and oversight	Ensuring generation, analysis and use of intelligence on:
	Trends and differentials in inputs, service access, coverage, safety;
	Responsiveness, financial protection and health outcomes, especially for vulnerable groups;
	The effects of policies and reforms;
	The political environment and opportunities for action; and
	Policy options.
Collaboration and coalition building	Across sectors in government and with actors outside government, including civil society, to:
	Influence action on key determinants of health and access to health services; and
	Generate support for public policies; keep the different parts connected—so-called 'joined up government'
Regulation	Designing regulations and incentives and ensuring they are fairly enforced
System design	Ensuring a fit between strategy and structure and reducing duplication and fragmentation
Accountability	Ensuring all health system actors are held publicly accountable
	Transparency is required to achieve real accountability

2 A policy process that engages key and competing interest groups on equal terms (given fair rules of competition), and allows negotiation and compromise among them;

3 Sufficient state capacity, power and legitimacy to manage policy making and implementation processes effectively; and

4 Engagement by non-state actors in policy processes, service delivery partnerships and in oversight and accountability.

Health system governance must, thus, seek to strengthen the critical processes through which norms and values are demonstrated, and rules established. Reflecting Table 2.2, such action might include: more effective engagement with policy actors and better use of information in the policy process (influencing interactions between citizen and state, and state and providers);

enhanced community participation (influencing interactions between citizen and state, and citizens and providers); and increased accountability and transparency, reducing corruption (influencing interactions among all three sets of actors).

2.4 Insights from wider theory relevant to health systems debates

The insights of three different and overlapping bodies of conceptual thinking are briefly presented in this section, and used both to examine the health system frameworks and think further about health system strengthening.

2.4.1 Understanding organizations

Although not a comprehensive theoretical overview (for that see, e.g. [15]), Table 2.3 summarizes three perspectives which illuminate different facets of organizational realities [16]. The machine perspective sees organizations as hierarchical arrangements of defined components that work together efficiently and reliably, as in an idealized bureaucracy. The variability of human behaviour is more or less written out of organizational life in this perspective. Instead, as Table 2.3 suggests, people working within an organization are assumed simply to comply with changes, responding to the exercise of organizational authority and related rules and procedures. The economic perspective, meanwhile, suggests that rather than controlling people through rules, 'the self-interested behaviour of people needs to be taken into account in the structuring of institutional arrangements... [and also]... provides a means of control and motivation' [16, p.15]. This perspective suggests that economic incentives rather than rules represent the institutional basis of organizations.

The WHO BB [1] and Roberts et al. [7] frameworks (Figures 2.1 and 2.5) seem to reflect the institutional understandings of some combination of these two perspectives; and the WHO HCF framework [6] (Figure 2.3) clearly reflects the economic perspective. Not surprisingly, therefore, the health sector reforms they emphasize (see Table 2.3) include standardized packages (such as decentralization, packages of care), those intended to encourage market-type relationships or strengthen financial incentives and the use of scientific evidence to identify the best technical solutions.

The sociocultural perspective, in contrast, sees organizations as networks or clans. It emphasizes that the behaviour of those working in organizations is fundamentally influenced by social relationships, and by both the norms and values *and* shared social meanings embedded in them. A growing body of empirical evidence also confirms this unpredictable human element within

Table 2.3 Three perspectives of organizational life

		Machine perspective	Economic perspective	Sociocultural perspective
Theoretical considerations	View of organization	Clearly defined parts working efficiently together in routinized ways	Atomistic economic actors engaged in market relations	Reflective, responsive people forming a complex social system
	View of human behaviour	Compliant: Humans simply comply with organizational changes	Calculating: Humans are individualistic and motivated by self-interest	Social: Human behaviour is influenced by social networks and relationships
	Organizational form	Hierarchy/bureaucracy	Market	Social network/community/clan
	Coordinating mechanisms	Formal rules and procedures Authority	Prices Competition Financial incentives	Norms Values Trust Shared meanings
	Institutional pillar	Regulative	Regulative	Normative Cultural-cognitive
Links to health system reform debates	Reforms of focus	Standardized packages such as: Restructuring, decentralization Scientific search for best technical solutions	Modify incentive structures through: Privatization, outsourcing, internal markets, competition, performance management	Strengthening norms and values Democratization

health systems. In Nepal, for example, the contradiction between the values-in-use of district health staff and the values expected to support bureaucratic functioning resulted in training interventions rarely improving performance [17]. Similarly, there is Indian evidence that the disjunctions between the ideals and practice of heath system supervision and disciplinary action reflect local level norms and power relations [18]; and evidence from Pakistan shows how societal gender norms infuse health system management, making working life difficult for female health workers [19].

This sociocultural organizational perspective is most clear in Brinkerhoff and Bossert's governance framework [14], although that tends to emphasize rights and responsibilities over shared social meanings as the institutional basis of health systems. The Frenk framework (Figure 2.4) also acknowledges social relationships, values and a range of institutional influences over behaviour, but the Roberts et al. framework (Figure 2.5) only hints at this perspective (in highlighting the importance of managerial changes in promoting better performance, in combination with economic incentives).

2.4.2 Understanding policy implementation

Policy analysis theory broadly considers how ideas, interests, and institutions play out in policy-making and includes theoretical perspectives on the processes of policy implementation. Understanding implementation as the interaction between policy and action, this body of theory is clearly relevant to thinking about how to strengthen health systems and has overlaps with organizational theory (see Table 2.4).

The mechanical model of implementation, for example, reflects the organizational machine perspective and both are rooted in reductionist thinking that simplifies complexity by dividing a problem into subproblems. In implementation this process is translated into a rational planning and management approach involving a linear sequence of activities controlled by policy actors at the centre or top of the organization [20]. Working through economic incentives rather than rules, the economic perspective on organizations also commonly assumes such a top-down approach to reform implementation [21].

In contrast, the cultural model of the policy-action relationship reflects the sociocultural perspective on organizations, illustrating the ways in which the human dimension of organizations plays out in policy implementation. This model and related work showing the influence of organizational culture on organizational performance [22,23], emphasize the influence of shared social meanings over policy implementation. The political model (Table 2.4), meanwhile, reflects a more political view of organizational life than so far discussed. It emphasizes the power relationships among actors between and within organizations,

Table 2.4 Models of policy implementation

The mechanical model
Central actors have power, working as controllers
Only central actors learn
Other components (departments, organizations, people) of a system are connected through static and predictable mechanisms
To bring about change central actors apply a new mechanism from above

The cultural model	The political model
Human beings are meaning makers and act on the basis of their own understandings, and interpretations of events	All system actors have their own interests and preferences, and seek to use their power to influence outcomes of system
In making meaning, they draw on a stock of shared social meanings about specific issues, including the language of politicians and policy makers	Actors at the bottom of the system, including citizens, always have discretionary power (actors at the top cannot control every action)
These social meanings shape how people respond to new ideas and policies	Power is not necessarily used for personal gain, but how it is used influences outcomes
Public managers and professionals draw on and use these meanings in making policy in their own environments	Policy and delivery is a result of power balances and of the strategies used by actors

Source: Derived from Open University teaching materials on the Policy-Action relationship. Available at: http://labspace.open.ac.uk/mod/resource/view.php?id=179001 (accessed 2 August 2009)

including the discretionary power of implementing actors who work at the local level, such as front-line providers [24], and of beneficiaries [25]. Environmental health officers in Ghana [26], for example, and community health workers in Brazil [27], exercised their power to support policy implementation; whereas in South Africa [28] and Tanzania [29] resistance from local level health workers and managers undermined the achievement of policy objectives.

These two implementation models suggest, therefore, that policy implementation is a much more negotiated and contested process than that envisaged in the mechanical model. Indeed, where this latter model suggests that implementation can essentially be commanded by those at the top, the bottom up perspectives of the other models indicate that implementation should be regarded as '…a policy-action dialectic involving negotiation and bargaining between those seeking to put policy into effect and those upon whom action depends… Policy may thus be regarded as a statement of intent by those seeking to change or control behaviour, and a negotiated output emerging from the implementation process' [21, p.253].

Given their largely mechanical and economic bases, health system frameworks are, however, often linked to a rational and top down perspective on how to implement change [30]—even when recognizing the importance of managing the politics of change. The institutional bases of resistance to, and so contested processes of, implementing change within health systems are essentially ignored.

2.4.3 Understanding systems

The ways in which 'systems thinking' see any system, including a health system, was highlighted in Chapter 1. Although more widely recognized in high-income countries, such thinking is only just beginning to influence work of relevance to health systems in other settings. The approach offers new insights into the complex and relational nature of health systems and their sociocultural bases, going well beyond the complexity presented in the Frenk [7] framework.

Of particular relevance to this discussion, and reflecting the sociocultural organizational perspective and the cultural model of policy implementation, is the insight that agents in a system respond to their environments using internalized rules, 'instincts constructs, and mental models' [31, p.626]. In the form of institutional memory, some rules are shared across a system, but others may not be shared and may change over time. Emerging from the interactions among its agents, the behaviour of the system is, therefore, often unpredictable, generating unexpected (and sometimes creative) outputs [32].

Further comparison of a systems thinking perspective on organizations with that of the machine and economic/market perspectives, shows different understandings of relationships and diversity (Table 2.5). It also makes clear the systems thinking contributions on learning, power and the importance of the local, rather than central, level. Reflecting bottom-up implementation theory, a systems thinking perspective suggests that efforts to implement policy through a top-down approach are 'doomed to failure because policy makers neither command nor control the whole of the system. Worse still attempts to impose command and control can end up destroying the system's ability to adapt—or, in other words, restrict its ability to learn and adapt in the face of a changing environment' [33, p.203].

Atun and Menabde [34] argue that the characteristics of health systems, such as the many interacting feedback loops and the unpredictability of intervention outcomes, clearly show the relevance of systems thinking to health systems. The health system barriers to TB DOTS implementation in the Russian Federation, for example, included the inherent disincentives created by existing financing and provider payment systems and organizational structures, as well as the political difficulties of required reductions or re-allocations of staff posts and the sociocultural norms which underpinned staff resistance

Table 2.5 Comparing systems thinking with other organizational perspectives [35, p.101]

Principle	Machine (linear hierarchy)	Market (linear network)	Ecosystem (non-linear network)
Relationships within the system	Simple, static, pre-set	Contractual; directed by price, supply and demand	Diverse and dynamic
Relationship to the environment	Closed	Relatively open	Open
Diversity of elements	Static diversity designed in	Some diversity of elements, little diversity of structure or process	Diverse elements, structure and processes continually changing
Knowledge management	Intelligence designed into the machine and remains fixed	A degree of learning	Learning perspective
Power	Power remains at the top of the hierarchy and is generally unresponsive	Power resides with the larger player and is responsive to resources	Power and influence are distributed locally and reside in relationships
Strategic focus	Little strategic focus	Some strategic focus, particularly by major players	Emphasis is on local level

to an externally developed programme. Thus, 'the context, the interaction between health system elements and context-health system interactions affect the way rules norms and enforcement mechanisms are interpreted to generate response that may not be easy to predict and may indeed be counter-intuitive' [34, pp.133–4]. Importantly, context is understood here as encompassing the values, norms, and understandings shaping the behaviours and relationships of heath system actors, rather than only referring to more material and structural factors [36].

2.4.4 **Summary**

All three bodies of theory presented here affirm the relational nature of health systems and the wide range of institutional influences embedded within them. The drivers of actor behaviour go beyond rules and financial incentives to include their relationships with others, the wider set of norms, values, and, importantly, shared meanings that underpin those relationships, and conflicting interests and relative power. Policy implementation theory and systems thinking also emphasize the importance of the local, rather than central, level in strengthening systems. Local level forces are the vital influences over system performance, and local actors, the ultimate implementers of any policy change.

In contrast, as Table 2.6 shows, current health system frameworks are imbued with a mechanical perspective on health systems, and a command and control approach to health system strengthening. The relational nature of the health system, its dynamic complexity, is perhaps most fully reflected in Frenk [7] and Brinkerhoff and Bossert [14] frameworks. However, neither offers much guidance on how to work with that complexity in seeking to strengthen health systems.

Table 2.6 Summary review of health system frameworks

Framework	Institutional drivers considered?	Recognizes relational nature of health system? (dynamic complexity)	Assumes command and control approach to HSS?	Recognizes role of local level?
Roemer [5]	None	No	n/a	No
WHO HCF [6]	Rules and incentives	Partially	Implicitly yes	Not clearly
Frenk [7]	Rules, incentives, sociocultural norms and values	Yes	Unclear	Not clearly
WHO BB [1]	None	No (though implied in text)	Largely; need for political management noted	No
Roberts et al. [8]	Rules and incentives emphasized; power acknowledged	Partially	Largely; notes need for political management and for participatory diagnosis and planning	Unclear
Brinkerhoff and Bossert [14]	Rules, socio-cultural norms & values, power influences	Partially	No	Partially

2.5 **Enabling system governance**

The bodies of theory examined in Section 4 suggest that health system strengthening will be better supported by participatory implementation approaches that seek to manage meaning and strengthen the norms and values shaping actor behaviour, rather than working primarily through rules, authority and economic incentives. But how can local level actors be engaged? Two complementary insights are drawn from the theoretical perspectives considered here.

First, a systems thinking perspective suggests that problem-solving must be based on testing and learning from action, rather than predominantly applying reductionist and rational approaches. The complexity of systems makes anticipating problems almost impossible. Instead systems must support local-level learning over time by encouraging open relationships and free exchange among system actors [32]. Such learning is 'more about problem coping than problem solving' [33, p.21].

Systems thinkers argue that whilst central planners ought to establish the general direction of the change they seek and the limits of the change they would find acceptable, they should allow local flexibility in achieving those goals and in resource use. Learning is fostered by encouraging experimentation, diversity, and reflection—and embracing both success and failure [37, 38].

Soft systems methodology (SSM) is an approach to such learning. It is particularly relevant where operational staff are seen to be influential and their ownership of improvements is essential for bringing about change [37], or where managers within organizations are willing to learn from the new ideas and perspectives of actors outside the system [33]. Undertaken by those directly involved in the area of concern, it involves groups of people working together to: explore the problem situation; develop an idealized model of how to transform it; identify the feasible and desirable changes required to bring about such transformation; taking any of those actions that they can; and, finally, reflecting and repeating the cycle of action and learning.

There are three key aspects of SSM analytical approaches and tools. They require iterative processes of action and learning. They allow multiple perspectives to be gathered about current challenges and ways of working differently. They seek to understand the complex chains of interactions underlying current problems as a basis for identifying the key points through which managerial action can leverage cycles of improvement. Some tools also allow consideration of who has to act differently in bringing about improvement. Hard analytical methods, such as cost-effectiveness analysis, may be used depending on the nature of the problem [39]. Nonetheless, the main strength of SSM 'is its ability to bring to the surface different perceptions of the problem and structure these in a way that all involved find fruitful. Because the process is strange to most participants, it also fosters greater openness and self-awareness. The process is very effective at team-building and joint problem-solving' [37, p.76]. On this basis, a ten-step approach to designing and evaluating health system strengthening interventions that is rooted in wide stakeholder involvement, including front-line providers, and knowledge sharing has been proposed [38].

Second, trusting relationships are commonly acknowledged as a critical basis for encouraging learning. 'For individuals to give of their best, take risks and develop their competencies, they must trust that such activities will be appreciated and valued by their colleagues and managers. In particular, they must be confident that should they err they will be supported, not castigated. In turn managers must be able to trust that subordinates will use wisely the time, space and resources given to them through empowerment programmes and not indulge in opportunistic behaviour. Without trust, learning is a faltering process' [40, p.65]. Trust is also identified, along with rules and contracts, as one of three possible bases for policy implementation and local management [41]. Indeed, given the distribution of power within them, implementation (or co-production) through local actor networks within and across organizations requires a more persuasive approach to management than that associated with rules or contracts.

Trust is often seen to be of particular importance to health due to the uncertainty and unpredictability of ill-health, and the influence of trusting relationships over caring behaviour [42, 43]. For instance, four detailed South African case studies of primary care facilities showed widespread distrust in the employer. Yet in the two better performing facilities (as assessed by healthcare managers, health facility users, and researcher observation), there was also higher staff motivation levels (assessed qualitatively), some degree of trust in colleagues and the manager was widely trusted. In contrast, in the worse performing facilities, there were lower staff motivation levels and little trust in colleagues or the managers [44].

Although not yet well developed, ideas about how to develop trust within health sector relationships highlight the importance of strengthening both inter-personal behaviours and the institutions shaping them. Relevant inter-personal behaviours include competence, sincerity, empathy, altruism, fairness and reliability; and these are enabled by institutions that allow the trustor to judge whether the trustee will act in her best interests or, at least, without malice. Such institutions encompass all three institutional pillars: organizational roles and procedures, rules and legal frameworks, and the communication and decision-making practices that generate shared meanings. They generate, in particular, information about how people are treated by others and the values driving their behaviour, and support the development of mutual understanding and shared interests. Indeed, it is often said that trust is constructed through use and worn out by dis-use [45].

In thinking about how to develop trust it is also necessary to acknowledge power: whilst trust may provide the basis for the exercise of legitimate power, trusting too much, without caution, may lead to the abuse of power [45]. Thus, where communication practices are strongly influenced by the underlying power relationships between actors, trust may be coerced and so illegitimate. Voluntary trust can only be generated when communication is 'sincere, open and directed towards achieving understanding and consensus' [46, p.437]. This represents a particular challenge for health systems given that the taken-for-granted power of the doctor or the system commonly results in 'instrumental and non-participatory communication based on the belief that the bio-medical approach is "right"' [47, p.1458].

Nonetheless, if managed carefully, participatory management approaches can provide opportunities to build trust. The application of soft system methodology, for example, may generate trust when based on open communication and dialogue among those involved, and the development of shared interests. Their use may, then, also, provide the basis for the co-production necessary to implement agreed actions. However, some initial trust will be needed to encourage open communication and draw in multiple perspectives. So in using these, or other participatory management, approaches it is important to pay particular attention to the procedures of dialogue, the provision of institutional guarantees of trust and to limiting the exercise of power during discussions [14, 47]. Other possible arenas and approaches for the trust-generation that can strengthen health system performance are summarized in Table 2.7.

2.6 **Implications for health system strengthening**

Health systems and health sectors within those systems comprise sets of relationships. However, the institutional foundations of these relationships are commonly seen through lenses that emphasize rules and economic incentives. Only the more recent governance frameworks give clearer attention to the norms and values that underpin systems, and there remains little consideration of the shared social meanings that shape individual and organizational performance.

Table 2.7 Generating trust

Relationship	How to generate trust (from health system perspective)
Provider-patient	Strengthening provider communication and listening skills and institutional strategies of communication (e.g. signage, interpreters, employing patient care advisors, working with expert patients, supporting peer support networks)
Health manager-citizen	Developing structures and approaches allowing health officials and communities to work together, supported by resource allocation to enable community engagement and procedures to protect deliberate dialogue
Health manager-health worker	Human resource management practices that offer institutional guarantees of fairness and transparency (e.g. checks on decision-making, opportunities for review, regularity, 360° appraisal systems), that are consistently implemented by managers with strong communication and listening skills and that are backed up by public messages from senior managers and politicians supporting staff without condoning abusive behaviour
Public-private health managers	Formally agreed and fairly enforced contracts, backed up by informal dialogue and engagement to support contract implementation
Health system-citizen	In terms of public health problems and interventions, for example: the provision of clear and consistent formal information messages through wide-ranging communication channels, backed up by consistent public messages (including actions) from senior managers and politicians

Sources: [45,47]

In low- and middle-income countries' health reform debates, action to strengthen health sectors has, meanwhile, often been portrayed as a centrally controlled intervention involving particular sets of structural or incentive reforms. In essence, the reformer is seen as an actor intervening from above and outside who adjusts the rules of the game (e.g. through control knobs) that other health actors play. Although there is growing recognition of the importance of adapting reforms to particular contexts on the basis of both careful diagnosis of the problems facing any health system and a deliberate process of managing change, the reformer is still commonly seen as a rational *deus ex machina* [8].

In contrast, this analysis argues that the complexity of health systems and sectors means that it is difficult to strengthen them through central action. Effectively implementing any change requires understanding implementation as the 'enculturation of change' [21, p.260]. It requires re-wiring the institutional drivers of local level behaviour and relationships to sustain new practices or activities. That means paying more attention to the inner workings of the system, and particularly to the overlooked institutions of norms and values, including trust, and shared social meanings, rather than to its outer structure of rules and incentives. Central level guidance for action must, therefore, be combined both with the local level learning that allows new ideas and interventions to be adapted effectively to local circumstances, and with deliberate action to build trusting relationships. This is the crux of health system governance, a critical leverage point for health system strengthening [38].

Soft systems methodology offers one concrete approach to local level learning and trust-building, and can be supported by other actions to generate trust. All such action also requires local leadership and engagement, and new ways of managing local relationships. The range of leadership strategies needed [48] include the ability to:

◆ Exercise authority through participation and negotiation, rather than control and command. Leaders must establish fair and transparent procedures that engage key stakeholders (political authorities, the scientific community, health professionals, civil society, and citizens) in the process of decision-making, generate legitimate decisions and contain the influence of particular interest groups.

◆ Use a wide range of data and information in decision-making, going beyond the statistics normally produced by health information systems and identifying operational and systemic constraints. This information must also be publicly accessible, flowing up the public bureaucracy through open knowledge networks that involve field level experimentation and adaptation, and learning-through-doing.

◆ Manage the political and implementation process actively, to secure high-level political support and the other resources needed to initiate reforms, and to bring about the changes in organizational structure and culture that sustain implementation and limit resistance to change.

To strengthen health systems, new attention must now be paid to how to develop these managerial leadership capacities, and enable the emergence of organizational cultures and structures that support local level learning and action.

References

1 World Health Organization (2007). *Everybody's Business: Strengthening health systems to improve health outcomes. WHO's framework for action.* WHO, Geneva

2 Shakarishivili G (2009). *Building on health systems frameworks for developing a common approach to health systems strengthening.* Prepared for the World Bank, the Global Fund

and the GAVI Alliance Technical workshop on Health System Strengthening. Washington, DC, June 25–27 2009. Available at: http://siteresources.worldbank.org/ INTHSD/Resources/376278-1114111154043/1011834-1246449110524/ HealthSystemFrameworksFINAL.pdf (accessed 14 May 2010).

3 Ben-Ner A, Putterman L (1998). Values and institutions in economic analysis. In Ben-Ner A, Putterman L (eds) *Economics, Values and Organization*, pp.3–69. Cambridge University Press, Cambridge.

4 Scott WR (2001). *Institutions and Organizations*. Sage Publications, Thousand Oaks, CA.

5 Roemer MI (1991). *National health systems of the world. Vol 1: The countries*. Oxford University Press, Oxford.

6 World Health Organization (1993). *Evaluation of recent changes in the financing of health services* (WHO Technical Report No. 829). WHO, Geneva.

7 Frenk J (1994). Dimensions of health system reform. *Health Policy*, 27, 19–34.

8 Roberts MJ, Hsiao W, Berman P, Reich MR (2008). *Getting health reform right: A guide to improving performance and equity*. Oxford University Press, New York.

9 Gilson L, Doherty J, Lowenson R, Francis V (2008). *Challenging inequity through health systems*. Final report of the Knowledge Network on Health Systems, WHO Commission on the Social Determinants of Health. Johannesburg: Centre for Health Policy, EQUINET, London School of Hygiene and Tropical Medicine.

10 Mills AJ, Ranson MK (2006). The design of health systems. In Merson MH, Black RE, Mills A (eds) *International public health: diseases, systems and policies*, pp.513–47. Jones and Bartlett Publishers, Sudbury.

11 Berman P (1995). Health sector reform: making health development sustainable. *Health Policy*, 32(1), 13–28.

12 Labonte R, Blouin C, Chopra M, *et al.* (2007). *Towards health-equitable globalisation: rights, regulation and redistribution - final report to the Commission on the Social Determinants of Health*. Globalization Knowledge Network. Institute of Population Health, University of Ottawa. Available at: http://www.who.int/social_determinants/ resources/gkn_final_report_042008.pdf (accessed 14 May 2010).

13 World Health Organization (2000). *The World Health Report 2000. Health systems: improving performance*. WHO, Geneva.

14 Brinkerhoff D, Bossert T (2008). *Health governance: concepts, experience and programming options* (Health Systems 2020 Policy Brief). Available at: http://www. eldis.org/assets/Docs/36831.html (accessed 14 May 2010).

15 Morgan G (1997). *Images of organizations*. Sage publications, London.

16 Blaauw D, Gilson L, Penn-Kekana L, Schneider H (2003). *Organisational relationships and the 'software' of health sector reform*. Background paper prepared for the Disease Control Priorities Project, Capacity Strengthening and Management reform. Available at: http://web.wits.ac.za/NR/rdonlyres/01AB730B-0E2E-44F7–955B-DC81DD64ACE2/0/b52.pdf (accessed 13 July 2009).

17 Aitken JM (1994). Voices from the inside: managing district health services in Nepal. *International Journal of Health Planning and Management*, 9, 309–40.

18 George A (2009). 'By papers and pens, you can only do so much': views about accountability and human resource management from Indian government health

administrators and workers. *International Journal of Health Planning and Management,* **24**(3), 205–4.

19 Mumtaz Z, Salway S, Waseem M, Umer N (2003). Gender-based barriers to primary health care provision in Pakistan: the experience of female providers. *Health Policy and Planning,* **18**(3), 261–9.

20 Green A (2002). *An Introduction to Health Planning in Developing Countries,* 2nd edn. Oxford University Press, Oxford.

21 Barrett SM (2004). Implementation studies: time for a revival? Personal reflections on 20 years of implementation studies. *Public Administration,* **82**(2), 249–62.

22 Grindle MS (1997). Divergent cultures? When public organisations perform well in developing countries. *World Development,* **25**(4), 481–95.

23 Mannion R, Davies HTO, Marshall MN (2005). *Cultures for performance in health care.* Open University Press, Maidenhead.

24 Lipsky M (1980). *Street-level bureaucracy: dilemmas of the individual in public services.* Russell Sage Foundation, New York.

25 Long N (2001). *Development sociology: actor perspectives.* Routledge, London.

26 Crook R, Ayee J (2006). Urban service partnerships: 'Street level bureaucrats' and environmental sanitation in Kumasi and Accra, Ghana: Coping with organisational change in the bureaucracy. *Development Policy Review,* **24**(1), 51–73.

27 Tendler J, Freedheim S (1994). Trust in a rent-seeking world: health and government transformed in Northeastern Brazil. *World Development,* **22**(12), 1771–91.

28 Penn-Kekana L, Blaauw D, Schneider H (2004). 'It makes me want to run away to Saudi Arabia': management and implementation challenges for public financing reforms from a maternity ward perspective. *Health Policy and Planning,* **19**(**Suppl. 1**), i71–i77.

29 Kamuzora P, Gilson L (2007). Factors influencing implementation of the Community Health Fund in Tanzania. *Health Policy and Planning,* **22** (2), 95–102.

30 Mackintosh M (2000). Do health care systems contribute to inequalities? In Leon D, Walt G. (eds) *Poverty, Inequality and Health: An International Perspective,* pp.175–94. Oxford University Press, Oxford.

31 Plsek PE and Greenhalgh T (2001). The challenge of complexity in health care. *British Medical Journal,* **323**, 625–8.

32 Kernick D (2004). An introduction to complexity theory. In Kernick D (ed.) *Complexity and health care organization,* pp.23–38. Radcliffe Medical Press, Oxford.

33 Hudson J (2007). Learns lesson from policy experience. In Bochel H, Duncan S (eds) *Making policy in theory and practice,* pp.191–210. The Policy Press, Bristol.

34 Atun R, Menabde N (2008). Health systems and systems thining. In Coker R, Atun R, McKee M. (eds) *Health systems and the challenge of communicable diseases: experiences from Europe and Latin America* (European Observatory on Health Systems and Policies Series), pp.121–40. Open University Press, Maidenhead.

35 Kernick D (2004). The search for the correct organisational solution for the NHS. Kernick D (ed.) *Complexity and health care organisation,* pp. 93–104. Radcliffe Medical Press, Oxford.

36 Pawson, R. (2006). *Evidence-based policy: a realist perspective.* London, Sage Publications.

37 Chapman J (2004). *System failure: why governments must learn to think differently*, 2nd edn. Demos, London. Available at: http://www.demos.co.uk/publications/systemfailure2, (accessed 14 May 2010).

38 de Savigny D, Adam T (eds) (2009). *Systems thinking for health systems strengthening*. Alliance for Health Policy and Systems Research, WHO, Geneva.

39 Powell J (2004). An introduction to systems theory from hard to soft systems thinking in the management of complex organisations. In Kernick D (ed.) (2004) *Complexity and health care organization*, pp.43–58. Radcliffe Medical Press, Oxford.

40 Davies H, Nutley S (2004). Organisations as learning systems. In Kernick D (ed.) (2004) *Complexity and health care organization*, pp.59–68. Radcliffe Medical Press, Oxford.

41 Hill M, Hupe P (2009). *Implementing Public Policy*, 2nd edn. Sage Publications, London.

42 Bloom G, Standing H, Lloyd R (2008). Markets information and health care: towards new social contracts. *Social Science and Medicine,* **66**(**10**), 2076–87.

43 Calnan M, Rowe R (2008). *Trust matters in health care*. Open University Press, Maidenhead.

44 Gilson L, Khumalo G, Erasmus E, Mbatsha S, McIntyre D (2004). *Exploring the influence of workplace trust over health worker performance. Preliminary national report: South Africa*. Report prepared for the Health Economics and Financing Programme, London School of Hygiene and Tropical Medicine, UK. Available at http://www.hefp.lshtm.ac.uk/publications/downloads/working_papers/06_04.pdf (accessed 14 July 2009).

45 Gilson L (2007). Acceptability, trust and equity. In McIntyre D, Mooney G (eds) *The Economics of Health Equity*, pp.124–48. Cambridge University Press, Cambridge.

46 Robb N, Greenhalgh T (2007). 'You have to cover up the words of the doctor': the mediation of trust in interpreted consultations in primary care. *Journal of Health Organization and Management,* **20**(**5**), 434–55.

47 Thiede M. (2005). Information and access to health care: is there a role for trust? *Social Science and Medicine,* **61**(**7**), 1452–62.

48 World Health Organization (2008). *The World Health Report 2008: Primary health care now more than ever*. WHO, Geneva.

The 'health sector': financing, purchasing, provision, and performance

Chapter 3

Measuring and evaluating performance

Ellen Nolte and Martin McKee

3.1 Introduction

There has been growing interest in comparisons of health system performance within and between countries. Early examples include the work of the Organisation for Economic Cooperation and Development (OECD) on benchmarking, in a series of international comparative studies published since the mid-1980s, focusing on inputs into healthcare such as healthcare expenditure and human resources [1], and the rankings of the World Health Report 2000 [2]. The latter especially has stimulated wide-ranging debate about approaches to performance assessment both nationally and internationally. Many commentators expressed concern that the report's use of composite indices took insufficient account of the multifunctional complexity of healthcare delivery, which requires trade-offs, for example between prevention and treatment or between primary and specialized care. It is thus unlikely that any health sector will perform well on all possible measures. Yet, while the main goals of a health sector may be easily defined, it is more difficult to identify measures of progress towards these goals and the extent to which apparent progress can be attributed to the health sector or to other factors.

This chapter examines some of the main conceptual issues and methodological challenges that underlie our understanding of, and approaches to, measurement of the performance of health sectors. It discusses the reasons behind performance measurement and its objectives, reviews selected conceptual frameworks that have been proposed to evaluate health sector performance, and examines some of the key challenges related to performance assessment in the context of existing frameworks. It then briefly explores a complementary approach to performance assessment that, drawing on the 'tracer' approach, makes it possible to identify weaknesses in elements of the health sector and so obtain more direct insight into its performance. It concludes with a brief overview of whether and how performance measurement actually makes a difference.

Much of the evidence presented in this chapter will inevitably relate to high-income settings where much of the conceptual work and development of indicators has been undertaken. However, many of the conceptual issues discussed here will apply equally to middle- and low-income settings. Where countries at different stages of development are likely to diverge is on the selection of actual indicators to measure performance, and, in particular, the availability of data.

3.2 **Why measure and report performance?**

Measuring the performance of health services is not new; indeed, in Britain early efforts can be traced back to at least the mid-19th century when Florence Nightingale advocated the systematic collection, analysis, and reporting of data on outcomes across hospitals to understand and improve performance [3,4]. Early examples have also been documented for the United States [4,5]; however, it is only recently that performance assessment has been put more firmly on national and international agendas.

The growing interest in performance assessment can be seen to be located within broader concerns about accountability of and within health sectors. Main issues centre on costs, quality of care, availability of, access to, and responsiveness of services [6]. Healthcare is a major element of national budgets everywhere and while actual levels vary across countries, systems have come under increased pressure to ensure that resources are spent efficiently. In particular, accelerating progress in medical technology offers considerable potential for advancing the delivery and organization of healthcare, with consequences for healthcare expenditure. There is thus a need to ensure that innovations in healthcare promote health objectives and avoid adverse side effects [7]. Growing evidence points to the use of new (and existing) interventions and procedures in the absence of demonstrable benefits for patients in a number of countries, such as the United States [8] and Germany [9]. Yet equally, there is increasing evidence of underuse and misuse of health services, further fuelling concerns about the quality and outcomes of healthcare. Thus in many settings patients do not receive interventions that are considered beneficial, because of restrictions on access or financial barriers, and/or because of fragmentation of services. Misuse of services reflects poor delivery, including medical errors and/or negligence, often symptoms of system failures. Examples of system failures include the deaths of children undergoing inadequate heart surgery at the Bristol Royal Infirmary in the United Kingdom in the late 1980s and early 1990s, highlighting the failings of existing internal quality assurance and professional regulation systems [10]. In the United States, the Institute of

Medicine estimated that at least 44,000 deaths annually (or 2% of all deaths) are caused by medical errors in hospitals that could have been avoided [11].

At the same time, the growth of the consumer society, coupled with increasing access to information available through new electronic media, is creating more empowered citizens who have become aware of medical errors and system failures and who are demanding evidence for value for money in their role as taxpayers [12]. Also, patients expect to make more informed choices about their treatment and are also increasingly prepared to challenge professional authority and to litigate. However, while these developments might increase the responsiveness of health services to those who use them, it may also compromise equitable access to care, as the digital divide enables those who are most privileged to take greatest advantage of the new opportunities provided while those in most need are left behind [13].

Finally, the increasing focus on performance measurement has been part of wider public sector management reform, borrowing ideas from the private sector, such as the New Public Management movement pioneered in Australia, New Zealand, and the United Kingdom during the 1980s [6]. The United Kingdom introduced performance monitoring as a means to measure the processes and outcomes of public services, and at the same time to establish a means for public accountability by the government for their stewardship of the public services, including the National Health Service (NHS) [14].

In the broader context of improving accountability of and within health sectors, performance measurement can thus be seen to inform the appropriate use of public resources and authority according to an existing regulatory framework, professional standards, and societal values; and to support and improve service delivery and management through feedback and learning [6]. Advances in information technology have made it possible to collect, store, and process vast quantities of data on the inputs and activities of the health sector, so offering substantial potential to inform and enable performance measurement and improvement [15], although of course this requires the availability of relevant data in the first place, an issue of concern for low-income countries in particular as we will see below.

3.3 Defining performance

The notion of performance in healthcare is often used interchangeably with healthcare quality, reflecting the key concern of many performance assessment frameworks to improve the quality of care (see below). However, it is important to recognize that these concepts are not identical. Indeed, performance data do not necessarily allow inferences about care quality [16], and earlier work on performance tended to focus on inputs such as healthcare expenditure and volume of activity rather than the quality of the care being delivered [1,17,18].

The World Health Report 2000 conceptualized performance as the extent to which the resources used by a given health sector achieve their objectives [19]. Quality was understood as a subset of overall attainment of objectives and measured as average levels of population health and responsiveness [20]. This reflected the beginning of a move away from a concept that emphasized inputs and activity to the interpretation of performance as a multidimensional concept that, along with efficiency, also incorporates dimensions of quality (safety; effectiveness; quality of services rendered, i.e. appropriateness and timeliness; and perceived quality of services, i.e. responsiveness) and equity [17]. The importance of this refined conceptualization of performance is not necessarily the recognition of the multiple dimensions of the concept as such but the growing interest in seeking to capture the various dimensions within the same performance assessment framework.

Subsequent work built on this conceptualization of performance. Drawing on work undertaken since the publication of the 2000 World Health Report, Smith and colleagues note that there is 'a fair degree of consensus' that health sector objectives can by summarized under a defined set of headings including health conferred on citizens; responsiveness to the legitimate expectations of the population; protection against the financial risk of illness; and productivity, i.e. the extent to which resources are used efficiently [15].

This conceptualization of performance has implications for measurement efforts. Thus, if performance is defined as the extent to which a given health sector meets its key objectives, a first step will require the identification and/or adoption of objectives against which to measure performance. While there may be general consensus about the overall goals that should be pursued, it is conceivable that the relative importance of objectives will vary among countries, in particular as they relate to equity objectives such as financial protection, which very much reflect political choices made by individual countries and so are likely to differ [21].

Similarly, the scope of what constitutes the 'health system' in a given setting is likely to vary, as outlined in Chapter 1. There are many activities contributing, directly or indirectly, to the provision of healthcare that, in different countries, may or may not be within what is considered to be the health system [22]. Arah et al. distinguish the *health system* from the *healthcare system* with the latter corresponding to the definition in Chapter 1 of a health sector: the 'combined functioning of public health and personal healthcare services' that are under the 'direct control of identifiable agents, especially ministries of health' [23]. The health system, in contrast, extends beyond these boundaries, consistent with Chapter 1, 'to include all activities and structures that impact or determine health in its broadest sense within a given society' [2]. Consequently, *healthcare performance* refers to the 'maintenance of an efficient and equitable system of healthcare', evaluating the system of healthcare delivery against the 'established public goals for the level and distribution of the benefits and costs of personal and public healthcare' [23]. *Health system performance*, in contrast, is based on a broader concept that also takes account of non-healthcare determinants of population health, principally building on the health field concept advanced by Lalonde [24] and thus subsuming healthcare performance.

While it is important to recognize this distinction, it is equally important to realize that, in practice, the concept of performance is likely to mean different things to different actors and that the precise boundaries of a health sector and health system are difficult to define. Nevertheless, reinforcing what was discussed in Chapter 1, any effort that aims to measure 'performance' will have to address the question on how to define the health sector or health system and its objectives, as this will determine the performance measures being used.

3.4 Objectives of performance measurement

As illustrated earlier, a key driver behind many efforts to measure and evaluate performance has been a growing concern about accountability. Thus, an important role of performance measurement and reporting is to help hold various actors to account by informing stakeholders and so enabling them to make decisions [15]. Other objectives of performance measurement include enabling the identification of areas of poor performance and centres of excellence; facilitating the selection and choice of providers by service users and purchasers of healthcare; encouraging provider behaviour change; and providing epidemiological and other public health data [25].

Depending on the objective(s), the target audience of performance measurement can include a range of actors and stakeholders, such as payers for/purchasers of health services, governments, regulators, healthcare providers, patients, the general public, and donors. The relationships between these various groups will vary, as will the scope and timeliness of information they require [15]. For example, purchaser organizations (such as insurance funds, national or local governments, health authorities) seeking to ensure that contracted services meet their populations' needs and expectations may require information on patient experience as well as on provider performance at the organizational level. Governments seeking to monitor the overall health of their population so as to inform policy development will look for information at the regional, national, and possibly international level on indicators of population health, access to and equity of care, and on service utilization. Citizens, in their role as service users, may need detailed information on the performance of local providers to inform their choice of care while, in their role as taxpayers, they may seek information on the overall performance of the system at the aggregate level to help them to hold governments to account at the ballot box [15].

However, performance measurement schemes have yet to address the various information needs of different stakeholders. Indeed, existing reporting systems have tended to address a wide range of (potential) users of performance data 'in the hope that some of the information collected will be useful to different parties' [15]. Thus, health sectors, and systems, will have to develop a more nuanced approach to the collection and presentation of performance data if the objective of performance measurement and reporting is to support the accountability function of performance assessment.

3.5 Frameworks for performance assessment

Since the late 1990s, several countries have been developing frameworks and/or indicator systems for monitoring and assessing performance, with improving the quality of care being at the core of many such approaches. Early initiatives include the 1998 NHS Performance Assessment Framework in the United Kingdom [26], the 2000 Canadian Health Information Roadmap Initiative Indicators Framework [27] and the subsequent Health Indicator Framework (2003) [28], the 2001 Australian National Health Performance Framework [29], the Danish National Indicator Project established in 2000 [30], and work by the US Agency for Healthcare Research and Quality [31]. More recent initiatives include work in the Netherlands [32,33], Sweden [34], Taiwan [35], renewed work in Australia to strengthen accountability through benchmarking [36], and the National Scorecard on US Health System Performance, an initiative by the Commonwealth Fund Commission on a High Performance Health System [37,38]. International initiatives include the work by the World Health Organization (WHO) and by the OECD mentioned earlier.

The nature and scope of existing frameworks and indicator systems varies, and so does the definition of performance and of what constitutes the health sector or system in a given context, with some indicator systems explicitly focusing on healthcare (e.g. [30,31,34,35]) while others take a broader approach that also encompass non-healthcare determinants of population health (e.g. [27–29]). Several of the performance assessment frameworks listed above have been reviewed in detail elsewhere [21,23,39–41]. We here focus on two international initiatives, the WHO framework for Health System Performance Assessment (HSPA) [42], and the OECD's Health Care Quality Indicators Project (HCQI) [43]. These two approaches to performance measurement differ in several ways, with the former attempting to achieve global coverage, with extensive use of imputed data, and covering overall performance, defined as health attainment, responsiveness, and equity. In contrast, the OECD's HCQI project focuses on more specific measures of healthcare processes and outcomes, utilizing databases collected by participating member states. Both approaches, however, face important problems of definition, methods, and interpretation, which we discuss later.

3.5.1 The WHO framework for Health System Performance Assessment

In 1998, WHO began to develop its framework for Health System Performance Assessment (HSPA), subsequently set out in the 2000 World Health Report, which was the first attempt to provide a comprehensive assessment of the performance of health systems of the then 191 Member States of the WHO [2,42]. The HSPA is based on 'all activities whose primary purpose is to promote, restore or maintain health' [2], with activities referred to as those which are under complete or partial control of governments. The definition also considers intersectoral actions 'in which the stewards of the health system [sector] take responsibility to advocate for improvements in areas outside their direct control, such as legislation to reduce fatalities from traffic accidents' [19].

The model underpinning the HSPA identifies three major social goals to which health sectors contribute: improving health, improving responsiveness to expectations of the population, and ensuring fairness in financial contribution [2]. However, in order to achieve these goals or objectives the health sector has to fulfil certain key functions; these are identified as financing, provision of personal and non-personal health services, resource generation, and stewardship or oversight function of the health sector (Figure 3.1).

The extent to which a given sector achieves the three goals was assessed using five indicators. Thus, health improvement was measured by two indicators of population health, considering both the average level of health in a given population using disability-adjusted life expectancy (DALE), and the distribution of health within that population, using child survival. The second goal, responsiveness, was conceptualized along two dimensions, respect for persons (dignity, autonomy, confidentiality) and client orientation (prompt attention, quality of basic amenities, access to social support networks during care, choice of provider), and assessed based on a survey of key informants in selected countries. As with the indicators of population health, responsiveness was

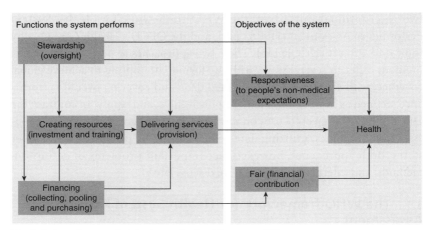

Fig. 3.1 Functions and objectives of a health system [2].
Source: Reproduced from [2] with permission of the World Health Organisation

measured as average level and as distribution within a given population. The third goal, fairness in financial contribution, was measured through a single indicator, the distribution of financial burden within the population, namely the fraction of disposable income that each household contributes to the health sector (including payments towards financing through income taxes, value-added tax, excise tax, social security contributions, private voluntary insurance, and out-of-pocket payments) [2].

Seeking to assess how well health sectors 'do their job', the report then produced two principal indices, goal attainment and performance. Goal attainment was measured for each of the five indicators and as a composite index from the weighted sum of components ('overall goal attainment'). Performance was assessed through relating achievement to expenditure, using two measures: performance on the level of health, defined as the ratio between achieved levels of health and the levels of health that could be achieved by the most efficient health sector; and overall health sector performance, which was assessed as overall achievements measured as a composite of the five indicators, compared with what might be expected given the country's level of economic and educational development. The 191 WHO member states were then ranked according to these performance measures, producing the highly controversial 'league table' (Table 3.1).

Prompted by the league table in particular, the 2000 World Health Report has stimulated a wide-ranging debate; much centred on the composite index of overall performance although, as illustrated in Table 3.1, rankings differed for different measures of performance, an issue which has received less attention. However, the various criticisms that the report engendered helped bring to light the methodological challenges inherent in conducting and interpreting international comparative analyses. Indeed, the publication of the report

Table 3.1 Health system performance in selected WHO Member States, estimates for 1997 [2]

	Overall performance (rank)	Performance on health level (DALE) (rank)	Overall goal attainment (rank)
France	**1**	4	6
Italy	2	3	11
Singapore	6	14	27
Oman	8	**1**	59
Japan	10	9	**1**
Colombia	22	51	41
United States	37	72	15
Philippines	60	126	54
Bulgaria	102	92	74
Zimbabwe	155	**191**	147
South Africa	175	182	151
Myanmar	190	129	175
Sierra Leone	**191**	183	**191**

stimulated a range of activities and consultations on conceptual, methodological, and data issues around performance assessment [44]. It is worth noting that the HSPA exercise has not been repeated although further developmental work is ongoing [45].

3.5.2 The OECD Health Care Quality Indicators (HCQI) Project

The OECD HCQI Project builds, to a considerable extent, on earlier work by the Commonwealth Fund sponsored International Working Group on Quality Indicators (CWF QI), which began in 1999 [46], and the Nordic Indicator Group Project set up by the Nordic Council of Ministers [47]. Its focus is on measuring the technical quality of healthcare with the aim to 'develop a set of indicators that reflect a robust picture of healthcare quality that can be reliably reported across countries using comparable data' [43]. The conceptualization of healthcare quality is based on the widely used definition by the US Institute of Medicine, which defines quality as 'the degree to which health services for individuals and populations increase the likelihood of desired health outcomes and are consistent with current medical knowledge' [48]; within the HCQI project, effectiveness, safety, and responsiveness are interpreted as the core components of healthcare quality [43]. A secondary aim of the work is to contribute to better coordination between major international organizations 'seeking to track healthcare quality indicators' with the ultimate aim to improve data comparability internationally [49].

HCQI's origins and history have been described in detail elsewhere [50]. However, it is important to highlight its rapid and continuing evolution, both in scope and number of participating countries, which has grown from 23 OECD countries in 2003 to 32 (including two non-OECD European Union countries) in 2007 [51]. The project involves a substantial methodological component in terms of indicator development and evaluation (Box 3.1), along with assessments of the feasibility to collect internationally comparable data that can be released publicly.

Following a two-stage process of indicator development, the 2006 HCQI indicator set included a total of 26 indicators in the areas of preventive and curative care as well as indicators of diabetes care and patient safety. Of these, seven indicators were evaluated as 'not fit', at that stage, for international comparison, because an insufficient number of countries (i.e. fewer than ten countries) was able to provide relevant data, data sources were not comparable (e.g. survey-based data vs. patient records), and/or countries differed in the definition of the relevant condition (e.g. variation in the definition of what is considered 'poor glucose control') [51].

However, as illustrated in Table 3.2, while a given indicator may not, at present, be considered suitable for international comparison, it may be included

Box 3.1 OECD HCQI project: indicator selection criteria

Indicators selected for inclusion in the OECD HCQI project are considered a tool for evidence-based policy decisions and therefore have to meet two conditions: they have to capture an 'important performance aspect' and they have to be scientifically sound [43]. Importance is assessed according to three dimensions: 1) the measure addresses areas in which there is a clear gap between the actual and potential levels of health; 2) it reflects important health conditions in terms of burden of disease, cost of care, or public interest; and 3) measures can be directly affected by the healthcare system. The second criterion, scientific soundness, requires indicators to be valid (i.e. the extent to which the measure accurately represents the concept/phenomenon being evaluated) and reliable (i.e. the extent to which the measurement with a given indicator is reproducible).

Table 3.2 OECD Health Care Quality Indicator Project: Indicator sets [51]

Indicator	Considered suitable for international comparison	
	2003–2005 HCQI set	**2006 HCQI set**
Breast cancer 5-year survival rate	✓	✓
Mammography screening rate	✓	✓
Cervical cancer 5-year survival rate	✓	✓
Cervical cancer screening rate	✓	✓
Colorectal cancer 5-year survival rate	✓	✓
Incidence of vaccine-preventable diseases (pertussis, measles, hepatitis B)	✓	✓
Coverage for basic vaccination programme, age 2 years (pertussis, measles, and hepatitis B)	✓	✓
Influenza vaccination rate, age >65 years	✓	✓
Annual HbA1c test for diabetics	No	No
Poor glucose control (identified by HbA1c level)	No	No
Annual retinal exam for diabetics	No	✓
Uncontrolled diabetes admission rate, age 15+	Not reviewed	No
Diabetes lower extremity amputation rate	No	No
Asthma mortality rate, ages 5–39	✓	✓
Asthma admission rate, age 15+	Not reviewed	✓
In-hospital mortality rate within 30 days of hospital admission for acute myocardial infarction	✓	✓
In-hospital mortality rate within 30 days of hospital admission for stroke	✓	✓
Hypertension admission rate, age 15+	Not reviewed	No
In-hospital waiting time for surgery after hip fracture, age >65 years	✓	✓
Postoperative hip fracture rate	Not reviewed	No
Transfusion reaction	Not reviewed	No
Smoking rate	✓	✓

in the future when, for example, the number of countries that can provide robust data on that indicator is considered large enough (a minimum of ten countries has to be in the position to provide data on the indicator in question) or data collection systems have been adapted to meet uniform standards set by the project.

The current focus of HCQI is on effectiveness and patient safety and indicator development is ongoing, especially in the areas of mental health and patient safety. Although patient-centeredness/responsiveness is also recognized as a key attribute of healthcare quality, work on this dimension is only beginning. Furthermore, because of the HCQI's methodological emphasis, the public release of international data has so far been limited to a small set of indicators covering selected areas in healthcare [52].

3.6 Conceptual and methodological challenges

As noted earlier, the WHO HSPA and the OECD HCQI Project represent two very different approaches to performance measurement; at the same time they face similar challenges, both conceptually and methodologically.

3.6.1 Underlying definitions

One of the more fundamental challenges relates to the definitions underlying the process of performance assessment, that is the conceptualization of performance and the definition of what constitutes the health sector or system and how these conform to each other. For example, as noted earlier, the 2000 World Health Report formulated three goals against which to assess performance: health improvement, responsiveness, and fairness of financial contribution [2]. Attainment of the first goal was measured as disability-adjusted life expectancy (DALE); i.e. the length of time that an individual can expect to live in good health. This measure has the advantage that it can be obtained for many countries. However it also has an important weakness: many of the determinants of (healthy) life expectancy lie outside the health sector. Thus, the measure of health attainment reflects not only those policies and resulting inputs whose primary intent is to improve health but also policies in a wide range of other sectors, such as education, housing, and employment, where the production of health is a secondary goal; that is, the health system as defined in Chapter 1. In contrast, the two other goals, responsiveness and fairness of financing, relate directly to the delivery of healthcare services.

We have previously examined how health sectors perform when health attainment can be more directly attributed to healthcare [53]. We have used

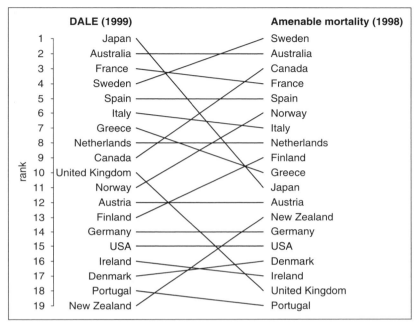

Fig. 3.2 Comparison of rankings based on DALE (1999) and from mortality amenable to health care (1998) in 19 countries. From [53].

the concept of 'amenable mortality' which is based on the notion that deaths from certain causes, and at certain ages, should not occur in the presence of timely and effective healthcare [54]. Conditions commonly considered 'amenable' to healthcare include bacterial infections, treatable cancers, diabetes, cardiovascular and cerebrovascular disease, and complications of common surgical procedures. We calculated death rates for these 'amenable' conditions for a total of 19 OECD countries for which data were available for the year 1998 and used this to produce a ranking on the level of 'amenable' mortality. We then compared our ranks with those by the 2000 World Health Report based on DALE for the year 1999 (Figure 3.2). Perhaps not surprisingly, rankings changed for several countries that were included in the analysis, illustrating that performance assessments very much depend on the concepts that underlie them.

In contrast to the WHO HSPA, the OECD HCQI project uses a narrower definition of what constitutes a health system, focusing performance assessment on the core components of healthcare quality set out in a proposed conceptual framework illustrated in Figure 3.3.

In figure 3.3, the HCQI project aims to develop a common set of quality indicators that 'are intended to help raise questions for further investigations

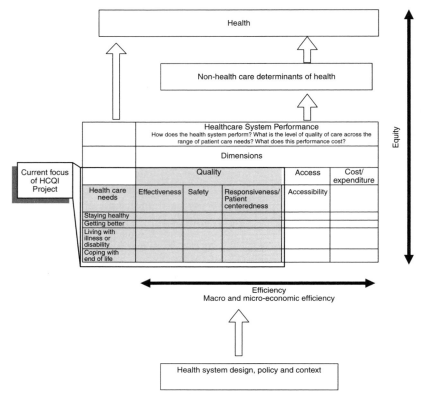

Fig. 3.3 Proposed conceptual framework for the HCQI project. From [43].
Source: Reproduced from Kelley, E and Hurst J (2006), Health Care Quality Indicators
Project: Conceptual Framework Paper, OECD Health Working Papers, 23. OECD,
Paris. http://dx.doi.org/10.1787/440134737301

of differences in quality of care across countries' [43]. Yet, the current set of
indicators selected to reflect the quality of care in participating OECD countries also includes smoking rates (Table 3.2). It is being acknowledged that
factors that determine smoking tend to lie outside the control of the health
sector and this indicator is therefore 'a relatively less valid indicator' of healthcare quality [51]. Work is being undertaken to explore the possible inclusion
of indicators of smoking cessation that are considered to more closely reflect
healthcare quality, based on evidence that advice and treatment provided by
physicians may impact on smoking cessation [46]. This line of reasoning
seems, however, slightly at odds with the rather narrow objective of evaluating
the technical quality of healthcare and in the light of the evidence that many of
the more effective strategies to reduce smoking rates lie clearly outside the
health sector as operationalized within the HCQI.

3.6.2 **Data availability**

One other key challenge to performance assessment is the absence of (uniform) data across different settings, a problem especially pertinent to low- and middle-income settings. Many parts of the world lack even basic vital statistics, because of fragmentary or non-existent vital registration systems. Routinely collected data on vital events such as deaths provide complete and representative information for only about 40% of countries in the world (or about 25% of its population). Recent work that aimed to measure maternal mortality in 171 countries with populations of over 250,000, demonstrated how over 30% of countries lacked appropriate empirical data that would allow for the assessment of maternal mortality in those settings; instead the indicator had to be estimated using statistical modelling procedures [55]. Maternal mortality is a largely avoidable cause of death and considered an essential indicator of progress of nations and a core indicator in the Millennium Development Goals. However, lack of adequate data poses substantial obstacles to assessing progress and identifying areas of concern to inform decision-making, highlighting the need to establish some form of vital registration system in those settings in order to enable performance measurement.

The challenges arising from lack of suitable data are further illustrated by the 2000 World Health Report which also had to draw, to considerable extent, on modelling techniques because of virtual absence of data from a majority of the countries involved [2]. In a critique of this approach, Musgrove showed that only 39% of the indicator values included in the report were based on existing data, the remainder being estimates imputed using regression analyses and other means [44]. Using complex models to generate estimates fails, however, to tackle the underlying problem.

Yet, even in countries with established vital registration systems significant gaps exist in coverage of some groups, for example native Americans or Australian aborigines, or selected geographical areas, such as Chechnya in the Russian Federation or the Transnistria region in Moldova [56]. Where data exist, their usefulness may be restricted due to lack of comparability, which poses particular challenges to international comparisons. The OECD HCQI seeks to overcome this by examining, in detail, data availability and comparability for each indicator considered for inclusion in the HCQI indicator set. Indeed, as noted above, one aim of the project is to improve data comparability internationally. However, as the work undertaken so far has demonstrated, comparability is often compromised because of lack of uniformity of data collection systems, differences in definitions, and data sources [51].

Accurate collection of indicator data relies on the existence of reliable and well-established health information systems, including vital registration systems to enable assessing basic indicators of population health such as infant and maternal mortality. The establishment of such systems poses challenges, in particular to low-resource settings. Efforts are underway to support the routine collection of core demographic and health data such as through the establishment of health and demographic surveillance systems that have been set up in a number of sites in low- and middle-income countries, with the INDEPTH network bringing together 37 sites in 2010, although issues around analytical and technical capacity remain a challenge [57]. The Health Metrics Network (HMN) was established in 2005 in partnership with the WHO to enhance the availability and use of health information through supporting the development of health information systems. The work of the HMN was found to be successful with regard to developing standards (the HMN Framework Toolset) for country health information systems and so raising awareness of information needs while detailed technical support activities as piloted in five countries were found to be unsustainable in the long run. Thus, while progress has been made, it remains slow, facing the continued challenge of resource constraints.

3.6.3 Developing performance measures

Given the challenges posed by the limited availability of data suitable for performance measurement, there is a risk that the selection and development performance indicators will be based on what is available and practical ('measurable') rather than what is meaningful, such as areas that need improvement and require prioritization or health system goals and values [58]. Thus, if performance measurement is to guide health sector and system improvement it will be important to develop a robust conceptual framework to inform the development of performance measures [15].

An important consideration for the design of individual performance indicators is the level at which assessment takes place. This can range from the primary process of patient care (micro level) to the organizational context (meso level) to the financing and policy, or health sector context within the wider health system (macro level) [59].

A further consideration is whether to use process and/or outcome measures to assess the effectiveness of healthcare. This consideration builds on the approach first developed by Donabedian in his work on quality of care [60], proposing that a system can be evaluated according to structure, process, and outcome [61]. Building on this work, most approaches to quality and performance assessment tend to use a combination of process and outcome measures, although the debate on the relative usefulness of each is ongoing [40]. Mant noted that the relevance of outcome measures is likely to increase with the broadening of the perspective, i.e. towards macro-level assessments of quality and performance because such measures tend to reflect the interplay of a range of factors, some of which are directly related to healthcare and these factors are more easily addressed at the national or system level [62]. Conversely, at the organizational or individual team level, process measures will become more useful as broader outcome measures are less easily influenced at this level.

Against this background, Kruk and Freedman presented a review of performance indicators for application to developing countries, which adapted Donabedian's framework to assess performance according to the dimensions inputs, process and outcomes as a means to guide indicator selection for performance assessments in relevant settings [63]. Table 3.3 illustrates this approach by also including examples of indicators most commonly used in developing countries.

Arguably, if performance measurement is to inform health sector improvement, any framework for assessment would aim to use a wide range of indicators covering major areas of the sector and dimensions of performance such as effectiveness, safety, access, responsiveness, equity, and efficiency. At the same time, however, such comprehensiveness may lead to information overload, which can make it difficult for the users of information on performance to make sense of the data being presented [15]. There is thus a persuasive argument to use composite indices, which bring together separate performance measures into one index or indicator, so helping to reduce a mass of complex information into a format that almost anyone can understand. One example of a composite measure includes the performance index used by the 2000 World Health Report as described earlier.

The use of composite measures has been challenged on conceptual and methodological grounds. Referring in particular to the methods employed by the 2000 World Health Report, Naylor and colleagues argued that composite indices of health system performance are, at best, of 'dubious precision' for they 'combine uncertain weighing systems, imprecision arising from the potential non-comparability of component measures, and misleading reliability in the form of whole-population averages that mask distributional issues' [12]. They further argued that even the use of disaggregated data in form of statistical means and medians could be misleading as such an approach is likely to conceal fluctuations at various levels within the health sector. Thus, composite indicators require careful design to avoid potential misuse for decision-making [64]. Given the complexity involved, Naylor et al. suggest abstaining from a single measure to capture performance altogether but instead applying a balanced approach that employs a range of indicators to address the varying information needs of the different stakeholders [12].

Table 3.3 Framework for health system performance indicators [63]

Inputs	Outputs/processes	Outcomes/impact
Policies	**Effectiveness**	
Legal framework (e.g. right to health)	Access to care	Health status improvement, e.g. *infant mortality, maternal mortality*
Composition of essential services package	Availability, e.g. *% population within 10 km of a clinic*	
Private sector regulation	Utilization, e.g. *TB case detection rates*	Patient satisfaction, e.g. *length of wait for care*
Funding/financing	Timeliness, e.g. *effective treatment for malaria within 24 hours*	
Level of health expenditure		
Modes of financing		
Fee schedules/provider payment	Quality of care	
Organization	Safety e.g. *infection and complication rates after surgery*	
Public/private mix		
Distribution of facilities/providers	Efficacy, e.g. *avoidable hospitalization rate*	
Management and information systems	Continuity e.g. *treatment completion rates (TB)*	
	Equity	
	Access for disadvantaged groups, e.g. *utilization of essential health services by disadvantaged groups*	Health status improvement for disadvantaged groups, e.g. *under-5 mortality rate for lowest income quintile*
	Quality for disadvantaged groups, e.g. *safety indicators analysed for disadvantaged groups*	Fair financing, e.g. *% government funding that reaches poorest income quintile*
	Participation/accountability, e.g. *perception of in/exclusion from health system*	Risk protection, e.g. *% population with catastrophic health expenditures*
	Efficiency	
	Adequacy of funding, e.g. *per capita health care spending*	Maximizing value of resources, e.g. *mortality rate per dollar invested in health care*
	Costs and productivity e.g. *average length of stay*	
	Administrative efficiency, e.g. *health worker attrition rates*	

3.7 **Moving beyond indicators**

A complementary approach to the frameworks presented thus far involves the use of tracer conditions [65], based on the premise that focusing on carefully selected health problems makes it possible to identify weaknesses in elements of the health sector and so to obtain more direct insight into its performance [66,67]. For a health problem to be used as tracer it should meet certain criteria; it should: 1) have a definitive functional impact, i.e. require treatment, with inappropriate or absent treatment resulting in functional impairment; 2) be relatively well defined and easy to diagnose; 3) have a prevalence high enough to permit collection of adequate data; 4) have a natural history which varies with utilization and effectiveness of healthcare; 5) have available techniques of medical management which are well defined for at least one of the following: prevention, diagnosis, treatment, rehabilitation; and 6) have a known epidemiology [65].

Diabetes mellitus has been proposed as a suitable 'tracer' condition and several analysts have examined its use as a measure of performance in high-, middle-, and low-income settings [66,68–70]. Diabetes meets the criteria for a tracer condition as effective treatment reduces the risk of specific complications that are disabling or potentially fatal [71,72], and premature onset of cardiovascular disease [73]. Consequently, several commentators have identified deaths from diabetes among young people as 'sentinel health events' raising questions about the quality of healthcare delivery [54,74]. Diabetes is also well defined, with internationally agreed criteria, and is easy to diagnose [75]. Furthermore, diabetes is common. Its prevalence worldwide in 2000 was estimated at 2.8%, projected to increase substantially by 2030, to 4.4% [76]. The total number of people with diabetes was estimated at 171 million in 2000, rising to 366 million in 2030, 284 million of whom will live in developing countries.

However, despite the availability of treatments of diabetes and the increasing evidence-base on effective management there remains substantial variation across countries in the standards of care people with diabetes actually receive. This is reflected dramatically in developing countries. Thus, life expectancy of a newly diagnosed child with type 1 diabetes in sub-Saharan Africa was recently estimated at 1.5–3.8 years, a figure seen in the United States only in the pre-insulin era before 1922 [77]. However, premature deaths from diabetes occur in all countries, although the extent to which this happens varies. Examining diabetes outcomes among young people measured as 'case-fatality', Nolte et al. [66] found a 10-fold variation on this measure across 29 high- and middle-income countries.

This and other work suggests gross differences in the ability of health sectors to provide adequate care for people with diabetes. However, it says little about why such differences exist. It is therefore necessary to examine in detail the specificities of the health sectors in question and so identifying possible underlying organizational and sectoral failures. One way of approaching this is the use of rapid appraisal which is increasingly being employed to provide a pragmatic assessment of the performance of complex systems, particularly where it is necessary to understand the interconnections between different policies.

Such an approach has been adapted by the International Insulin Foundation to develop a Rapid Assessment Protocol for Insulin Access (RAPIA) [77]. It provides a multi-level assessment of the different elements that influence the access of patients to insulin in a given country. Its focus is the analysis of the path of insulin from its arrival in the country to the point where it reaches (or fails to) to treat the patient effectively. Applying the RAPIA protocol to Mozambique and Zambia, Beran et al. noted that insulin supplies were available in both countries and in sufficient quantities; yet, there were considerable challenges at the various levels of both sectors that impacted on the appropriate distribution of insulin according to patient need, along with supporting measures such as providing for sufficient supplies and monitoring equipment such as syringes and testing strips, adequately trained healthcare workers, and knowledge about the condition among both healthcare workers and patients [69]. As a consequence, there was substantial risk of misdiagnosis or failure to detect diabetes.

A variation of the rapid appraisal approach was also used in Kyrgyzstan, which sought to understand the state of diabetes services and the challenges people with diabetes are facing in obtaining appropriate care after the breakdown of the Soviet Union in 1991 [70]. This study also identified an array of weaknesses but the overriding problem was one of integration. Thus, individual health professionals would be trained abroad in the methods of foot care but would be unable to obtain the inexpensive equipment required to provide it on their return. Newly diagnosed patients would be discharged from hospital without a supply of insulin and would become ill while they waited for the distribution system to make it available in their local pharmacy. Similar findings were obtained in Georgia [78].

These studies demonstrate how a single intervention, for example, providing adequate supplies of insulin, as in Mozambique and Zambia [69], or training health professionals in foot care [70], may be necessary but by no means sufficient to improve diabetes care in these settings. More broadly, using the tracer approach they show how, while many of the inputs are in place, there are often critical gaps and a failure to integrate them, so that the end result is that the patients receive treatment that is far from optimal. Although such studies focus on a single tracer, the problems they identify are often generic. Thus, diabetes can be seen as an example of a much larger group of complex chronic diseases requiring long term treatment by multi-professional teams with active involvement by informed and empowered patients.

3.8 **Does performance assessment make a difference?**

We have noted earlier that the reporting of performance indicators can have different objectives, such as increasing patient choice and facilitating change in provider behaviour, and, ultimately, improving performance. There are, however, relatively little data to assess whether and how well performance indicators achieve any of these objectives [79].

A recent review of the impact of annual performance ratings of NHS providers in England between 2001 and 2005 indicated that the assessment system did improve reported performance on key targets such as hospital waiting times [80]. However, the analysis also revealed that in some cases these improvements were made at the expense of clinical areas where performance was not measured or were undermined by different forms of gaming such as data manipulation.

The evidence of whether the public release of performance data improves quality of care remains somewhat inconsistent [81]. This is, in part, because of lack of rigorous evaluation of many major public reporting systems. Evidence from the United States suggests that users as well as purchasers or payers rarely search out publicly available information and do not understand or trust it [82]. Also, physicians appear to be rather sceptical about the data and only a small proportion apparently uses them. In contrast, there is growing evidence suggesting that managers and some providers do use comparative information, with again data from the United States indicating that hospitals appear to have been most responsive to publicized data with some evidence pointing towards improvements in care where public reporting occurred [82,83]. Indeed, Hibbard and colleagues have demonstrated how hospitals improved in clinical areas following the public release of performance data on those areas [84]. Moreover, they also found that reporting impacted on hospitals' reputation among service users.

3.9 **Conclusion**

This chapter has examined some of the main conceptual issues and methodological challenges that underlie our understanding of, and approaches to, performance assessment. It finds that there is growing interest in assessing and comparing performance at the various levels of healthcare. It takes place in the wider context of pressures to increase transparency and accountability to payers and citizens, not only in the health sector but in public services overall.

Performance measurement remains at a fairly early stage [85]. However, there is considerable potential for performance measurement to contribute to health improvement and advances in technology are likely to play a considerable role in the process [86]. It is important to recognize though that performance measurement does not come free; indeed, it can be a costly undertaking that is likely to divert valuable resources from health services. This is likely to pose a particular challenge in settings where there is little infrastructure to support the routine collection of data suitable for performance measurement. However, if performance measurement is set in the context of an overall goal to promote accountability and so providing assurance that public finances are used effectively, it may contribute to government and citizens' willingness to invest additional resources into the health sector.

Arguably, while performance measurement is an important means to check whether a given health sector achieves its goals, it is only one instrument for improvement. In a recent comprehensive overview of the experiences and challenges of performance measurement, Smith et al. noted that for performance measurement to be effective it needs to be aligned with other levers for improvement such as financing, market structure, accountability arrangements, and regulation [86]. To support this process they identify a set of recommendations for decision-makers to consider for policy development, highlighting that a key requirement will be to develop a clear vision and framework of how performance measurement sits within the overall accountability relationships if performance measurement is to improve ultimate performance.

References

1 OECD (1985). *Measuring health care, 1960–1983 expenditure, costs and performance.* OECD, Paris.

2 World Health Organization (2000). *The World Health Report 2000. Health systems: improving performance.* World Health Organization, Geneva.

3 Smith P (2002). Measuring health system performance. *European Journal of Health Economics,* **3**, 145–8.

4 Spiegelhalter D (1999). Surgical audit: statistical lessons from Nightingale and Codman. *Journal of the Royal Statistical Society,* **22**, 45–58.

5 McIntyre D, Rogers L, Heiei E (2001). Overview, history, and objectives of performance measurement. *Health Care Financing Review,* **22**, 7–43.

6 Brinkerhoff D (2004). Accountability and health systems: toward conceptual clarity and policy relevance. *Health Policy and Planning,* **19**, 371–9.

7 Smith P (2002). Editor's preface. In Smith P (ed) *Measuring up. Improving health system performance in OECD countries*, pp.7–9. OECD, Paris.

8 Becher EC, Chassin MR (2001). Improving the quality of health care: who will lead? *Health Affairs*, **20**, 164–79.

9 Advisory Council for the Concerted Action in Health Care (2001). *Appropriateness and efficiency. Volume III: Overuse, underuse and misuse. Report 2000/2001. Executive summary*. Advisory Council for the Concerted Action in Health Care, Bonn.

10 Smith R (1998). Regulation of doctors and the Bristol inquiry. *British Medical Journal*, **317**, 1539–40.

11 Kohn LT, Corrigan JM, Donaldson MS (1999). *To err is human. Building a safer health system*. National Academic Press, Washington, DC.

12 Naylor CD, Iron K, Handa K (2002). *Measuring health system performance: problems and opportunities in the era of assessment and accountability, in Measuring up. Improving health system performance in OECD countries*, pp.13–34. OECD, Paris.

13 Stroetmann VN, Hüsing T, Kubitschke L, Stroetmann KA. (2002). The attitudes, expectations and needs of elderly people in relation to e-health applications: results from a European survey. *Journal of Telemedicine and Telecare*, **8**(Suppl 2), 82–4.

14 Working Party on Performance Monitoring in the Public Services (2005). Performance indicators: good, bad, and ugly. *Journal of the Royal Statistical Society*, **168**, 1–27.

15 Smith P, Mossialos E, Papanicolas I (2009). Introduction. In Smith P, Mossialos E, Papanicolas I, Leatherman S (eds) *Performance measurement for health system improvement*, pp.3–24. Cambridge University Press, Cambridge.

16 Campbell S, Braspenning J, Hutchinson A, Marshall MN (2003). Research methods used in developing and applying quality indicators in primary care. *British Medical Journal*, **326**, 816–19.

17 Girard J-F, Minvielle E (2002). Measuring up: lessons and potential. In *Measuring up. Improving health system performance in OECD countries*, pp.337–47. OECD, Paris.

18 OECD (1990). *Health care systems in transition*. OECD, Paris.

19 Murray CJL, Evans DB (2003). Health systems performance assessment: goals, framework and overview, In Murray CJL, Evans DB (eds) *Health Systems Performance Assessment. Debates, methods and empiricism*, pp.3–18.World Health Organization, Geneva.

20 Murray C, Frenk J (2000). World Health Report 2000: a step towards evidence-based health policy. *Lancet*, **357**, 1698–700.

21 Hurst J, Jee-Hughes M (2000). *Performance measurements and performance management in OECD health systems*. OECD, Paris.

22 Nolte E, McKee M, Wait S (2005). Describing and evaluating health systems. In Bowling A, Ebrahim S (eds) *Handbook of health research methods: investigation, measurement and analysis*, pp.12–43. Open University Press, Maidenhead.

23 Arah O, Westert GP, Hurst J, Klazinga NS (2006). A conceptual framework for the OECD Health Care Quality Indicators Project. *International Journal for Quality in Health Care*, **18**(Suppl 1), 5–13.

24 Lalonde M (1974). *A new perspective on the health of Canadians*. Government of Canada, Ottawa.

25 Nutley S, Smith PC (1998). League tables for performance improvement in health care. *Journal of Health Services Research and Policy*, **3**, 50–7.

26 NHS Executive (1998). *The NHS performance assessment framework*. Department of Health, London.

27 Canadian Institute for Health Information and Statistics Canada (2000). *Canadian Health Information Roadmap Initiative Indicators Framework*. Canadian Institute for Health Information, Ottawa.

28 Canadian Institute for Health Information (2003). *About health indicators*. Available at http://www.cihi.ca/indicators/en/about.shtml (accessed 16 June 2009).

29 National Health Performance Committee (2001). *National health performance framework report*. NHPC, Brisbane.

30 Mainz J, Krog BR, Bjørnshave B, *et al.* (2004). Nationwide continuous quality improvement using clinical indicators: the Danish National Indicator Project. *International Journal for Quality in Health Care*, **16**(Suppl.1), i45–i50.

31 Agency for Healthcare Research and Quality (2009). *Measuring healthcare quality*. Available at: http://www.ahrq.gov/qual/measurix.htm (accessed 16 June 2009).

32 Westert, G., van den Berg M, Koolman X, Verkleij H (2008). *Dutch health care performance report 2008*. National Institute for Public Health and the Environment, Bilthoven.

33 Westert G, Verkleij H (2006). *Dutch health care performance report*. National Institute for Public Health and the Environment, Bilthoven.

34 Heugren M, Aberg A, Koester M, Ljung R (2007). Performance indicators in Swedish health care. *BMC Health Services Research*, **7**(Suppl), A10.

35 Chiu WT, Yang CM, Lin HW, Chu TB (2007). Development and implementation of a nationwide health care quality indicator system in Taiwan. *International Journal for Quality in Health Care*, **19**, 21–8.

36 National Health and Hospitals Reform Commission (2008). *Beyond the blame game: accountability and performance benchmarks for the next Australian Health Care Agreements*. National Health and Hospitals Reform Commission, Canberra.

37 The Commonwealth Fund Commission on a High Performance Health System (2006). *Why not the best? Results from a national scorecard on U.S. health system performance*. The Commonwealth Fund, New York.

38 The Commonwealth Fund Commission on a High Performance Health System (2008). *Why not the best? Results from the national scorecard on U.S. health system performance*. The Commonwealth Fund, New York.

39 Arah OA, Klazinga NS, Delnoij DMJ, Ten Asbroek AHA, Custers T (2003). Conceptual framework for health systems performance: a quest for effectiveness, quality and improvement. *International Journal of Quality in Health Care*, **15**, 377–98.

40 Nolte E (2009). *International benchmarking of health care quality. A review of the literature*. RAND Corporation, Santa Monica.

41 Tawfik-Shukor A, Klazinga NS, Arah OA (2007). Comparing health system performance assessment and management approaches in the Netherlands and Ontario, Canada. *BMC Health Services Research*, **7**, 25.

42 Murray C, Frenk J (2000). A framework for assessing the performance of health systems. *Bulletin of the World Health Organization*, **78**, 717–31.

43 Kelley E, Hurst J (2006). Health care quality indicators project. Conceptual framework paper. In *OECD Health Working Papers 23*. OECD, Paris.

44 Musgrove P (2003). Judging health systems: reflections on WHO's methods. *Lancet*, **361,** 1817–20.

45 Valentine N, Prasad A, Rice N, Robone S, Chatterji S (2009). Health systems responsiveness – a measure of the acceptability of health care processes and systems from the user's perspective. In Smith P (ed) *Performance measurement for health system improvement: experiences, challenges and prospects*, pp.138–86. Cambridge University Press, Cambridge.

46 Hussey PS, Anderson GF, Osborn R, *et al.* (2004). How does the quality of care compare in five countries? *Health Affairs*, **23,** 89–99.

47 Idänpään-Heikkilä U (2003). The Nordic Indicator Group Project. Presentation at the OECD Health Care Quality Indicators Meeting, 13–14 January, 2003, Paris.

48 Lohr K (1990). *Medicare: A strategy for quality assurance*. National Academy Press, Washington, DC.

49 Mattke S, Kelley E, Scherer P, *et al.* (2006). *Health Care Quality Indicators Project: Initial indicators report*. OECD, Paris.

50 Mattke S, Epstein A, Leatherman S (2006). The OECD Health Care Quality Indicators Project: history and background. *International Journal for Quality in Health Care*, **18,** 1–4.

51 Garcia Armesto S, Gil Lapetra ML, Wei L, Kelley E, Members of the HCQI Expert Group (2007). Health care quality indicators project 2006 data collection update report. In *OECD Health Working Papers No. 29*. OECD, Paris.

52 OECD (2007). *Health at a glance 2007 – OECD indicators*. OECD, Paris.

53 Nolte E, McKee M (2003). Measuring the health of the nations: how much is attributable to health care? An analysis of mortality amenable to medical care. *British Medical Journal*, **327,** 1129–32.

54 Nolte E, McKee M (2004). *Does healthcare save lives? Avoidable mortality revisited*. The Nuffield Trust, London.

55 Hill K, Thaomas K, AbouZhar C, *et al.* (2007). Estimates of maternal mortality worldwide between 1990 and 2005: an assessment of available data. *Lancet*, **370,** 1311–19.

56 World Health Organization Regional Office for Europe (2009). *European health for all database. Updated January 2009*. World Health Organization Regional Office for Europe, Copenhagen.

57 Kinyanjui, S, Timaeus IA (2010). *External review of the INDEPTH Network: Report to SIDA and other funders. Swedish International Development Cooperation Agency*, Stockholm.

58 Walshe K (2003). International comparisons of the quality of health care: what do they tell us? *Quality and Safety in Health Care*, **12,** 4–5.

59 Plochg T, Klazinga NS (2002). Community-based integrated care: myth or must? *International Journal for Quality in Health Care*, **14,** 91–101.

60 Donabedian A (1966). Evaluating the quality of medical care. *Milbank Quarterly*, **44,** 166–203.

61 Donabedian A (1988). The quality of care: how can it be assessed? *Journal of the American Medical Association*, **260,** 1743–8.

62 Mant J (2001). Process versus outcome indicators in the assessment of quality of health care. *International Journal for Quality in Health Care*, **13,** 475–80.

63 Kruk M, Freedman L (2008). Assessing health system performance in developing countries: A review of the literature. *Health Policy*, **85,** 263–76.

64 Smith P (2002). Developing composite indicators for assessing health system efficiency. In Smith P (ed) *Measuring up. Improving health system performance in OECD countries*, pp.295–316. OECD, Paris.

65 Kessner DM, Kalk CE, Singer J (1973). Assessing health quality: the case for tracers. *New England Journal of Medicine*, **288**, 189–94.

66 Nolte E, Bain C, McKee M (2006). Chronic diseases as tracer conditions in international benchmarking of health systems: the example of diabetes. *Diabetes Care*, **29**, 1007–11.

67 Nolte E, Bain C, McKee M (2009). Population health. In Smith P (ed) *Performance measurement for health system improvement: experiences, challenges and prospects*, pp.27–62. Cambridge University Press, Cambridge.

68 Adeyi O, Smith O, Robles S (2007). *Public Policy and the challenge of chronic noncommunicable diseases*. World Bank, Washington DC.

69 Beran D, Yudkin J, de Courten M (2005). Access to care for patients with insulin-requiring diabetes in developing countries: case studies of Mozambique and Zambia. *Diabetes Care*, **28**, 2136–40.

70 Hopkinson B, Balabanova D, McKee M, Kutzin J (2004). The human perspective on health care reform: coping with diabetes in Kyrgyzstan. *International Journal of Health Planning and Management*, **19**, 43–61.

71 Diabetes Control and Complications Trial Research Group (1993). The effect of intensive treatment of diabetes on the development and progression of long-term complications in insulin-dependent diabetes mellitus. *New England Journal of Medicine*, **329**, 977–86.

72 United Kingdom Prospective Diabetes Study Group (UKPDS) (1998). Intensive blood-glucose control with sulfonylureas or insulin compared with conventional treatment and risk of complications in patients with type 2 diabetes (UKPDS33). *Lancet*, **352**, 837–53.

73 Laing SP, Swerdlow AJ, Slater SD, *et al.* (2003). Mortality from heart disease in a cohort of 23,000 patients with insulin-treated diabetes. *Diabetologia*, **46**, 760–5.

74 McColl AJ, Gulliford MC (1993). *Population health outcome indicators for the NHS. A feasibility study*. Faculty of Public Health Medicine and the Department of Public Health Medicine, United Medical and Dental Schools of Guy's and St Thomas' Hospitals, London.

75 World Health Organization (1999). *Definition, diagnosis and classification of diabetes mellitus and its complications. Part 1: diagnosis and classification of diabetes mellitus*. World Health Organization, Geneva.

76 Wild S, Roglic G, Green A, Sicree R, King H (2004). Global prevalence of diabetes. *Diabetes Care*, **27**, 1047–53.

77 Yudkin JS, Beran D (2003). Prognosis of diabetes in the developing world. *Lancet*, **362**, 1420–1.

78 Balabanova D, McKee M, Koroleva N, *et al.* (2009). Navigating the health system: diabetes care in Georgia. *Health Policy Planning*, **24**, 46–54.

79 Loeb J (2004). The current state of performance measurement in health care. *International Journal for Quality in Health Care*, **16**(Suppl 1), i5–i9.

80 Bevan G, Hood C (2006). Have targets improved performance in the English NHS? *British Medical Journal*, **332**, 419–22.

81 Fung, C., Lim YW, Mattke S, Damberg C, Shekelle PG. (2008). Systematic review: the evidence that releasing performance data to the public improves quality of care. *Annals of Internal Medicine*, **148**, 111–23.

82 Marshall MN, Shekelle PG, Leatherman S, Brook RH (2000). The public release of performance data: what do we expect to gain? A review of the evidence. *Journal of the American Medical Association*, **283**, 1866–74.

83 Chassin MR (2002). Achieving and sustaining improved quality: lessons from New York State and cardiac surgery. *Health Affairs*, **21**, 40–51.

84 Hibbard J, Stockard J, Tusler M (2005). Hospital performance reports: impact on quality, market share, and reputation. *Health Affairs*, **24**, 1150–60.

85 Leatherman S (2002). Applying performance indicators to health system improvement. In Smith P (ed) *Measuring up. Improving health system performance in OECD countries*, pp.319–33. OECD, Paris.

86 Smith P, Mossialos E, Papanicolas I, Leatherman S (eds) (2009). *Performance measurement for health system improvement*. Cambridge University Press, Cambridge.

Chapter 4

Revenue collection and pooling arrangements in financing

Di McIntyre and Joseph Kutzin

4.1 Introduction

There are three key functions in a health financing system: revenue collection, pooling, and purchasing. Revenue collection refers to the sources of funds for healthcare or who healthcare funding contributions are collected from, how these funding contributions are structured, and which organizations collect these funds. Pooling of funds refers to accumulating prepaid healthcare revenues on behalf of a population, with a particular emphasis on the population coverage and composition of groups which are covered by a specific pool [1]. Pooling can be seen as both an instrument of financing policy (i.e. the arrangements used for the accumulation of prepaid funds) and as an objective, i.e. risk pooling. Risk pooling addresses the unpredictability of illness, particularly at the individual level, and the inability of many individuals to be able to mobilize enough resources to cover healthcare costs without forewarning, and hence the need to spread these risks over as broad a group as possible and over time. Purchasing refers to the process of transferring pooled funds to healthcare providers to ensure that appropriate and efficient services are available to the population. The purchasing function includes considerations such as what type of services should be provided, the route by which different services should be accessed (i.e. the benefit package), and the mechanism(s) by which providers are paid.

This chapter focuses on two of the key functions of a health sector financing system; revenue collection and fund pooling. Other chapters touch on issues related to purchasing (e.g. provider payment mechanisms for non-state providers) and on healthcare delivery. The starting point in considering alternative approaches to undertaking these two functions is the World Health Assembly's resolution calling for healthcare financing systems to provide universal coverage and protection against the financial risks associated with using health services [2]. Financial protection has become a key concern internationally, not least of all due to the mounting evidence on the extent to which households (particularly, but not exclusively, low income) incur catastrophic costs when using health services which can (further) impoverish them [3]. It is now widely accepted that 'prepayment and pooling of resources and risks are basic principles in financial-risk protection' [2]. It is also apparent that policy should seek to protect needed service utilization in addition to protecting households against the costs of such use.

We go further and argue that, in order to achieve equitable, efficient, and sustainable universal coverage, it is necessary to reduce fragmentation between funding pools. From an equity perspective, there is wide agreement that individuals and households should contribute to funding healthcare according to their ability to pay, and should benefit from health services according to their need for healthcare [4]. This requires that the health sector financing system promotes both income and risk cross-subsidies, from the wealthy to the poor and the healthy to the ill respectively [5]. Maximizing income cross-subsidies relates to the mix of contribution mechanisms used to raise funds, while promoting risk cross-subsidies is more related to pooling arrangements. In each case, expanding the scope for cross-subsidies to flow in the health sector requires that fragmentation between funding pools is minimized. Reduced fragmentation also limits duplication in administration of the financing system and in some cases (where provision and financing are vertically integrated) can also reduce similar fragmentation in service provision and will promote efficiency. Thus, our focus is also on how to minimize fragmentation in the financing system.

Although some countries may be exploring ways of changing their existing financing system in order to generate additional revenue for health services, changing the financing system may equally be pursued as a mechanism for addressing inequities and inefficiencies in the existing system. Our intention is to provide insights into how both of these objectives can be achieved.

We review the complex array of alternative ways of collecting and pooling health sector resources. Progress towards the policy objective of universal financial risk protection and access to needed health services [1] can be promoted through different combinations of revenue collection and fund pooling mechanisms. How best to achieve this policy objective within each country's specific context should be the primary focus when reviewing these alternative financing mechanisms.

4.2 Revenue collection

Two specific aspects of revenue collection are considered here:

- ◆ Funding sources, and
- ◆ Contribution mechanisms.

While both aspects are important, the structure of financing contributions is fundamental to promoting appropriate income cross-subsidies in the health sector and, thus, receives particular attention here.

4.2.1 Sources of funds

All funding for health services ultimately comes from households or firms. All tax revenue, all health insurance contributions, and all direct payments for healthcare come from one or both of these sources. What is important to note is that, frequently, the burden of payments which appear to be made by firms are in fact passed on to households. For example, if employers are required to contribute towards health insurance contributions, they may offset the cost of these contributions through smaller salary increases than would have been paid in the absence of these contributions.

In addition to these domestic sources of healthcare revenue, many low- and middle-income countries (LMICs) also benefit from external or donor funding. This may take the form of loans (e.g. from the World Bank) or grants from bilateral and/or multilateral organizations. There are considerable debates about the advantages and disadvantages of donor funding and about the form that it should take; these issues are taken up in Chapter 9. The concerns about the predictability and long-term sustainability of donor funding highlights the importance of giving serious consideration to ways of mobilizing more domestic funds, as is done in this chapter, even in countries that are currently aid dependent.

4.2.2 Contribution mechanisms

Households and firms can contribute to funding health services either through direct payments or through prepayment mechanisms. For households, direct or out-of-pocket (OOP) payments take the form of user fees at public sector health facilities, 'informal' or not legally sanctioned payments to health workers or for treatment inputs in public sector health facilities [6], or fees paid to a private provider (ranging from formally qualified health professionals working in private practice to traditional healers and informal drug sellers). In the latter case, these payments may be for the full fee or may be a co-payment where the service user is covered by some form of prepayment, but which does not cover the total cost of the service. OOP payments generally have to be made at the time of using the health service.

There are two broad categories of prepayment mechanisms: compulsory and voluntary. Compulsory prepayment includes various forms of taxation or mandated contributions to funding services. Taxes can be used to fund health services through allocations from general revenues (i.e. personal income tax,

Value Added Tax (VAT), etc. which are collected to fund a wide range of government sponsored services) and/or through collecting certain taxes which are earmarked or dedicated to the funding of healthcare. The most common form of such dedicated taxes are payroll taxes for 'social' or mandatory health insurance (MHI). Other forms include a specific tax from which all or some revenues are earmarked for the health sector, such as excise taxes on tobacco products. Earmarking may also relate to a specific percentage of a more general tax to the health sector. For example, in Ghana, VAT of 15% is charged on most goods and services; 10% is for general government revenue, 2.5% is an earmarked tax for the health sector, and 2.5% is an earmarked tax for the education sector [7]. Similarly in Latvia between 1998 and 2003, 28.4% of personal income tax was dedicated to health insurance [8].

The distinction between MHI and an earmarked health tax is often very blurred. This is because the groups who are required to make contributions in either form are specified in legislation and that health service benefits will flow to contributors, and in some countries also to non-contributors, from these payments.

The main form of voluntary pre-payment is voluntary private health insurance. Although the name implies that it is entirely at the individual's discretion as to whether or not they choose to contribute to a health insurance scheme, scheme membership is often a condition of employment in countries such as South Africa and the United States which have a large private health insurance market.

The precise prepayment mechanism(s) used differs from country to country and there are advantages and disadvantages to each mechanism. It is helpful to explore these issues through considering empirical evidence on alternative prepayment mechanisms from a range of countries.

4.3 Empirical evidence on alternative financial contribution mechanisms

Over the past two decades, a number of studies have been undertaken to quantify the relative progressivity of alternative healthcare financing mechanisms. The results of the first major project of this kind (the 'ECuity project') were published in the early 1990s and focused on European countries and the USA [9]. These findings were updated and extended to include additional OECD (Organisation for Economic Cooperation and Development) countries in the late 1990s [10]. More recently, the same methods have been applied in a range of Asian countries [11]. Similar studies are underway in some African [12,13] and Latin American countries.

Although some of this data does not reflect the current funding situation within individual countries due to substantial health sector reform in recent years, such as in Switzerland, they do provide accurate insights into the general trends in terms of relative progressivity of different healthcare financing mechanisms. Relative progressivity is represented in terms of the Kakwani Index,[1] and a summary of the most recently published Kakwani Index values for individual financing mechanisms in different countries is provided in Table 4.1.

4.3.1 Direct payments

Before considering empirical evidence on prepayment mechanisms, it is important to note that direct payments for health services by households have been found, with few exceptions, to be regressive (i.e. these payments account for a greater share of household income among poorer groups than richer groups) [10]. Moreover, they have been found to be more regressive than any other healthcare financing contribution mechanism.

However, recent research in LMICs in Asia has shown that direct payments may be progressive. The Kakwani Index for direct payments was positive in countries such as Bangladesh, Hong Kong, Indonesia, Korea, and the Philippines, but was negative (i.e. regressive) in China, Japan, Kyrgyzstan, and Taiwan. A key reason for this is 'the constrained ability of poor households to pay for healthcare. The poorest of the poor simply cannot afford to pay' [14: p.15]. Thus, the so-called progressivity of direct payments is simply attributable to the fact that the poorest do not use health services if they are required to pay. Nevertheless, even where direct payments were found to be 'progressive', they are less progressive than other healthcare funding mechanisms.

4.3.2 General public revenues

General revenues may come from direct or indirect taxes (or from public enterprise revenues such as oil production). Direct taxes are levied either on

---

[1] The Kakwani index is a measure of the relative progressivity of a financing mechanism and considers the distribution of the burden for contributing to healthcare funding relative to the distribution of income or ability-to-pay for healthcare. A negative Kakwani reflects that a funding mechanism is regressive (i.e. poorer households contribute a greater share of their income than richer households), a positive Kakwani indicates that a funding mechanism is progressive (i.e. richer households contribute a greater share of their income than poorer households), while an index of zero indicates that the funding mechanism is proportional (i.e. all households contribute the same proportion of their income). The greater the negative (positive) number is, the more regressive (progressive) the financing mechanism.

Table 4.1 Kakwani Indices for selected OECD and Asian countries

	Direct taxes	Indirect taxes	General taxes	Mandatory insurance	Total public	Private insurance	Direct payments	Total private	Total payments
OECD countries [10]									
Denmark (1987)	0.0624	−0.1126	0.0372		0.0372	0.0313	−0.2654	−0.2363	−0.0047
Finland (1990)	0.1272	−0.0969	0.0555	0.0937	0.0604	0.0000	−0.2419	−0.2419	0.0181
France (1989)				0.1112	0.1112	−0.1956	−0.3396	−0.3054	0.0012
Germany (1989)	0.2488	−0.0922	0.1100	−0.0977	−0.0533	0.1219	−0.0963	−0.0067	−0.0452
Ireland (1987)	0.2666	N/A	N/A	0.1263	N/A	−0.0210	−0.1472	−0.0965	N/A
Italy (1991)	0.1554	−0.1135	0.0343	0.1072	0.0712	0.1705	−0.0807	−0.0612	0.0413
Netherlands (1992)	0.2003	−0.0885	0.0714	−0.1286	−0.1003	0.0833	−0.0377	0.0434	−0.0703
Portugal (1990)	0.2180	−0.0347	0.0601	0.1845	0.0723	0.1371	−0.2424	−0.2287	−0.0445
Spain (1990)	0.2125	−0.1533	0.0486	0.0615	0.0509	−0.0224	−0.1801	−0.1627	0.0004
Sweden (1990)	0.0529	−0.0827	0.0371	0.0100	0.0100		−0.2402	−0.2402	−0.0158
Switzerland (1992)	0.2055	−0.0722	0.1590	0.0551	0.1389	−0.2548	−0.3619	−0.2945	−0.1402
UK (1993)	0.2843	−0.1522	0.0456	0.1867	0.0792	0.0766	−0.2229	−0.0919	0.051
US (1987)	0.2104	−0.0674	0.1487	0.0181	0.1060	−0.2374	−0.3874	−0.3168	−0.1303

Asian countries [11]

Bangladesh (1999–2000)	0.5523	0.1110			0.2192	0.2142
China (2000)	0.1521	0.0398	0.2348		−0.0168	0.0404
Hong Kong SAR (1999–2000)	0.3940	0.1102		0.0403	0.0113	0.1689
Indonesia (2001)	0.1962	0.0741	0.3057		0.1761	0.1729
Japan (1998)	0.0950	−0.2232	−0.0415		−0.2691	−0.0688
Korea Rep. (2000)	0.2683	0.0379	−0.1634		0.0124	−0.0239
Kyrgyz Rep. (2000)	0.2395	0.0508	0.1422		−0.0520	0.0087
Nepal (1995–96)	0.1436	0.1143			0.0533	0.0625
Philippines (1999)	0.3809	0.0024	0.2048	0.1199	0.1391	0.1631
Sri Lanka (1996–7)	0.5693	−0.0100		With direct payments	0.0687	0.0850
Taiwan (2000)	0.2601	0.0296	−0.0305	0.1961	−0.0962	−0.0119
Thailand (2002)	0.5101	0.1819	0.1803	0.0039	0.0907	0.1972

Other countries [32]

Estonia (2006)	0.245	−0.146	0.157		−0.377	

income such as salaries, wages, and interest from investments, or on wealth, and mainly take the form of personal and corporate income tax. Indirect taxes are levied on items that are consumed by households, such as excise taxes on tobacco and alcohol products and VAT on a wide range of goods and services.

All published empirical studies indicate that direct taxes are progressive (see Table 4.1) [9–12,14]. In almost all countries, personal income taxes are explicitly structured progressively where the percentage of income due in tax increases as incomes increase.

In contrast, indirect taxes tend to be regressive. This has been found to be the case in those high-income countries for which there are published results [10]. This was also found to be the case in high-income countries in Asia, such as Japan, and in some middle-income countries on different continents such as Sri Lanka and South Africa [11,12]. Indirect taxes have, however, been found to be progressive in many LMICs in Asia, largely due to the fact that most food items in these countries are exempt from VAT and other indirect taxes and that poorer households purchase goods that are produced in the local informal sector and which escape these indirect taxes [14]. Even where indirect taxes have been found to be progressive, they are far less progressive than direct taxes.

Overall, general revenues tend to be progressive, but this depends on how progressive (or regressive) direct and indirect taxes are within a particular country, as well as the relative mix of each type of tax.

In summary, progressivity of general taxes can be strengthened by placing a relatively greater emphasis on direct as opposed to indirect taxes. Clearly, the extent to which direct income taxes are progressively structured is also important. However, the limited size of the formal employment sector in many low-income countries means that it may not be feasible to increase the share of direct taxes in overall tax revenue. For this reason, care should also be taken to protect the poorest groups from the impact of key indirect taxes, e.g. exempting all basic foodstuffs from VAT. The challenges of increasing general tax revenue in countries with a small formal employment sector are considered later.

4.3.3 Compulsory contributions for mandatory health insurance

Typically, but not always, these contributions are in the form of a fixed percentage tax on salaries or wages, and hence referred to as a payroll tax. The relative progressivity of payroll taxes for mandatory (or social) health insurance varies considerably from country to country. In general, these contributions tend to be less progressive than direct tax payments, but may be more progressive than overall general taxes (i.e. direct and indirect taxes combined) (see Table 4.1). This makes intuitive sense given that MHI contributions are levied on salaries and wages only, and are frequently a fixed percentage contribution of the payroll, whereas direct taxes are levied on all sources of income and on wealth and are almost always structured as an increasing percentage as income increases. Salaries and wages as a proportion of total income tends to decrease as income levels increase [11].

What is particularly important to note is that where MHI is the major healthcare financing contribution mechanism within a country, such as in France (accounting for 74% of all healthcare financing), Germany (65%), the Netherlands (65%), Japan (54%), and Taiwan (52%), these contributions tend to be regressive. An important contributor to this is the existence in most countries of a ceiling or *cap* on contributions which effectively mean that higher-earning persons pay a lower percentage of their income than those earning an amount that is not subject to the cap. France, which completely phased out its contribution cap by 1983, and in 1998 switched the contribution base from salaries to all income [15], is the only country in this group where mandatory insurance contributions are progressive.

In summary, the evidence suggests that the progressivity of compulsory contributions for MHI depends critically on whether the tax is levied on salaries only or all forms of income, and whether or not contributions are capped. Because overall progressivity depends on the mix of revenue sources, it is the mix of total public funding between general tax revenue and MHI that is of particular importance. Key lessons from France, which has a progressive mandatory insurance system even though it accounts for nearly three-quarters of all financing, include:

- Not permitting high income earners to opt out of the mandatory insurance scheme (in Germany, the highest income groups do not participate in the mandatory insurance scheme).

- Not having a contribution cap because this reduces the effective contribution rate of higher income persons.

- Minimal contributions for some of the lowest income groups, such as pensioners and the unemployed [10].

4.3.4 Voluntary health insurance (VHI) contributions

In the case of voluntary (typically private) health insurance, the relative progressivity of contributions varies considerably across countries, depending largely on the role of VHI in a particular health system [16]. VHI is strongly regressive in Switzerland and the United States (see Table 4.1), the two countries that had the largest shares of total healthcare financing attributable to VHI contributions (accounting for 41% and 29% respectively in the late 1990s—this has now changed in Switzerland). It is also regressive in France. However, VHI contributions are progressive in most countries.

The major factor that seems to determine whether VHI contributions are regressive or progressive is the proportion of the population making these contributions. Where the majority of the population make VHI contributions, such as the United States and formerly in Switzerland, this financing mechanism is regressive because these contributions are typically not income related [16]. This is also the case in France where a large portion of the population takes out VHI to cover the relatively high copayments required by the universal mandatory insurance scheme. In contrast, where VHI is limited to those who opt out of social insurance, as is the case in Germany, it tends to be the highest income earners who opt out, resulting in positive Kakwani indices. Similarly, where VHI is taken out in addition to having an entitlement to benefit from publicly funded services (i.e. supplemental cover) it is essentially a luxury good accessible only to the richest households [10]. This is the case in many LMICs (see Asian countries in Table 4.1), including South Africa [12].

Although there is no empirical evidence on its relative progressivity, it is important to briefly refer to a form of VHI that is growing in popularity in LMICs, particularly in Africa and Asia, namely community-based health insurance (CBHI). These schemes exist within localized communities, most frequently in rural areas, where members make small payments (often on an annual basis after the harvest time) to the scheme, which then covers fees charged at local health services. Given that CBHI schemes focus on rural areas and sometimes informal sector workers in urban areas, they are a mechanism to collect revenue from poorer groups in society and would, thus, tend to be a regressive contribution mechanism. CBHI tends to place a burden on those with the least ability to pay, and may end up being a mechanism whereby 'the poor simply cross-subsidize the healthcare costs of other poor members of the population' [17]. They also tend to have very high collection and other administration costs relative to the revenue they generate. However, CBHI is often introduced as an alternative to OOP payments for these poor communities and the progressivity (or regressivity) of CBHI contributions should be assessed relative to OOP payments. Given the growing popularity of these schemes, it is concerning that there is little or no evidence on the extent to which they provide risk protection, and this should be a key area for future research.

4.3.5 Overall financing

The relative progressivity of overall healthcare financing is determined by aggregating the weighted indices of each contribution mechanism, where the weight is the percentage share of each mechanism to total healthcare funding. The OECD countries with the most regressive healthcare financing systems in the late 1990s were Switzerland and the United States. The majority of financing in both of these countries at that time was attributable to private funding mechanisms; private insurance accounted for 41% in Switzerland and 29% in the United States while direct payments accounted for 24% and 22% respectively [10].

In contrast, OECD countries with the most progressive financing systems in the late 1990s (United Kingdom and Italy) were those which are very largely publicly funded. At that time, 84% of healthcare financing in the United Kingdom was through public mechanisms, 64% from general tax revenues and a further 20% from national insurance contributions. In Italy, public financing mechanisms accounted for 77% of all funds, which was evenly split between general tax revenue (38%) and MHI contributions (39%) [10].

Findings from Asia are less clear cut, not least of all because many of the poorest households in these countries do not contribute, but also do not manage to benefit from health services. For example, Bangladesh appears to have the most progressive healthcare financing system, despite the fact that 65% of funding is attributable to direct payments [11]. The other country with a very progressive financing system is Thailand, where public funding accounts for the major share of overall financing (56% from general government revenue and 5% from MHI contributions). This is more in line with the findings for the United Kingdom and Italy.

However, Japan has an even higher share of public finance (87%), with 33% from general government revenue and 54% from mandatory insurance contributions, but is the most regressive of the Asian countries. This is largely because the MHI scheme is regressive, highlighting the importance of appropriate structuring of mandatory insurance contributions. The other Asian country whose healthcare financing system is strongly regressive is the Republic of Korea. It is similar to Japan in the sense that MHI contributions account for a larger share of financing (34%) than general government revenue (16%) and that mandatory insurance contributions are strongly regressive (partly due to the cap on insurance contributions for the highest income groups, which was abolished in 2002). Interestingly, a full 50% of healthcare financing in Korea are attributable to direct payments, largely in the form of very high co-payments. However, these are somewhat progressive as many of the poorest are unable to pay these co-payments and so have much lower utilization levels than higher income groups [18].

4.3.6 Key lessons from empirical evidence

Direct (OOP) payments impose a regressive financing burden; the only instance where this does not occur is where the poorest households do not make such payments, usually because they do not seek care because they cannot afford it [11]. There is now overwhelming evidence that high levels of direct payments can have catastrophic effects on households, leading to impoverishment in many cases [4,19].

This issue is of considerable importance. While a growing number of countries are moving away from patient cost sharing (either in the form of user fees for public sector health services or co-payments required by many health insurance schemes, both mandatory and voluntary), they continue to prevail in many countries. In addition, patients in many LMICs face high OOP costs to get needed services, regardless of official policy on user fees or co-payments. This may be in the form of informal payments to health workers or for inputs needed for treatment, high levels of spending for medicines purchased from private pharmacies or other sellers, or the costs of transport to health facilities.

Regressivity can also be minimized by both clearly defining and limiting the role of voluntary health insurance in the health system. The ability to 'opt out' of a compulsory insurance system should be prohibited, as this facilitates an explicitly multi-tiered system whereby it becomes more difficult to enable cross-subsidies to flow (see next section on pooling). There may be some scope for complementary VHI (including in the form of CBHI), but this requires explicit linkage between the entitlements afforded under the publicly mandated system and the VHI benefit package (e.g. covering part/all of the cost sharing obligations). From an equity perspective, this option makes sense only if the VHI substitutes for OOP spending. If instead it substitutes for public funding, the consequences would be regressive. VHI in the form of supplemental 'double-cover' is a lesser cause for concern, as this can be seen as a luxury good for those who are willing to pay to secure services over-and-above what they could use in the publicly funded health system. In contexts of very scarce health human resources, however, there remains a risk that even supplemental VHI can have harmful effects on service availability for the majority of the population, if it contributes to staff shortages in the publicly mandated system by attracting health workers to spend more time serving insured patients in the private sector.

There is indisputable evidence that in order to achieve progressive, universal healthcare, public funding should account for the major share of healthcare financing. Funding from general tax revenue has the potential to be the most progressive, though this depends on the underlying mix of taxes (direct vs. indirect) as well as the progressivity of the rates imposed on direct income and corporate taxes. Mandatory or social health insurance can also be progressive or (more commonly) at least proportional, with the following features promoting progressivity in such schemes:

- The rich should not be permitted to opt out of the scheme.
- The contributions of vulnerable groups (e.g. the unemployed, pensioners, the poor) should be fully or partially subsidized.
- A cap should not be placed on contributions as this results in those earning above the threshold paying a lower percentage of their earnings than those earning below the threshold [20].

4.4 **Key issues relating to public healthcare financing**

This section attempts to address briefly two key issues, namely: How much public funding should be made available to the health sector? How can one optimize public funding levels if there is a mix of allocations from general revenues, compulsory MHI contributions, and any dedicated health taxes?

4.4.1 **How much public funding should be made available to the health sector?**

The reason for posing the question of appropriate levels of public funding is that relatively regressive forms of financial contributions such as direct payments and private insurance have developed primarily in response to inadequate public funding of the health sector.

There is no existing, generally accepted target for the 'optimal' level of public funding for healthcare. Potentially an appropriate target would be public spending on health as a percentage of the country's gross domestic product (GDP). The attraction of such a target is that it is linked to a country's level of economic development, which implies that the target could be 'affordable'. One way of going about determining an appropriate target is to attempt to identify levels of public spending that translate into universal coverage, in the sense of the extent to which the population is protected from OOP payments and particularly catastrophic spending.

As shown in Figure 4.1, public health spending as a proportion of GDP explains a remarkable degree of the variation in the share of OOP spending in total healthcare expenditure. Even with the strong R^2, however, there remains substantial variation around the trend. A simple way to interpret this variation (apart from data shortcomings) is the recognition that policy

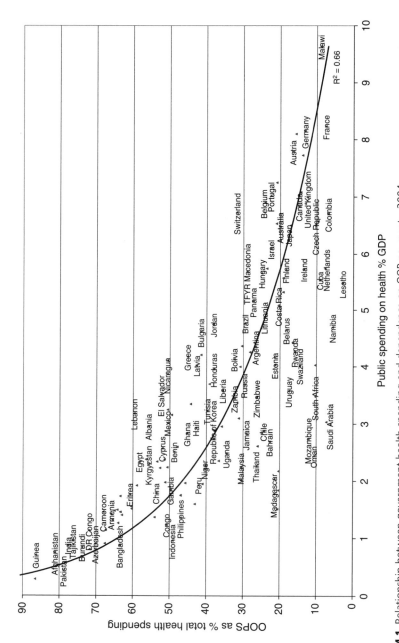

Fig. 4.1 Relationship between government health spending and dependence on OOP payments, 2004.

Source: WHO health expenditure database. Only countries with populations greater than 600,000 included in the data, and of these, only selected countries identified by name in the figure.

Source: Reproduced from [4] with permission of the World Health Organization.

matters—while the level of public spending on health is important, it is not the entire story.

The dependence of a health sector on OOP payments is important because of its link to concerns about financial protection. Further international comparative analysis [21] shows that there is a strong correlation between the share of OOP payments in a country's total healthcare spending and the percentage of families that face catastrophic health expenditures. Hence, reducing the share of health spending coming from OOP payments is a policy objective for most countries that are concerned to improve financial protection for their populations.

Figure 4.1 clearly shows that there are almost no countries where governments spend at least 5% of GDP on health that have OOP spending representing 30% or more of total healthcare expenditure. This strongly suggests that attaining universal coverage with public expenditures below this level will be difficult for any country. This is based on an 'eyeballing' of the data, and of course demands deeper analysis of the basic data as well as methodological development with regard to the definition and measurement of coverage.

4.4.2 Optimizing public funding with a mix of general tax revenue and MHI

The next issue is that of how one can optimize public funding levels if there is a mix of allocations from general tax revenue and a payroll tax for MHI. Revenue collection can be described as the 'art of the possible' rather than a 'technical choice of the optimal'. This is because much of the decision making around public funding for healthcare is outside of the control of the health sector. Nevertheless, there is a need for the health sector to engage more with the Ministry of Finance/Treasury to advocate for a fair share of resources for the health sector as well as to learn from the experiences of other countries with respect to how to optimize overall public funding where there is a mix of general revenue allocations and payroll tax for MHI. Issues related to this are covered in later chapters, especially Chapter 12.

Many countries that introduce a payroll tax for MHI do so as a means of generating additional funds for health services [22]. Given that these contributions are made by the same individuals who contribute to direct taxes (personal income tax in particular), some may ask why this approach is adopted rather than simply increasing personal income tax rates.

There are several reasons why some experts have a preference for a health specific payroll tax or insurance contribution mechanism, a key one being that it is a payroll deduction for which there is a specific package of healthcare benefits [23]. A potential advantage of this financing mechanism is that if formal sector employment and/or salary levels are increasing, a dedicated health tax levied on income or wages can be stable and sustainable [24] relative to general tax allocations which are subject to the vagaries of budget decision making. Other reasons may be ideological, such as a desire by some ex-USSR countries to move away from the inherited Soviet budgeting system, or the desire of many central European countries to return to the type of system they had been developing prior to World War II [22].

Counterbalancing these apparent advantages of a payroll tax for MHI are two important potential disadvantages. Firstly, employment levels and salary levels may not increase as rapidly as overall GDP growth and tax funded government expenditure. For example, in Estonia health services are almost entirely funded through mandatory insurance contributions, resulting in the health sector's share of total public spending declining considerably [22]. Also, in times of economic difficulty, unemployment grows and people may lose their entitlements to healthcare benefits (as occurred in some countries during the 'Asian economic crisis').

Secondly, additional revenue generated from the mandatory insurance contributions or dedicated payroll tax may displace general tax revenue allocations to the health sector. However, two precautions could be taken to limit the potential for general tax funding for healthcare to be displaced. The first precaution is that it appears to be easier to control the impact of introducing payroll taxes on the level of general revenue funding for healthcare where government health spending decisions are centralized. In fiscal federal systems, where considerable autonomy is granted to decentralized government levels in decision making around healthcare funding, there is a greater likelihood of mandatory insurance displacing tax funding. This was found to be the case in both Russia and Kazakhstan. In Kazakhstan, there was a dramatic decline in tax revenue allocations to the health sector, which 'reflected, in many instances, a withdrawal from health system funding and a shift to other priorities by the local governments in reaction to the loss of direct hierarchical control implied by the creation of the MHIF [Mandatory Health Insurance Fund]' [22].

The other strategy that could be adopted, to limit the likelihood of general tax revenue allocations to the health sector being reduced, is to tie general tax funding to partially or fully subsidized contributions on behalf of those with limited ability to pay mandatory insurance contributions. Given the relatively low levels of formal sector employment in many LMICs, it can be argued that general tax funds should be used to fund the contributions of those outside of the formal sector to ensure universal coverage or entitlements via the mandatory insurance system. The level of contributions on behalf of those outside the formal sector should be specified. This could either take the form of a specific percentage of average salaries or wages (as in the Czech Republic) or of the minimum wage (as in Serbia), which would be similar to the percentage contribution by formal sector workers, or a flat amount per person which may be linked to the average cost of providing the benefit package (as in Lithuania and Moldova) [22].

Although decision-making around some of these issues may remain outside the control of the health sector, awareness of the experience of other countries when introducing payroll taxes for MHI can assist in strategic negotiations with those who do have decision-making power to ensure that overall public funding for the health sector is maximized irrespective of the precise mix of allocations from general tax revenues and payroll tax for MHI.

4.5 Fund pooling

Healthcare costs are unpredictable; it is difficult for individuals to know when they will fall ill, what healthcare they will require and what this healthcare will cost. Sometimes the cost of care can be very high, particularly for hospitalization or long-term serious illness such as cancer or AIDS, and most people are unable to cover these unexpected costs drawing on resources that they have available at one point in time. While it is difficult to predict healthcare needs and costs for an individual, it is more feasible to predict these for a group of people drawing on epidemiological and actuarial data. This is the core of the concept of risk-pooling; individuals contribute on a regular basis to a pooled fund so that when they fall ill, the pool will cover their costs. Essentially, at any one point in time, the healthy members of the pool are helping to pay for the healthcare costs of those who are ill; those who are healthy and those who are ill will change over time. The risk of falling ill and incurring unexpected and high healthcare costs is shared between those in the pool. There is also a time element to risk pooling in that individuals draw on contributions that they made when healthy to pay for healthcare costs when ill [25].

The larger the group pooling their risks, the easier it is to predict healthcare expenditure requirements. Where there is more than one funding pool, it is important to consider the market structure, including the number of pools, whether or not there is competition between the different pools and the extent to which there are inter-pool financial flows.

The key issues that are considered in this section are:

- The size, or population coverage, and composition of risk pools, and
- Allocation mechanisms for distributing pooled resources.

4.5.1 Coverage and composition of risk pools

There is considerable variation between countries with respect to the nature, number, and composition of risk pools. This section provides an overview of some of these variations, evaluated relative to the goal of achieving universal coverage. Universal coverage is commonly defined as all citizens having access to adequate healthcare at an affordable cost [26]. This implies that universal coverage can be achieved through a combination of different financing mechanisms within one country, where different groups are covered by different mechanisms but all are 'adequately' covered in some way. However, universal coverage is much more costly and difficult to attain in sectors with fragmented risk pools which do not allow for income and risk cross-subsidies in the overall health sector. As indicated previously, these cross-subsidies are critical to achieve an equitable, efficient, and sustainable healthcare financing system. Pooling is particularly important in creating the conditions for redistribution of resources according to individuals' need for healthcare and thereby promoting equitable utilization of health services.

It is particularly notable that in the United States, the country with the highest level of total health spending (including one of the highest levels of public spending on health in the OECD), the highly fragmented arrangement of risk pools is a major reason why universal coverage has not yet been attained. This country has a large number of voluntary private health insurance schemes, and also has two state funded schemes to cover the poor and the elderly (Medicaid and Medicare). Nevertheless, 28% of adults (50 million Americans) were either completely uninsured or uninsured for part of the year in 2007 [27]. One-third of adult Americans spent 10% or more of their income on health insurance premiums and direct healthcare payments in 2007, suggesting the financial burden on families is widespread. Risk-selection is also a problem, with those with the greatest risk of ill-health being excluded from coverage.

Other countries have what some would term 'universal coverage', in the sense that all citizens have at least legal entitlement, and varying degrees of access, to some form of healthcare, but where there are completely separate risk pools for different sections of the population resulting in a tiered health system. This is particularly the case where there is mandatory or social health insurance covering only those working in the formal sector and general tax revenue funded health services covering the rest of the population, as exists in Mexico and many other Latin American countries [28]. A further tier may be introduced into these systems by allowing individuals to opt out of the social health insurance, such as occurred in Chile.

Some argue that a tiered system is the only way to move towards universal healthcare based on mandatory insurance. This is based on the fact that, historically, most universal mandatory insurance systems have begun by covering only formal sector employees, and often their dependents. Coverage was gradually extended over many years as the formal sector expanded and as efforts were made to include the self-employed and informal sector workers [26].

However, we would argue that simply because this is the route that has been historically adopted by countries with compulsory contributions for MHI does not mean that it is the only way to achieve universal coverage in this context. Indeed, creating a two-tier system can become an obstacle to achieving universal coverage which includes comprehensive income and risk cross-subsidies. This has certainly been the experience of a number of Latin American countries that initiated mandatory insurance by covering formal sector workers and their dependents, and where this group has remained the focus of mandatory insurance initiatives for many decades. These countries have found that a two-tier health sector has become entrenched and have encountered considerable difficulties in extending coverage, not least of all because the vocal and powerful formally employed groups have opposed moves towards universal coverage for fear of losing their preferential benefits [29].

Turning now to universal systems which are more integrated and less explicitly tiered, there are several countries that have achieved universal mandatory insurance systems but with a number of smaller schemes acting as the financing intermediaries. In some cases, these smaller schemes may compete with each other for members, as is the case in the Netherlands. One drawback of this approach is the high administrative costs involved with having a number of separate schemes and the high marketing costs incurred as schemes compete for members. There could also be problems with ensuring income and risk cross-subsidies, which require risk-equalization mechanisms that are costly to maintain. Indeed it is for these and other reasons that, in 2000, Korea integrated 139 separate private insurance associations, 227 insurance associations for the self-employed, and numerous other insurance associations into a single National Health Insurance Corporation.

Other countries have embarked on MHI systems through non-competing insurance schemes. This generally occurs where these schemes are geographically defined, as in the case of Ghana and Bosnia-Herzegovina which have an insurance scheme for each district or 'canton'. One of the problems with this approach is that some schemes may have relatively small risk pools. For example, the smallest cantonal scheme in Bosnia-Herzegovina has only 35,000 members [30]. Multiple small pools also result in inefficiently high administrative costs when measured at the national level. Other problems that have arisen in Bosnia-Herzegovina include inequities due to differences in participation, contribution rates, and total revenues between the cantonal schemes combined with the lack of a mechanism to redistribute funds across them to ensure that each scheme's resources reflect the relative healthcare needs of the covered population. Instead, each cantonal scheme's resources are determined by the socioeconomic status of the resident population, and hence the contribution rate that is considered affordable in that territory, which has resulted in very different benefit packages being offered in each canton [30].

The Ghanaian national health insurance has attempted to avoid some of these problems by specifying a uniform benefit package for all district schemes and a uniform contribution schedule [7]. The contributions for all formal sector workers are deducted from the payroll, sent to the NHI fund, and then distributed to each district scheme according to the number of registered formal sector workers. The innovative element of the Ghanaian NHI is that they have built on their extensive historical experience of community-based health insurance schemes as the basis of drawing in the large population not in the formal sector, which created the requirement for district-based insurance schemes. One problem, however, is that differences have arisen in the contribution rates for those in the informal sector between districts; some districts are charging all residents outside of the formal sector the mandated minimum contribution while other districts, with higher socioeconomic status, have been able to implement the full range of income-related contributions mandated under the NHI. As in Bosnia-Herzegovina, there is no mechanism for ensuring that district schemes have the resources required to provide for the resident population's health needs which is likely to result in differences in the benefit package available in reality. More importantly, there is complete fragmentation between funding which flows via the Ministry of Health and that which flows via the NHI fund and its district-based schemes, i.e. there are parallel funding flows to the same healthcare providers with no coordination between the two funding streams.

There are some recent examples of countries that have successfully overcome the problem of parallel funding streams, particularly Moldova and Kyrgyzstan. The process of moving towards an integrated system was gradual in Kyrgyzstan. The initial step was the creation of a mandatory health insurance fund (MHIF) in 1997, which received payroll contributions from formal sector employees, contributions from pension and unemployment funds for these two groups and contributions from general tax funds for children under 16. Members of the MHI received care from hospitals and primary healthcare providers that also received tax-funded budgets, and the MHIF paid these providers on a case-based and capitation basis respectively (i.e. additional payments above the basic budget). An integrated hospital information system incorporating both the insured and non-insured population was also established. In 2000, the oblast (province or region) level of the health (and other) ministries was eliminated. It was decided to allocate all local government health budgets to the local offices of the MHIF, which then purchased healthcare on behalf of the entire population in their area whether so-called insured on uninsured. This effectively created a purchaser–provider split, a single-payer mechanism, and a complete shift from budgets for providers to case-based and capitation reimbursement for hospitals and primary care providers respectively [30,31].

A similar approach was adopted in Moldova, but the implementation was not phased as in Kyrgyzstan. Instead, a MHI was introduced in 2004 and at the same time, government health budgets were centralized and allocated to the National Health Insurance Company (NHIC) where they were pooled with payroll NHI revenues. About one-third of the NHIC revenues were attributable to payroll contributions while two-thirds came from an allocation from general tax revenues. As in Kyrgyzstan, this created a single-payer system with a purchaser-provider split [30,31].

Where it is for some, usually political, reason not possible to completely integrate general tax and payroll tax for MHI revenues into a single pool, it is essential to ensure that there is close coordination between the funding flows in the two pools. A key lesson from country experience is that when a payroll tax for MHI is introduced, it is essential to concurrently reform the flows and pooling arrangements for general budget revenues.

4.5.2 Allocation mechanisms

The other key component of risk pooling is the mechanism for ensuring an equitable distribution of resources relative to the need for healthcare, or risk of incurring healthcare costs. Risk-adjusted allocation mechanisms can be applied to any system with multiple pools regardless of whether the funds come from compulsory contributions or general tax revenues.

With respect to decentralized and typically budget-funded pools, risk-adjusted, also called needs-based, mechanisms are used to allocate resources from central level to decentralized health authorities. In general, a formula that includes indicators of relative need for healthcare is used to determine resource allocations to each geographic area [32]. The indicators most frequently used internationally are:

◆ Population size.
◆ Demographic composition, as young children, the elderly and women of childbearing age tend to have a greater need for health services.

- Levels of ill-health, with mortality rates usually being used as a proxy for morbidity.
- Socioeconomic status, given that there is a strong relationship between ill-health and low socioeconomic status and that the poor are most reliant on publicly funded services.
- Cost factors that are outside the influence of the health sector (e.g. relative population density, percentage of the population living at high altitude, etc.).

A similar approach to promoting equitable resource allocation is used in the case of competing health insurers, though typically under a different label called risk-equalization. This generally occurs where a MHI scheme offers people a choice among different insurance funds. In broad terms, the risk profile of each fund or scheme is assessed using a range of factors such as the age and gender profile of members, the disability status of members, and the number of members with specific chronic illnesses [32]. A risk-adjusted capitation amount, which is the average amount of money required to cover the likely healthcare costs per member for a uniform, specified benefit package given the scheme or fund's risk profile, is calculated. The risk-adjusted capitation is multiplied by the number of members in that scheme with each type of risk profile to calculate the total allocation for that scheme. The importance of introducing risk-equalization is that it changes the behaviour of schemes so that they are not competing on the basis of attracting the lowest risk members to their scheme but rather have to compete on the basis of efficient purchasing of health services so that they can offer the best possible benefit package within the constraints of the risk-adjusted capitation revenue they receive.

4.6 Conclusion

In this chapter, we have placed the emphasis firmly on public funding of health services in the form of general revenue allocations to the health sector and compulsory contributions (usually in the form of payroll tax) for MHI. This is where we believe the focus should lie if we are to achieve equitable, efficient and sustainable healthcare financing systems that offer universal financial risk protection.

The precise mix between these revenue sources will vary from country to country, depending on its specific context. It may be feasible for some countries to rely entirely on allocations from general tax revenue, i.e. introducing MHI contributions is not a pre-requisite for universal publicly-funded healthcare. Indeed, a MHI system may introduce unnecessary complexities and importantly, will not necessarily generate additional revenue for the health sector. Individual countries seeking ways to strengthen public funding of health services should, therefore, seriously consider whether a MHI is necessary in order to achieve the policy objective of achieving universal financial risk protection, distinguishing the need for raising more revenues from other reasons why the establishment of a new agency for pooling funds and purchasing services may be desirable. It is also important to recognize that while health services may be entirely funded from general tax revenue, it is not possible to fund universal healthcare entirely through MHI contributions. Even in the richest countries, there will be some who do not have the ability to pay MHI contributions, and universal coverage can only be achieved if government contributes on their behalf from general tax funds.

Where a combination of MHI contributions and allocations from general tax revenue are used, it is important to integrate these into a single pool wherever possible, or as a minimum to explicitly coordinate the funding flows of the two funding mechanisms. Fragmentation between different funding pools can lead to considerable inequities, as it reduces the potential for income and risk cross-subsidies in the overall health sector, as well as to inefficiencies in financial administration and in the purchasing and delivery of health services. There are a number of recent examples of general tax allocations being transferred to the MHI fund, which then purchases services on behalf of the entire population.

There is enormous potential for countries to achieve equitable, efficient and sustainable universal health financing systems. The key requirement is a demonstrated commitment to public funding of health services.

Acknowledgements

Our thanks go to Kara Hanson for very helpful comments on an earlier version of this chapter. DM is supported by the South African Research Chairs Initiative of the Department of Science and Technology and National Research Foundation. The usual disclaimers apply.

References

1 Kutzin J (2001). A descriptive framework for country-level analysis of health care financing arrangements. *Health Policy*, **56**, 171–204.

2 World Health Organization (2005). *Sustainable health financing, universal coverage and social health insurance: World Health Assembly resolution WHA58.33*. World Health Organization, Geneva.

3 Xu K, Evans D, Kawabata K, Zeramdini R, Klavus J, Murray C (2003). Household catastrophic health expenditure: A multicountry analysis. *Lancet*, **362**(362), 111–17.

4 Wagstaff A, Van Doorslaer E (1993). Equity in the finance and delivery of health care: Concepts and definitions. In Van Doorslaer E, Wagstaff A, Rutten F (eds) *Equity in the*

finance and delivery of health care: An international perspective, pp.2–19. Oxford University Press, New York.

5 Baeza CC, Packard TG (2006). *Beyond Survival: Protecting Households from Health Shocks in Latin America*. Stanford University Press and the World Bank, Palo Alto, California and Washington, DC.

6 Gaal P, McKee M (2004). Informal payment for health care and the theory of 'INXIT'. *International Journal of Health Planning and Management*, **19**(2), 163–78.

7 Government of Ghana (2003). *National Health Insurance Act (Act 650)*. Government of Ghana, Accra.

8 Tragakes E, Brigis G, Karaskevica J, *et al.* (2008). Latvia: Health system review. In Avdeeva O, Schäfer M (eds) *Health Systems in Transition*, Volume 10(2), pp.1–251. World Health Organization on behalf of the European Observatory on Health Systems and Policies, Copenhagen.

9 Van Doorslaer E, Wagstaff A (1993). Equity in the finance of health care: Methods and findings. In Van Doorslaer E, Wagstaff A, Rutten F (eds) *Equity in the finance and delivery of health care: An international perspective*, pp.7–97. New York: Oxford University Press, New York.

10 Wagstaff A, van Doorslaer E, van der Burg H, *et al.* (1999). Equity in the finance of health care: some further international comparisons. *Journal of Health Economics*, **18**, 263–90.

11 O'Donnell O, Van Doorslaer E, Rannan-Eliya R, *et al.* (2008). Who pays for health care in Asia? *Journal of Health Economics*, **27**, 460–75.

12 Ataguba J, McIntyre D (2009). *Financing and benefit incidence in the South African health system: Preliminary results. Health Economics Unit Working Paper 09/1*. Health Economics Unit, University of Cape Town, Cape Town.

13 McIntyre D, Garshong B, Mtei G, *et al.* (2008). Beyond fragmentation and towards universal coverage: Insights from Ghana, South Africa and Tanzania. *Bulletin of the World Health Organization*, **86**, 871–6.

14 EQUITAP (2005). *Who pays for health care in Asia?* Institute of Policy Studies, Colombo.

15 Busse R, Saltman R, Dubois H (2004). Organization and financing of social health insurance systems: current status and recent policy developments. In: Saltman R, Busse R, Figueras J (eds) *Social health insurance systems in western Europe*, pp.33–80. Open University Press, for World Health Organization on behalf of the European Observatory on Health Systems and Policies, Maidenhead.

16 Mossialos E, Thomson S (2004). *Voluntary health insurance in the European Union*. World Health Organization, Copenhagen.

17 Bennett S, Creese A, Monasch R (1998). *Health insurance schemes for people outside formal sector employment: ARA Paper No. 16*. Division of Analysis, Research and Assessment, World Health Organization, Geneva.

18 Yang B (1991). Health insurance in Korea: Opportunities and challenges. *Health Policy and Planning*, **6**(2), 119–29.

19 Van Doorslaer E, O'Donnell O, Rannan-Eliya R, *et al.* (2006). Effect of payments for health care on poverty estimates in 11 countries in Asia: an analysis of household survey data. *Lancet*, **368**, 1357–64.

20 McIntyre D (2007). *Learning from experience: health care financing in low- and middle-income countries*. Global Forum for Health Research, Geneva.

21 Xu K, Evans D, Carrin G, Aguilar-Rivera A (2005). *Designing health financing systems to reduce catastrophic health expenditure* (Technical Briefs for Policy-Makers Number 2. WHO/EIP/HSF/PB/05.02). World Health Organization, Geneva.

22 Sheiman I, Langenbrunner J, Kehler J, Cashin C, Kutzin J (2009). *Sources of funds and revenue collection: reforms and challenges.* In Kutzin J, Cashin C, Jakab M (eds) *Implementing Health Financing Reforms. Lessons from countries in transition*, pp.87–118. World Health Organization, on behalf of the European. Observatory on Health Systems and Policies, Copenhagen.

23 Normand C, Weber A (1994). *Social Health Insurance: A guidebook for planning.* World Health Organization and International Labour Office, Geneva.

24 Zschock D (1982). General review of problems of medical care delivery under social security in developing countries. *International Social Security Review*, **35**, 3–15.

25 Normand C (1999). Using social health insurance to meet policy goals. *Social Science and Medicine*, **48**, 865–9.

26 Carrin G, James C (2004). *Reaching universal coverage via social health insurance: key design features in the transition period* (Discussion Paper Number 2–2004). World Health Organization, Geneva.

27 Collins S, Kriss J, Doty M, Rustgi S (2008). *Losing ground: How the loss of adequate health insurance is burdening working families. Findings from the Commonwealth Fund Biennial Health Insurance Surveys, 2001–2007.* The Commonwealth Fund, New York.

28 Frenk J (1995). Comprehensive policy analysis for health system reform. *Health Policy*, **32**(3), 257–77.

29 Ensor T (2001). *Transition to universal coverage in developing countries: An overview.* Centre for Health Economics, University of York, York.

30 Kutzin J, Shishkin S, Bryndová L, Schneider P, Hrobo P (2009). Reforms in the pooling of funds. In Kutzin J, Cashin C, Jakab M (eds) *Implementing Health Financing Reforms. Lessons from countries in transition*, pp.119–54. World Health Organization, on behalf of the European Observatory on Health Systems and Policies, Copenhagen.

31 Kutzin J (2007). Current reforms aiming at the extension of social protection in health: Linking up mixed health financing sub-systems. In: ILO GTZ, WHO (eds) *Extending social protection in health: Developing countries' experiences, lessons learnt and recommendations*, pp.86–121. Deutsche Gesellschaft fur Technische Zusammenarbeit (GTZ), Eschborn.

32 Rice N, Smith P (2002). Strategic resource allocation and funding decisions. In Mossialos E, Dixon A, Figueras J, Kutzin J (eds) *Funding health care: Options for Europe.* Open University Press, Buckingham.

Chapter 5

Delivering health services: incentives and information in supply-side innovations

Kara Hanson

5.1 **Introduction**

While Chapters 1 and 10 indicate the wide range of environmental, social, and behavioural influences on population health, it remains the case that preventive and curative services delivered through the health sector are the primary means by which societies act to improve population health. Yet coverage of these services among the populations that can most benefit from them remains low, and there is growing evidence of stark socioeconomic differences in intervention coverage, with the poor most likely to miss out [1,2], contributing to persistent inequalities in health outcomes [1,3]. The reasons for these low levels of coverage and poor equity outcomes lie within the health sector and beyond. The framework for classifying the constraints to expanding service delivery that was developed by the Commission for Macroeconomics and Health identifies challenges at six different levels [4,5]:

1 Community- and household-level constraints limiting demand for effective services and their use.

2 Constraints at the service delivery level such as lack of staff, drugs and weak information systems.

3 Health sector strategic policy and management constraints, including inappropriate policies, lack of incentives to use resources efficiently and respond to users' preferences, and lack of intersectoral collaboration.

4 Public policies cutting across sectors, including those that relate to human resources management and fiscal space.

5 Environmental and contextual factors, including systems of governance, accountability, and characteristics of climate and geography that impede service delivery.

6 Global level constraints relating primarily to aid effectiveness, but also including problems arising from cross-border flows of health workers (see Chapter 8).

The cumulative impact of these factors, which obviously vary in the ways in which they affect different countries, is to limit the coverage of these health interventions. Table 5.1 summarizes evidence of coverage of priority health interventions targeted at maternal, neonatal, and child survival; these data show the extent to which opportunities for improving population health are being missed, and indicate the need for improvements in the performance of the health sector.

Throughout the last decades there have been continuous efforts to strengthen health sector performance (see Chapter 1). This chapter focuses on one

Table 5.1 Coverage of priority health interventions for maternal, neonatal and child health, 49 low-income countries

Median coverage level	Intervention
≥80%	Vitamin A supplementation (2 doses)
	Protection against neonatal tetanus
	DPT3 vaccination
	Hib3 vaccination
50–79%	Measles vaccination
	Complementary feeding (6–9 months)
30–49%	Careseeking for pneumonia
	Skilled attendant at delivery
	Early initiation of breastfeeding
	4+ antenatal visits
	Diarrhoea treatment
	Exclusive breastfeeding
	Condom use at last high-risk sex (females)
	Malaria treatment
	Antibiotics for pneumonia
<30%	Contraceptive prevalence
	Prevention of mother-to-child transmission of HIV
	Children sleeping under ITN
	Intermittent preventive treatment for malaria in pregnancy

Source: Task Force report, using data from Countdown Working Group (2008). *Tracking progress in maternal, newborn & child survival: the 2008 report*. United Nations Children's Fund, New York; and UNICEF (2008). *The state of the world's children*. New York, United Nations Children's Fund, New York.

particular set of supply-side reforms aimed at strengthening health service delivery: those that target incentives for provider performance. These reforms include creating autonomous public agencies to deliver services; 'pay for performance' initiatives linked to the delivery of specific services; and a range of models for working with private healthcare providers, such as contracting and franchising. The chapter begins with an overview of incentives in organizations, located in the conceptual framework of principal-agent theory. It then examines four major types of reform, framing them in terms of a principal agent model which interprets these reforms as measures designed to align more closely the incentives of government and providers; and reviewing the current evidence about their effectiveness. The evidence does not come from a new or fully systematic review, but rather draws on existing reviews, supplemented by the author's research. The conclusions highlight the challenges of introducing stronger incentives for healthcare provider performance in the context of information problems, and the implications for both broader system performance and for the evaluation of such interventions.

5.2 Conceptual framework: principal agent theory, incentives, and information

Because of the multitude of market failures in health and healthcare, the government remains a critical provider of priority public health interventions in many low- and middle-income countries (LMICs), and efforts to increase service coverage have, in the first instance, addressed performance issues in the public sector. The traditional, bureaucratic model of public service provision has adopted planning approaches within hierarchical organization. The centre (e.g. the Ministry of Health) seeks to achieve a number of objectives (in healthcare, often described in terms of high levels of service coverage, high quality and responsiveness to patients' preferences, equity, and efficiency; see Chapter 3). The centre assumes that actors at different levels share their objectives and are adequately motivated. Provided they have sufficient information, supplies, equipment, and infrastructure, they will apply these to the objective of delivering needed services. Improving service delivery is therefore a matter of better planning and management: increasing the resources available for service delivery (if these are in short supply), providing more technical guidance to improve providers' knowledge, decentralizing decision-making authority if this will improve the flow and use of information, and strengthening the systems that deliver needed inputs and track information.

During the 1980s and 1990s, against a political background of neoliberalism, this view of the public sector was increasingly challenged. Public choice theorists argued that government production of goods and services would be intrinsically inefficient due to politicians' (rational) pursuit of their own self-interest. Others pointed to the critical failures of information and incentives in large bureaucracies, which would be more severe in the public sector because of the absence of a clear 'bottom line' against which to track performance and the lack of competitive pressure from other firms [6]. Improvements in public services would be achieved through greater competition, achieved either through privatization (transferring ownership of assets from the state to the private sector) or, where this was not feasible, through the creation of 'internal markets' to mimic the operation of private markets within the public sector. This agenda became known as the New Public Management, and was adopted in the 1990s by the United Kingdom and a number of other Organisation for Economic Co-operation and Development (OECD) countries [7].

Others have argued that neither state nor market production of services is intrinsically superior, but that provider performance is primarily determined by the specific institutional features of an organization and its environment, including the incentives that providers face together with the quality of management and oversight. An incentive is defined as 'any factor (financial or non-financial) that enables or motivates a particular course of action. . . it is an expectation that encourages people to behave in a certain way' [8]. A further useful distinction is between those incentives that work through a material reward (either in the form of money or in-kind benefits) and those which operate through a moral imperative—in the form of social pressure (how one ought to behave) or altruism. One commentator on the reforms of the United Kingdom National Health Service distinguished the treatment of public sector workers along these lines, differentiating models of reform which assume that workers are motivated by altruism and a sense of public service ('knights') from those which assume self-interested behaviour by individuals concerned primarily by material rewards ('knaves') [9].

Principal-agent theory provides one formulation of how incentives might operate to influence provider behaviour. This characterizes the challenge faced by a principal (e.g. government) who delegates the responsibility for producing a service to its agents (healthcare providers), and seeks for them to behave in a way which will secure the government's social objectives. Principal-agent theory postulates that: 1) the motivations and objectives of principals may not be entirely shared by agents, and that this divergence may impede the performance that the principal seeks; 2) the outcomes of interest in the health sector require 'costly' effort (motivation) on the part of the agent/provider; 3) both this effort, and the outcome of interest are difficult to observe or measure and therefore are difficult to contract; and 4) there is some uncertainty which affects the achievement of the outcome. The mechanism or 'contract' that is needed to induce the agent to act in the best interests of the principal therefore needs to encourage effort on the part of the agent by creating the appropriate incentives, but also address uncertainty and accommodate imperfect information.

Principal-agent theory thus places incentives and information at the centre of the challenge of performance, and therefore provides a useful conceptual lens through which to examine the health sector strengthening interventions reviewed in this chapter. A further useful element of incentive theory is the distinction between 'low powered incentives', in which there is little or no relationship between what a provider does and how much they are paid [10,11] and 'high-powered' incentives, in which a provider receives a high proportion of any profit or efficiency gain that they generate, which is assumed to motivate them to expand their output and to use resources efficiently. In the public sector context, paying providers on the basis of salary (for individuals) or historical budgets (for institutions) provides low-powered incentives because these payments are received regardless of whether or not the individual/institution works hard to achieve its objectives. This can be contrasted with incentives facing a for-profit private organization (e.g. individual clinical practice or for-profit hospital), where because the owner has a residual claim on any profits generated, they are assumed to exert effort to maximize their return. Many of the reforms reviewed here can be seen as efforts to introduce higher-powered incentives in the public sector; they also generally assume that providers are more responsive to financial incentives than to non-financial ones.

In addition to incentives, the principal-agent model identifies the challenge posed by information problems in efforts to improve provider performance. As has been widely recognized, healthcare suffers from a variety of information problems:

1 Problems in measuring health: the output of interest—health itself—is difficult to measure, with little consensus on the appropriate weights to give to length and quality of life, and which dimensions of quality are most relevant.

2 Lack of information about the production process: the ways in which healthcare inputs are transformed into the output of ultimate interest (health) is ill-understood; there is very limited evidence about the effectiveness of many health interventions in common use.

3 Information asymmetry between patients and providers: patients generally have less technical knowledge about healthcare than their providers, delegating decision-making to them, and potentially leaving them vulnerable to 'supplier-induced demand' in which providers order excess tests or procedures because of financial incentives.

Together, the challenges of incentives and information problems create a fundamental dilemma when trying to use incentives to strengthen provider performance: how to balance strengthened incentives for improved performance with the risk that incentives can become too high powered and have negative consequences. Where payments are too closely related to simple measures of quantity of services or target achievement, providers may resort to supplier-induced demand or engage in strategic behaviour to manipulate targets or the data used to measure their achievement. Where incentives to reduce healthcare costs are too powerful, providers may skimp on care or avoid more complicated and therefore more costly cases. In addition, the output of health services is frequently multidimensional and relies on teamwork, making it very difficult to identify individuals' contributions to the production process (and indeed, if non health sector inputs to health are allowed for, even greater difficult in rewarding these). Patients are often vulnerable and poorly placed to challenge providers and demand appropriate services. Indeed, it is in the very nature of the traditional public sector, with its lower powered (financial) incentives, that it has been relied upon to provide those services that were believed to be subject to market failure where incentives in the private sector might be too powerful given information asymmetries.

Despite these challenges of incentives in a context of imperfect information, health sector reform programmes from the 1980s onwards drew on models that relied more heavily on financial incentives to encourage improved provider performance. The New Public Management model for public services in the United Kingdom and other high income settings proposed that introducing higher powered incentives into the public sector, and liberalizing health provider markets to allow a greater degree of competition either within the public sector or between public and private providers, would create stronger incentives for efficiency and responsiveness in service provision. In parallel, there was a growing recognition of the role played by private industry in health sectors in LMICs, and interest in taking advantage of the opportunities this offered to expand coverage while also addressing the some of the problems of private sector quality. These ideas were quickly transferred to low- and middle-income settings via the influence of the World Bank and other funding agencies, and translated into a series of service delivery innovations aimed at increasing coverage, improving efficiency and quality of services provided.

In the remainder of this chapter, the framework provided by principal-agent theory and the role of high-powered and low-powered incentives, provides a lens through which a number of different types of supply-side reform are examined. Two main groups of reforms are distinguished: first, those which seek to strengthen incentives in the public sector through, e.g. strategic purchasing, pay-for-performance and the creation of autonomous agencies; and second, those which seek to build on the perceived advantages of higher powered incentives in the private sector but at the same time to draw these resources into the service of the broadest population (e.g. by contracting private providers to provide services to underserved groups) and measures to improve the quality of services provided in the private sector. In the next section, these measures and the evidence about their effectiveness in LMICs are reviewed.

5.3 Public sector purchasing and results-based financing

5.3.1 Strategic purchasing by the public sector

Chapter 4 outlined the arguments in favour of greater pooling of funding (through public tax-based funding or insurance contributions) for health service provision in order to support more equitable cross-subsidies. However, a second advantage of pooled funding for health services is the opportunity it presents to introduce strategic purchasing of services [12,13]. The concept of strategic purchasing starts with the idea of separating the functions of purchasing and providing services, which allows for a more active consideration of which interventions should be purchased, how they should be purchased, and from whom. Strategic purchasing is distinguished from a more 'passive' approach to commissioning services which is primarily about allocation of resources to provider organizations. Contracting (see below) can be seen as a specific component of purchasing, describing the details of the agreement that is negotiated between purchasers and providers, including a specification of the contracted services, tendering processes, and procedures for monitoring and reviewing contract performance [12].

Strategic purchasing provides the opportunity to specify more precisely the package of services to be provided with the pooled funds, as well as to introduce higher powered incentives in the form of payment mechanisms and/or performance review, to encourage providers to deliver these services more efficiently and at higher level of quality. Services can be purchased from public or private providers, though there is relatively little experience in LMICs of purchasing from private providers (though see below on contracting in LMICs). In terms of the principal-agent framework, purchasing involves three layers of actor (purchaser/provider/consumer), and a more complex web of principal agent relationships [12]:

◆ Purchaser/consumer—with purchaser acting on behalf of consumers to secure needed services.

- Purchaser/provider—with purchaser acting as principal to secure services from providers.
- Purchaser/government—with purchaser acting on behalf of the government to meet national health strategies/targets.

Although the idea of purchasing as a way to strengthen health system performance was highlighted in the 2000 World Health Report [14], there has been quite limited uptake of this approach in LMICs, and even less empirical evidence of its effectiveness. Box 5.1 describes the experience of purchasing health services in Thailand.

Box 5.1 Health service purchasing in Thailand [37]

In Thailand, there are three main purchasers of services under the Universal Coverage system—the Civil Service Medical Benefits Scheme, which contracts with public and private providers for care provided to civil servants; the Ministry of Labour, which purchases services for those insured through the Social Health Insurance scheme (those in formal employment); and the National Health Security Office for those whose cover comes through the UC scheme. The main elements of the purchasing strategy under these schemes are specification of the benefit package and the payment mechanisms for providers. Under the UC scheme, there is a well-defined benefit package which excludes some treatments that have been deemed either not cost-effective or unaffordable to the scheme; and payment is made through capitation to primary care contractor units for outpatient care and DRG for inpatient care. Cost-effectiveness criteria are an important consideration in determining which interventions are included in the benefit package. For example, a review by the Technology Assessment Program (HITAP) concluded that the vaccination against human papillomavirus (HPV) as a means of prevention of cervical cancer, was not cost-effective at the current vaccine price level and advised against its inclusion in the UC benefit package. However, equity concerns also play a part in decisions about what should be included, with the decision taken in 2006 to cover second-line antiretroviral therapy and renal replacement therapy for those with end-stage renal disease, neither of which meets conventional cost-effectiveness thresholds but both of which can lead to financial impoverishment. While the UC scheme purchases only from public providers, the CSMBS purchases services from public and private providers, and uses fee-for-service as the means of provider payment; consequently the scheme has suffered from problems of cost escalation.

The experience to date is still too limited to conclude on the effectiveness of purchasing as a way of sharpening provider incentives and improving quality and efficiency. The addition of a new layer in the principal agent relationship—the purchaser who acts both on behalf of both the government and the population—complicates matters as they must deal with multiple objectives which may be in conflict, and raises questions about the optimal institutional arrangements. Finally, the effectiveness of purchasing systems will undoubtedly depend on both the specific form of purchasing arrangements—including the nature of the contracts and payment mechanisms—and the broader economic and political context.

5.3.2 Pay for performance

Results-based financing or 'pay-for-performance' has been defined as the transfer of money or material goods conditional on taking a measurable action or achieving a predetermined performance target [15]. Performance-based payments can be made to health service users (e.g. linking cash payments to the utilization of specific services, such as in the *Opportunidades* programme in Mexico), or to providers (where they receive additional payment for meeting population coverage targets for specified services). Some programmes have combined the two, such as the Safe Delivery Incentive Programme in Nepal, in which cash payments are made to both women who deliver in health facilities and trained providers who attend deliveries, either at home or in a health facility [16]. The discussion here is restricted to supply side payments.

Results-based financing is directly linked to the principal agent framework: it uses financial incentives to align the interests of principal and agent by paying for a specified output or target. It can be used in conjunction with strategic purchasing (see above) or contracting (below) as part of a mechanism for compensating providers. While pay-for-performance schemes are being implemented in a wide variety of contexts, there is still very little robust evaluation evidence of their impact in low- and middle-income settings [17], although a Cochrane review is currently underway [18]. Rwanda is one exception, where a quasi-experimental evaluation was undertaken (Box 5.2).

There is, however, ample evidence that healthcare providers respond to financial incentives (including the provision of excessive services if incentives are too high powered), and a growing literature reviewing the experience of implementing these schemes in low- and middle-income settings [15,19]. This literature identifies a number of key design features of pay-for-performance when applied in the health sector, many of which address directly the principal agent problem:

- ◆ Whether payments are to individuals, teams, or facilities: schemes have used a variety of different arrangements. In the health sector, it is important

Box 5.2 Pay-for-performance in Rwanda [38]

Building upon the experience of small-scale NGO projects, in 2006 the Rwandan government introduced a performance-based pay scheme for primary care facilities. The scheme rewards performance for 14 maternal and child healthcare output indicators, together with an overall quality score. The indicators are a combination of number of visits of specific types (e.g. antenatal care or delivery) and services provided during those visits (vaccinations given). Indicators are assessed quarterly through the routine health facility monitoring system, employing an unannounced visit by district level supervisors who review facility records and assess quality through direct observation. To evaluate the impact of the scheme a quasi-experimental study was undertaken, with random assignment of matched health facilities to an intervention or control group. The incentive effect of tying payment to performance was isolated from the income effect of higher revenue by giving the control facilities a payment equivalent to the average performance-based payment. A baseline household and facility survey was conducted, with a follow-up survey after 24 months of implementation.

Mothers in the intervention group saw a 21% increase in the probability of an institutional delivery, and there were positive effects of the scheme on the quality of antenatal care, although there was no effect on the likelihood of receiving any antenatal care or of completing at least four visits. Large and positive effects were also seen on the probability of preventive health service visits by children under 5 years, but no impact on immunization coverage. In general, larger effects were seen for services associated with larger payments (confirming that providers do respond to financial incentives) and for those outputs that were provider, rather than patient, determined.

These effects were measured 2 years after the launch of the intervention, so it is not likely that these were short-lived effects, though their sustainability over time will depend on how targets and payment levels are revised, and on whether health workers eventually learn how to game target levels or distort the information used to monitor their performance. However, the evaluation did not appear to measure effects on non-targeted services, so it is difficult to assess the diversion of effort away from these activities and therefore to comment on the magnitude of any unintended consequences.

to find a means of payment that recognizes the joint nature of production and encourages teamwork.

◆ Form of payment: as with all payment schemes, different mechanisms embody different incentives. It is essential to consider a form of payment that will encourage increases in coverage, but which does not incentivize supplier-induced demand.

◆ Form and level of target: targets can be in the form of reaching a certain threshold, achieving a certain percentage improvement, or a given percentage point improvement (which implies a greater relative improvement for those operating at lower levels of achievement). Thought needs to be given to how to provide encouragement to those facilities whose level of performance is still low in absolute terms, but which have seen a significant improvement; and how to encourage high performing facilities to continue to improve.

◆ The share of remuneration that is performance-related: this needs to be large enough to induce effort and creativity in finding new solutions to service delivery challenges, but not so great that providers bear so much risk that they withdraw from the process altogether.

◆ Method of verification of output: some early pay-for-performance programmes used independent groups (e.g. NGOs) to undertake independent verification of performance (e.g. [20]). This may have been due to poor quality of routine health management information system data, or alternatively, in recognition of the potential for providers to manipulate routine data to ensure that coverage targets are reached (see below). But such independent verification adds to the administrative costs of the system.

Pay-for-performance also raises a series of policy concerns linked to the question of whether the incentives are too high powered, which is, in turn, closely related to issues of information. These include the following:

◆ 'Tunnel vision' and myopia: fears that providers will focus excessively on the service targets that carry a financial incentive and short-term measures, to the detriment of other services that are more difficult to measure or require longer-term action [21].

◆ Crowding out of altruistic incentives: providers who do not meet the performance targets may be demoralized by the linking of financial payments to performance, or financial incentives might undermine altruistic ones [9].

◆ Strategic behaviour and gaming: risk that providers will engage in strategic behaviour around target setting, for example, under-performing in the run-up to the setting of performance targets so that their targets are easy to achieve.

◆ Risk selection, or 'cherry-picking': to dissuade enrolment of groups or individuals who might undermine target achievement.

◆ Corruption in performance measurement: collusion between providers and those who are assessing performance achievement, or deliberate manipulation and misreporting of the data that are used to measure performance.

The potential for these unintended consequences of high powered incentives means that evaluations of performance-based pay arrangements must take particular care to measure the spillover effects (positive and negative) on services other than those that are incentivized, and consider other incentive effects.

Recent reviews of the effectiveness of pay-for-performance have concluded that while the evidence is limited, performance-related payments to providers appears to be an effective way of increasing service coverage. However, more robust evidence is needed to fully explore its impact in different contexts, the management support and oversight systems needed to ensure its effective implementation, the extent of unintended consequences, and the cost-effectiveness of pay-for-performance compared with, other approaches to improving public sector performance [5].

5.4 **Creation of autonomous agencies**

Provider autonomy, which involves transforming the governance of public institutions through management by an autonomous board allowing them to be de-linked from civil service rules and other public sector constraints, was fashionable in a range of countries in the 1990s. Under New Public Management arrangements, large referral hospitals were encouraged to become 'Trusts' (in the United Kingdom) or 'Crown Health Enterprises' (in New Zealand). This practice was also adopted for secondary and tertiary hospitals in a number of low-income countries, including Zimbabwe [22], Ghana [23], Zambia [24], and Indonesia [25]. National drug stores have also been a target for this type of institutional change, with autonomous drug supply agencies being created in a number of settings [26].

The extent of provider autonomy can be classified along a spectrum which runs from full budgetary control (least autonomy), through to institutions which are autonomous, corporate, or fully private. Harding and Preker locate hospitals on this continuum depending on the degree of control they exercise over decision rights, residual claims, market exposure, accountability, and extent of social function [27].

In the principal-agent framework described above, the shift from budgetary control to autonomy can be seen as a form of transformation from a hierarchical arrangement of direct control to a more arms-length relationship in which the principal (MOH) restructures arrangements to induce the agent (hospital board) to fulfil its mission. Generally speaking these new arrangements have taken the form of greater managerial freedom (for example, to hire and fire staff, to manage their own budgets with greater autonomy) aimed at encouraging efficiency and quality improvements, together with greater exposure to parts of the healthcare market through which hospitals can compete to attract additional revenue. In predominantly public systems, such as the United Kingdom in the 1990s, this took the form of competition for contracts with local health authorities and fundholding GP practices. In some low- and middle-income settings, this has usually meant competing for private (fee-paying) patients.

The challenge for the principal in this context has been to create a set of operating rules and guidelines that aligns the incentives of the hospital management board with its own objectives of meeting its public service mission (providing hospital services to the catchment population) and doing so in a way which encourages improved efficiency and quality. These arrangements, however, can create two quite different problems. In one, the incentives are too high powered, and equity suffers; in the other, incentives are not powerful enough, and the desired efficiency and quality gains are not realized.

The first situation arises because of the multiple and competing objectives of hospitals and problems of measuring output (see above), which means that the 'contracts' that govern their relationship with the Ministry of Health can be incomplete, in the sense that they do not fully specify all of the desired outcomes in a clear and measurable way. This gives the hospital management the latitude to interpret its contract in the way that best suits its interests. This means that the incentive to generate revenue can come to dominate and thereby undermine the achievement of the hospital's public service mission.

In the second situation, the key issue is whether the incentives are strong enough to elicit the managerial reforms needed to improve hospital performance. For instance, public accounting rules may preclude the hospital from being the residual claimant for any surpluses generated; or its decision-making over the use of any surplus may be highly constrained. In both cases, the hospital (as agent) may decide that the effort required to improve a service is greater than any gains from generating a surplus. A further issue is the extent to which the changes in the incentives facing the hospital as an organization can be transmitted to those at the frontline of service delivery, whose actions ultimately influence determinants of hospital performance, such as efficient resource use.

As with many of these supply-side arrangements, there has been little robust evaluation of the effectiveness of hospital autonomy. However, studies of hospital policy in Zambia and Indonesia (Boxes 5.3 and 5.4), conducted in the 1990s are instructive about how 'high-powered' incentives can come to dominate hospital behaviour. These studies also illustrate that hospital managers can and do respond to incentives. However, they also illustrate a further characteristic of incentive-led interventions, which is their potential for unintended consequences arising from the interactions between different

Box 5.3 Hospital autonomy in Zambia

Following a change in government in 1991, the Zambian health ministry initiated a wide ranging reform of the health sector. The reforms created a 'purchaser-provider split' structure by which a Central Board of Health acted as national purchasing agency, contracting with district health boards for services up to the level of the district hospital, and with referral hospital boards (public and private not-for-profit) for services at that level. This created hospital autonomy at secondary and tertiary level in the sense that the management relationship between the Ministry of Health and the hospitals was intended to be mediated through the contract rather than operate directly.

The Zambian hospital reforms were affected by a number of other features of the policy context. First, there were a number of changes in leadership at the Ministry of Health, leading to frequent interruptions in implementation. Second, the contracts with the hospitals never developed beyond 'block contracts' in which a global budget was agreed in exchange for meeting the demand for hospital services. The opportunities to make purchasing more strategic were largely missed. Attempts to 'de-link' hospital staff from the Public Services Commission and have them become Board employees, and therefore subject to local control over 'hiring and firing' decisions, were heavily resisted by the public services union. Some strategic posts, such as accounting staff, were created by the hospitals, however.

It was the health financing policy, which while never formally adopted, was widely acknowledged to guide hospital actions, which provided the main opportunity for hospitals to respond to market forces and generate revenue. The core of the financing policy was the distinction between services in the 'basic service package', for which nominal 'cost-sharing' fees would be levied; and those outside the package for which 'cost-recovery' fees could be charged. In the absence of a full specification of the basic service package, hospitals interpreted this as meaning that cost recovery fees could be charged for 'high-cost', 'fast-track', and 'private' wards and clinics which hospitals increasingly developed during the reform period. These offered patients the choice of a higher priced service with some characteristics superior to those on ordinary wards or clinics, for example shorter waiting time or access to a consultant of choice. As the main hospital contract was unresponsive to patient numbers, these 'cost recovery' services offered the hospitals the only opportunity to earn additional, discretionary revenue.

In practice, therefore, the implication of greater hospital autonomy in Zambia and the form which greater exposure to market forces took was most clearly witnessed in the development of two-tier charging [39]. While the stated aim of introducing these private services was to charge more for higher quality 'hotel' (i.e. non-clinical) services, and thereby generate a surplus to subsidise the 'public' wards, in practice we observed differences in access to staff, drugs, and diagnostic facilities which suggested that private patients were also receiving superior clinical services [40].

Box 5.4 Hospital autonomy in Indonesia [42]

The propensity for higher-powered incentives to undermine equity outcomes was also observed in Indonesia, where a policy of hospital autonomy was implemented in 1991. This allowed for hospitals to be granted autonomy on the basis of meeting a set of criteria in relation to cost recovery, bed occupancy, and length of stay, and the prosperity of the surrounding economy. The major objective of hospital autonomy was to encourage hospitals to generate revenue [25]. Swadana (autonomous) hospitals enjoyed the following freedoms: the hiring and firing of hospital staff; setting fees; distribution of beds among fee levels, except class III (set aside for the poor and charged at the lowest rates); purchasing drugs and supplies; selecting incentive systems for use of a specified portion of own source revenue; and contracting with the private sector. This suggests that Indonesian autonomous hospital managers had considerably greater room for manoeuvre than their Zambian counterparts. Perhaps the most important source of greater autonomy was in relation to their own generated revenues, which constituted a high share of total hospital revenue—between 30% and 80% [25], and 40% was set as the minimum to achieve Swadana status [41].

Two small-scale studies assessed the consequences of autonomy in Swadana hospitals: one conducted in ten hospitals, five of them Swadana,

Box 5.4 Hospital autonomy in Indonesia (continued)

three public, managed by either provincial or district authorities, and two private (one small, one large) in 1996, assessing trends in relation to levels of fees, pattern of service provision (bed availability by class), unit costs, staffing patterns, length of stay, bed occupancy, and management systems [25]; and one conducted analysis of six Swadana hospitals and one traditional district hospital in 1998 [41]. Both evaluations found that fees in Swadana hospitals increased substantially after their change in status, though fees increased in the non-Swadana public hospitals to similar degrees—a finding that might have been related to the requirement to increase cost recovery rates in order to qualify for Swadana status. Fees increased in private hospitals too, although more gradually. Both studies found a reduction in the number of Class III (low cost) beds in Swadana hospitals, potentially compromising access to care for the poorest. Evidence on the direction of cross-subsidy was mixed; one finding a cross-subsidy in favour of the higher-paying beds (regressive) [25] and one finding a subsidy in the opposite (progressive) direction [41].

healthcare system components. Links between health financing policy, human resources, and service delivery can be seen, in both instances, to have undermined equity.

5.5 Contracting private providers

Contracting private providers to deliver healthcare services also has its origins in the New Public Management reforms described above. The splitting of the functions of purchasing and provision of services opens up the opportunity for public funds to be used to purchase services from private (non-profit or for-profit) providers. The rationale for contracting private providers combines elements of greater provider autonomy, focus on measurable results and performance, and the positive effects of competition and market exposure. Contracting therefore has elements of both of the reforms described above, in addition to higher powered incentives combined with a greater reliance on private providers. Early experience with contracting was based on very small scale operations. More recently, NGOs have been contracted to provide services to much larger populations, particularly in post-conflict settings where public sector infrastructure is very weak or non-existent.

A number of papers review the experience of contracting in LMICs, nearly all of which involve contracting non-profit providers. An examination of ten schemes with at least before-and-after comparisons concluded that contracting was a promising way of expanding service coverage, though more evaluation was needed [28]. Another study reviewing a larger number of schemes also found a generally positive effect on utilization, but argued that there was insufficient evidence to reach conclusions about the effect of contracting on other outcomes, such as quality of care, efficiency, and equity [29]. A recent Cochrane review of contracting in low- and middle-income settings applied more restrictive inclusion criteria (only studies which used experimental or quasi-experimental methods) and identified only three eligible studies [30]. The authors concluded that contracting may increase health service access and utilization, but the evidence base is extremely weak.

A more extensive literature points out some of the implementation challenges with contracting, in particular capacity needed to design contracts and monitor their implementation [31]. The potential challenges with contract monitoring are closely related to information issues: in addition to the standard difficulties with all performance monitoring systems, the fact that the population being served is often remote further amplifies the difficulties of effective oversight. This remoteness also means that there may be no effective competition for contracts, undermining one of the key theoretical mechanisms of action. Finally, contracting is itself a multidimensional process, involving additional management and technical resources, making it very difficult to isolate the effect of the changed incentives per se on provider performance.

5.6 Improving quality in the private sector

Private healthcare providers play an extensive role in many low- and middle-income settings, often more convenient and accessible than public health facilities. They are frequently perceived to give higher quality, reflecting the higher powered incentives that private providers face arising from their status as residual claimant to any surplus they generate and their greater exposure to market forces. However, a number of studies of private providers have demonstrated worryingly low levels of technical quality in areas such as treatment for malaria, sexually transmitted infections, and tuberculosis. Enthusiasm for expanding the role of private providers, and drawing on their resources to extend population coverage with key interventions, is therefore often accompanied by recognition of the need to work with them to improve their quality and, in some cases, their affordability by applying subsidies.

A number of approaches to working with private providers have been developed, largely in the context of donor-funded programmes. These include

Table 5.2 Results of systematic review of effectiveness of interventions working private providers to improve utilization of quality services by the poor

Intervention	Number of references retrieved	Number of interventions subject to robust evaluation*
Social marketing	472	14
Franchising	906	5
Training	599	29
Regulation	276	2
Accreditation	150	1
Contracting Out	80	3

*Criterion was inclusion of any form of comparison group (before/after, intervention/control). This systematic review comes from reference 32 (Patouillard et al).

training programmes, franchising, social marketing, voucher schemes, regulation, accreditation, and regulation [32]. A recent systematic review found that even applying a very low threshold for evaluation methodology (an intervention group compared with any type of control group) there was very limited evidence of the effectiveness of these interventions (Table 5.2)—somewhat surprising given the huge amount of investment in these providers by some donor agencies. However, the review demonstrated that there is strong evidence of the feasibility of working with these providers to improve quality and access, in a wide range of low-income settings.

5.7 Implications for strengthening health systems

This chapter has reviewed the experience of health sector interventions which attempt to alter incentives (usually financial) for healthcare provider performance, in a policy environment characterized by severe information problems. The interventions themselves have been classified into two main groups—-those which change incentives in the public sector (through strategic purchasing, pay-for-performance and the creation of autonomous units), and those which involve making greater use of private providers, who are assumed to face higher-powered incentives (through contracting or other interventions to increase utilization or improve quality). These interventions have been characterized using a principal-agent framework, which emphasizes the use of incentive mechanisms to align the interests of a principal (e.g. the Ministry of Health) and the agents to whom it delegates responsibility for providing services.

At first glance, the review of experience presented here indicates much that is promising—these interventions are being implemented in a wide variety of low- and middle-income settings. However, the evidence about their potential for achieving health sector change is extremely weak.

First, many of these interventions have only operated at a small scale, in a small number of individual facilities (for autonomous hospitals) or in limited geographic areas. Exceptions include the large-scale purchasing of services through the various insurance schemes in Thailand that make up the national Universal Coverage arrangements; the scaling up of performance-based payment in Rwanda; and the large scale contracting of primary care services in some post-conflict settings such as Afghanistan and Southern Sudan. Scaling up these interventions to the national level may require new and different implementation processes [33,34], and it remains unclear whether the capacity exists to implement them on a large scale.

Second, where such schemes have been subject to rigorous evaluation, this has usually taken place after a relatively short period of time, making it difficult to ascertain the longer-term consequences of these interventions and their adaptive nature. For instance, the long-term success of pay-for-performance schemes will depend critically on the way in which payment targets and levels are adjusted from one period to the next, and the feedback loops through which providers and patients respond to changed incentives, in order to reward appropriately and to continue to generate sufficiently powerful incentives.

Most importantly, both the conceptualization and the evaluation of these interventions need to take a more 'systems' approach (as outlined in Chapter 1), looking at the multiple ways in which changing incentives in one part of the health sector can have broader effects, both positive and negative. At a narrow level, the introduction of higher powered incentive schemes through pay-for-performance, purchasing or contracting can lead to strategic behaviour on target setting, efforts to distort information that is used for monitoring performance, or supplier induced demand. Changed incentives can also affect the availability and quality of non-targeted/contracted services, potentially leading to adverse health consequences. Greater autonomy for public institutions or increased reliance on the private sector creates new needs for regulatory capacity, and may generate labour market effects that influence the availability of trained health workers in other sectors. Describing and characterizing these wider effects is therefore essential both for implementation and for evaluation.

More generally, because of their multiple interactions and sector-level effects, many of these supply-side measures that address incentives should be seen as 'complex interventions' and adopt appropriate evaluation methods [35,36]. At a minimum, this should involve characterizing the causal pathway in a way which encompasses the wider effects of intervention, and including the most important of these effects in the evaluation framework. Such approaches will help to ensure that experience with interventions of this type is able to contribute evidence to guide further action in this area.

Acknowledgements

Material on hospital autonomy draws extensively from unpublished work undertaken in collaboration with Barbara McPake.

References

1 Victora C, Wagstaff A, Schellenberg JA, Gwatkin D, Claeson M, Habicht JP (2003). Applying an equity lens to child health and mortality: more of the same is not enough. *Lancet*, **362**, 233–41.

2 Countdown 2008 Equity Analysis Group (2008). Mind the gap: equity and trends in coverage of maternal, newborn, and child health services in 54 Countdown countries. *Lancet*, **371**, 1259–67.

3 UNICEF (2010). Progress for Children. *Achieving the MDGs with equity*. UNICEF, New York.

4 Hanson K, Ranson MK, Oliveira-Cruz V, Mills A (2003). Expanding access to priority health interventions: A framework for understanding the constraints to scaling-up. *Journal of International Development*, **15**, 1–14.

5 Task Force on Innovative International Financing for Health Systems (2009). *Constraints to scaling up and costs: Working Group 1 Report*. Available at: http://www.internationalhealthpartnership.net//CMS_files/documents/working_group_1_-_report_EN.pdf.

6 Walsh K (1995). *Public services and market mechanisms: Competition, contracting and the New Public Management*. Macmillan, Basingstoke.

7 Preker AS, Harding A (2003). *Innovations in health service delivery: The corporatization of public hospitals*. World Bank, Washington DC.

8 http://en.wikipedia.org/wiki/Incentives (accessed 26 August 2010).

9 Le Grand J (2003). *Motivation, Agency and Public Policy: Of Knights and Knaves, Pawns and Queens*. Oxford University Press, New York.

10 Williamson O (1985). *The economic institutions of capitalism: firms, markets, relational contracting*. Free Press, New York.

11 Frant H (1996). High-powered and low-powered incentives in the public sector. *Journal of Public Administration Research and Theory*, **6**(3), 365–81.

12 Figueras J, Robinson R, Jakubowski E (eds) (2005). *Purchasing to improve health systems performance*. Open University Press, Maidenhead.

13 Yip W, Hanson K (2009). Purchasing health care in China: experiences and challenges. In Chernichovsky D, Hanson K (eds) *Innovations in Health System Finance in Developing and Transitional Economies*. Emerald, Bingley.

14 World Health Organization (2000). *The World Health Report 2000. Health systems: improving performance*. WHO, Geneva.

15 Eichler R, Levine R (2009). *Performance Incentives for Global Health: Potential and Pitfalls*. Center for Global Development, Washington DC.

16 Powell-Jackson T, Neupane B, Tiwari S, *et al.* (2009). The impact of Nepal's Safe Delivery Incentive Programme in the district of Makwanpur. In Chernichovsky D, Hanson K (eds) *Innovations in Health System Finance in Developing and Transitional Economies.* Emerald, Bingley.

17 Oxman A, Fretheim A (2008). *An overview of research on the effects of results-based financing.* Norwegian Knowledge Centre for the Health Services, Oslo.

18 Witter S, Kessy F, Fretheim A, Lindahl AK (2009). Paying for performance to improve the delivery of health interventions in low and middle-income countries. *Cochrane Database of Systematic Reviews*, **3**, CD007899.

19 Eldridge C, Palmer N (2009). Performance-based payment: some reflections on the discourse, evidence and unanswered questions. *Health Policy and Planning*, **24**, 160–6.

20 Eichler R, Auxila P, Pollock J (2001). *Performance based payment to improve the impact of health services: Evidence from Haiti.* Management Sciences for Health, Center for Health Reform and Financing, Arlington, VA.

21 Goddard M, Mannion R, Smith P (2000). Enhancing performance in health care: A theoretical perspective on agency and the role of information. *Health Economics*, **9**, 95–107.

22 Needleman J, Chawla M, Mudyarabikwa O (1996). *Hospital Autonomy in Zimbabwe.* Data for Decision Making Project, Harvard School of Public Health, Boston, MA.

23 Govindaraj R, Obuobi AAD, Enyimayew NKA, Antwi P, Ofosu-Amaah S (1996). *Hospital autonomy in Ghana: The experience of Korle Bu and Komfo Anokye Teaching Hospitals.* Data for Decision Making Project, Harvard School of Public Health, Boston, MA.

24 Hanson K, Atuyambe L, Kamwanga J, McPake B, Mungule O, Ssengooba F (2002). Towards improving hospital performance in Uganda and Zambia: Reflections and opportunities for autonomy. *Health Policy*, **61**(1), 73–94.

25 Bossert T, Kosen S, Harsono B, Gani A (1997). *Hospital autonomy in Indonesia.* Data for Decision Making Project, Harvard School of Public Health, Boston, MA.

26 Hanson K, Palafox B, Anderson S, *et al.* (2010). Pharmaceuticals. In Merson M, Black R, Mills AJ (eds) *Global health: Diseases, interventions, systems, programs, 3rd edition.* Jones and Bartlett, Sudbury MA.

27 Harding A, Preker AS (2003). A conceptual framework for the organizational reforms of hospitals. In Harding A, Preker AS (eds) *Innovations in health care delivery: The corporatization of public hospitals.* The World Bank, Washington DC.

28 Loevinsohn B, Harding A (2005). Buying results? Contracting for health service delivery in developing countries. *Lancet*, **366**, 676–81.

29 Liu X, Hotchkiss DR, *et al.* (2008). The effectiveness of contracting-out primary health care services in developing countries: a review of the evidence. *Health Policy Plan*, **23**(1), 1–13.

30 Lagarde M, Palmer N (2009). The impact of contracting out on health outcomes and use of health services in low and middle-income countries (Review). *Cochrane Database of Systematic Reviews*, **4**, CD008133.

31 Mills A, Bennett S, *et al.* (eds) (2000). *The challenge of health sector reform: what must governments do?* Palgrave Macmillan, London.

32 Patouillard E, Goodman C, Hanson K, Mills A (2007). Can working with the private sector improve access of the poor to quality health services? A systematic review of the literature. *International Journal for Equity in Health*, **6**, 17–28.

33 Gilson L, Schneider H (2010). Commentary: Managing scaling up—What are the key issues? *Health Policy and Planning*, **25**, 97–8.

34 Mangham L, Hanson K (2010). Scaling up in international health: A review. *Health Policy and Planning*, **25**(2), 85–96.

35 Craig P, Dieppe P, Macintyre S, *et al.* (2008). *Developing and evaluating complex interventions: new guidance.* Medical Research Council, London. Available at: www.mrc.ac.uk/complexinterventionsguidance.

36 de Savigny D, Adam T (eds) (2009). *Systems thinking for health systems strengthening.* Alliance for Health Policy and Systems Research and WHO, Geneva.

37 International Health Policy Programme (2010). *Effectiveness of public health insurance schemes on financial risk protection: the assessments of purchasers' capacities, contractors' responses and impact on patients.* Consortium for Research on Equitable Health Systems, London School of Hygiene and Tropical Medicine, unpublished mimeo.

38 Basinga P, Gertler P, Binagwaho A, Soucat A, Sturdy J, Vermeersch C (2010). Paying primary health care centres for performance in Rwanda. *Policy Research Working Paper 5190.* The World Bank, Washington DC.

39 McPake B, Hanson K, Adam C (2007). 'Two-tier' charging strategies in public hospitals: implications for intra-hospital resource allocation and equity of access to hospital services. *Journal of Health Economics*, **26**(3), 447–62.

40 McPake B, Nakamba P, Hanson K (2004). *Incentives and the allocation of resources within public tertiary hospitals in Zambia.* London, Health Economics and Financing Programme WP 05/04, London School of Hygiene and Tropical Medicine.

41 Lieberman SS, Alkatiri A (2003). Autonomization in Indonesia: the wrong path to reduce hospital expenditures. In Harding A, Preker AS (eds) *Innovations in health care delivery: The corporatization of public hospitals.* The World Bank, Washington DC.

42 McPake B, Hanson K (2006). Implementation of hospital reform policies: Lessons of experience. WIDER Conference on Advancing Health Equity, Helsinki.

Chapter 6

Human resources and the health sector

Barbara McPake

6.1 Introduction

As outlined in Chapter 1, the health workforce constitutes one of the 'building blocks' of the health sector. However, it is this component of the health sector that determines the efficiency with which all others function. Conceived broadly to include all those who are 'primarily engaged in actions with the primary intent of enhancing health', the health workforce includes those who directly deliver health services and determine what should be delivered; what can be delivered given available resources and what will be delivered in reality; identify health information requirements, make plans, implement plans, and collect data; identify what medical products, vaccines, and technologies are purchased, stored, and distributed, and the standards applied at all stages; identify financing strategies and put them into practice at all levels; and establish leadership and governance systems, lead, and govern. It includes civil servants, researchers, and teachers of health-related subjects as well as doctors, nurses, and midwives.

It is therefore critical to examine issues concerning the political economy of human resource management within the health sector, especially in light of concerns over retention and migration. This chapter therefore outlines the current state of play concerning human resources in health, the role of migration and response of high- and middle/low-income countries, and then focuses on two case studies of Kenya and Ghana, before concluding with policy implications.

6.2 Human resources in crisis? A mixed picture

The human resources for health situations in low-income countries are widely reported to be in crisis. Indicators used to support this position include vacancy rates in specific countries and comparisons amongst countries, specifically

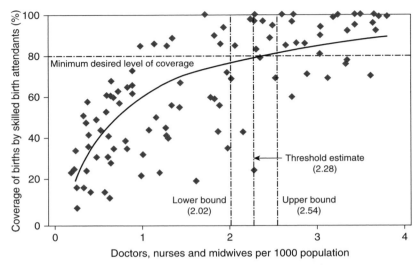

Fig. 6.1 Population density of healthcare professionals required to ensure skilled attendance at births. Reproduced from [4] with permission.

across the low-income–high-income country divide. Comparisons can also be made with specified 'norms'.

For example the World Health Organization's (WHO's) report in 2006 [1] defined 'critical shortage' as falling below the threshold of 2.28 doctors, nurses, and midwives per 1000 population which was derived, following the Joint Learning Initiative [2] from an analysis of the level of workforce density associated with 80% coverage of deliveries with skilled birth attendants (see Figure 6.1) and an analysis suggesting similar density associated with 80% coverage of measles immunization.

Using this definition, countries were classified as in critical shortage or not, as in Figure 6.2.

There are problems with these approaches to identifying 'crisis'. Figure 6.1 shows considerable dispersion around the regression line and eight countries achieve more than 80% coverage at levels of health worker density between one and two per thousand population, indicating that this threshold of 'critical shortage' is not an absolute boundary beyond which no country can reach adequate public health coverage. Vacancy rates are contingent on the level at which funded posts have been established. Both Kenya and Nigeria for example, have low vacancy rates, significant numbers of unemployed health workers, but are still deemed to be in 'critical shortage' because the number of funded posts does not match WHO's estimation of the minimal number of health workers required. Furthermore, an exercise such as that conducted by

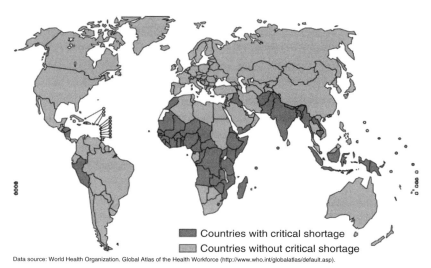

Data source: World Health Organization. Global Atlas of the Health Workforce (http://www.who.int/globalatlas/default.asp).

Fig. 6.2 Countries with a critical shortage of health service providers (doctors, nurses, and midwives).
Source: Reproduced from [4] with permission of the World Health Organization.

WHO requires a standard doctor, nurse, or midwife who does not exist in reality. Training differs in curricula, length of study, and standards applied. Many countries do not recognize a separate category of midwife and some have additional categories of clinical worker such as clinical officer or medical assistant which are not counted in a total of 'doctors, nurses, and midwives' but whose contribution can be significant.

Using comparative data will always highlight variation. There has never been an even distribution of skilled health workers between rich and poor countries without it being clear what levels constitute excess and what constitute crisis. Table 6.1 shows the numbers of physicians and nurses per 100,000 population in a selection of countries in or around 2004.

In some low-income countries, numbers are thought to have been declining, suggesting that inequities are worsening. While data are lacking to confirm trends, the situation is generally considered a crisis in some very low-income countries such as Ghana, where 43% of doctor posts and 26% of nurse posts are vacant and Malawi, where 36% of doctor posts and 18% of nurse posts are vacant. [3] It is worth noting that most but not all low-income countries face a critical shortage of skilled health staff. Countries such as Namibia, Sudan, and most of the countries of South America are judged not in this situation. [4]

Inequalities within countries may be as or more important than inequalities between countries in constraining access to care for the majority of the world's

Table 6.1 Physician and nurse densities in selected countries, 2004 or most recent year available

Country	Physicians per 10,000 population	Nurses per 10,000 population
Ghana	2	9
Kenya	1	12
Malawi	<1	12
Sierra Leone	<1	5
South Africa	8	41
Chile	11	6
Jamaica	9	17
Colombia	14	6
Bangladesh	3	3
India	6	13
Cambodia	2	9
Papua New Guinea	21	5
United States	26	94
Netherlands	37	146
United Kingdom	23	128

Source: WHOSIS: core health indicators at http://www3.who.int/whosis/core/core_select_process.cfm (accessed 21 July 2010).

Table 6.2 Estimates of geographical workforce imbalance from a range of settings

Country	Measure of imbalance	Source
Nicaragua	50% of health personnel in Managua where 20% or population lives	[6]
Mexico	15% of doctors unemployed, underemployed, or inactive, but rural posts remain unfilled	[7]
Indonesia	Health staff reluctant to locate in remote islands and forest locations	[8]
Bangladesh	35% of doctors; 30% of nurses live in metropolitan areas where 15% of population live	[9]
Brazil	Physicians per 1000 population by region varies from 0.52 to 2.05	[10]
Ghana	87% of general physicians worked in urban regions, while 66% of population lives in rural areas	[11,12]

Source: [5]

population. Skewed distributions favouring urban over rural and richer over poorer parts of most countries is well documented. For example, Dussault and Franceschini [5] cite the data in Table 6.2 from a wide range of sources.

This suggests that the so-called 'medical carousel' [13] operates within as well as between countries to render the lowest level and most peripheral services most difficult to staff and implies that primary care workers are likely to be in greatest shortage.

6.3 **The role of migration**

Migration of health professionals is not a new phenomenon. For example, Canada aggressively recruited from overseas in response to a perceived shortage of medical professionals between 1954 and 1975, and during the 1960s, there was active encouragement of medical staff from India and the West Indies to migrate to the United Kingdom. However, rates of emigration of skilled health professionals from low-income countries increased markedly in the 1990s and early 2000s, especially from sub-Saharan Africa.

Rates of emigration from low-income countries seem to be increasing [14]. There have been rising intakes of foreign medical and nursing graduates to the United Kingdom [15] where one-third of doctors were trained overseas, 9152 in sub-Saharan Africa, and where the proportion of nurses added to the United Kingdom register and trained overseas exceeded 50% for the first time in 2001–2 [16] and to the United States and Canada where 30% of doctors trained in Ghana and 20% of doctors trained in Kenya now work [17]. The United Kingdom has been an important destination for migrating skilled health staff, but since 2006 its recruitment rates have declined due to financial crisis, and the situation is changing [18].

One factor implicated seems to be globalization, or the increasingly easy linkages between people and economies. Marchal and Kegels [19] report that 27,000 highly qualified Africans emigrated between 1960 and 1975, an average of 1800 people per year. This annual rate had risen to 8000 by 1987, and to 20,000 during the 1990s.

In some countries, the export of health workers has been a deliberate strategy to earn foreign remittances. India, Cuba, Egypt, and the Philippines purposefully export health workers, and some people train in the health professions with the intention of acquiring an internationally marketable skill [20].

Others have pointed to a set of specific health sector 'push' and 'pull' factors that have driven unplanned migration. For example, Buchan [21] and Labonté et al. [22] have produced similar tables, as adapted in Table 6.3.

Table 6.3 Push and pull factors in international market for skilled health workers

Push factors	Pull factors
Low pay/late and non-payment	Higher pay; opportunities for remittances
Low job availability	Vacancies
Poor working conditions (inadequate resources; high workload; poor human resources planning)	Better working conditions
Lack of resources to work effectively	Better resourced health systems
Limited career opportunities	Career opportunities
Limited educational opportunities for worker and children	Provision of post-basic education; good general education system
High prevalence of HIV/AIDS	Low prevalence of HIV/AIDS
Unstable/dangerous work environment	Political stability
Unstable general political environment: risks of political and criminal violence	Low crime rates
Economic instability	Economic stability

Adapted from [14,15].

6.4 **What can low-income country governments do?**

These identified push and pull factors are almost entirely features or direct consequences of the macro-economic and geo-political circumstances that separate low- from high-income countries. If these are the only points of leverage over the situation, there is little prospect of action to solve this particular one of the many problems these factors are implicated in.

However, it is also clear that from a low-income country perspective, there are more tractable sets of factors implicated in the human resource crisis in the form of the management practices that govern health workers in low-income countries. For example, in Kenya and Benin it was found that a significant source of demotivation and frustration for health workers was inadequate or inappropriately applied human resource management tools [23]. Research in South Africa linked the problem of poor management to health workers' work location choices [24]. Health workers considered that better management in their working location was more important than a 15% increase in pay (but less than a doubling of pay). This suggests that if Ministers of Health in low-income countries can improve the management system within the health sector in ways that enable health workers to pursue their vocation and satisfy their professional conscience, higher rates of retention can be expected. The kinds of measures that might be taken have been suggested by Stilwell and colleagues [25]. While action in high-income countries will still be important, this is perhaps the single most important area for attention within low-income countries themselves.

This is still a relatively neglected intervention in countries' strategies to deal with the human resource crisis. However South Africa launched its National Human Resources Plan for Health in 2006 whose central objective was to stem the tide of migration. South Africa has been estimated to lose between a third and a half of its medical graduates to emigration [26]. The South African strategy placed more effective human resource management at the centre of its approach. For example Principle 6 of the plan is: 'Work environments must be conducive to good management practice in order to maximise the potential for the health workforce to deliver good quality health services' [27].

Low-income country governments can also support the principle of task shifting to ensure that those human resources available are able to have the maximum impact on improving access to essential interventions. Huicho et al. [28] provide a comprehensive study of this issue, comparing results across four countries and finding that health workers with shorter duration of training performed at least as well and sometimes significantly better than those with longer duration of training in assessing, classifying, and managing episodes of routine childhood illness, and counselling the children's care takers.

6.5 What can high-income country governments do?

High-income country governments can influence the situation by mitigating the problems caused by migration of skilled health personnel and through aid programmes. It has been argued that the critical factor driving health worker migration has been health sector policies in high-income countries [29]. Far from being at the mercy of market forces such as salary differentials between countries and the growing demands of ageing populations, policy measures largely unrelated to these trends have created staff shortages in four Organisation for Economic Co-operation and Development (OECD) countries that have consequently increased the extent to which they have called on trained health staff from elsewhere. In the United Kingdom, the policy measure was a decision to significantly increase spending on the National Health Service after a Labour government took power in 1997. In France, restrictive quotas for nursing and medical training operated until the late 1990s, threatening to result in a decline in health worker density. After this point, new policies increased the quotas and relaxed restrictions on foreign educated doctors. In Germany, at unification there was first a consensus that there was an over-supply of doctors which resulted in reductions in numbers in training. Shortages of doctors emerged in some regions and the number of foreign doctors working in Germany increased by 36% between 1995 and 2003. In the United States, attitudes to managed care arrangements that seek to contain the costs of the healthcare system have waxed and waned in government, and nursing short- ages have periodically been experienced each time cost containment has been relaxed [30]. The current nursing shortage in the United States is more severe and will likely have longer-term repercussions than previous ones.

However, rather than examine the forces that have created shortages of health staff and could presumably eliminate them within local labour markets, emphasis has instead been put on the development of ethical recruitment poli- cies, in identifying measures that high-income governments can take to amel- iorate the migration crisis. The first international code to be adopted was the Commonwealth Code of Practice for the International Recruitment of Health Workers, but this code has not been signed by Australia, Canada, and the United Kingdom, reputedly because it recommends compensation for the loss of investment in low-income countries [31,32]. At national level, the United Kingdom developed the first code of practice and revised it in 2004 in an attempt to close some loopholes that had become apparent, for example seek- ing to extend its reach to the private sector, and temporary/locum staff [33]. The code restricts the specific targeting for recruitment of a list of developing countries, including some African and Asian Commonwealth countries, but does not preclude acceptance of individual applications from those countries.

The codes and intergovernmental agreements that have been set up with similar intent are widely viewed as having been largely ineffective. For exam- ple, in 2003–4, more than a quarter of newly registered nurses (or approxi- mately half of newly registered foreign nurses) in the United Kingdom, originated from proscribed countries [23], and these numbers continued to increase in several proscribed countries after the code should have taken effect [24]. Some have even suggested that ethical recruitment codes could have the detrimental effect of appearing to address a problem and deflecting attention from more effective strategies [34].

High-income countries benefit from a significant subsidy from low-income countries when a health professional moves from the latter to the former. One source estimated in 1996 that Africa lost US$184,000 for each migrating pro- fessional [35]. The cost of obtaining an adequate supply of health staff from within a high-income population includes not only the training costs but the costs of maintaining pay and conditions at a level attractive to the home work- force. Depending on the domestic elasticity of labour supply, this cost might be considerable, perhaps even considered prohibitive by those countries. When the United Kingdom sought to expand its health workforce at the end of the 1990s, several strategies were enumerated to achieve the increase: 1) retention of current staff and return of those working elsewhere; 2) recruitment of newly qualified health professionals into the NHS from United Kingdom training institutions and 3) recruitment of doctors and nurses into the NHS from international sources [36]. In the event, the dominant source was (3) [21].

If beneficiary countries such as Australia, Canada, and the United Kingdom are unwilling to consider relatively modest compensation of the training cost of the health staff recruited, it is unlikely that they will be willing to underwrite the considerably greater expense of achieving increases in health staff from their own populations. The policy constraints in high-income countries go still further. As Arah [37] points out, health professional migration is one component of globalized migration trends, and it may not be tenable to achieve control over a single professional group.

Traditionally, aid programmes have excluded core funding for remuneration of health personnel on the grounds that there are serious sustainability problems associated with subsidising this core component of recurrent cost and that a country's sovereignty is undermined when its civil service is no longer remunerated by the national government. These grounds had lost cogency as human resource shortage increasingly figured as the main explanation of failure of all kinds of development initiative and mechanisms of supporting health personnel remuneration in all but name (through a range of per-diem, allowance and bonus arrangements) had become ubiquitous.

In Malawi, the Emergency Human Resources Programme has channelled international development assistance funds to the supplementation of the salaries of some cadres of health personnel among other interventions designed to support the human resources situation, including training and recruitment initiatives. Here, the concerns with respect to sustainability and sovereignty have been mitigated by the use of the funding mechanism associated with the Sector Wide Approach, a mechanism that pools development assistance and government finances under a joint administrative framework [38].

6.6 **Case studies**

Case studies reviewing the HRH situations in Kenya and Ghana were conducted in 2007 as part of an evaluation of the Department of Health, England, Code of Practice on International Recruitment [39]. The case studies involved the identification and analysis of secondary data and interviews with multiple stakeholders in Ministries of Health, training institutions, development partner organizations and support agencies. Groups of health workers were also interviewed to establish their insights and experiences.

6.6.1 Kenya case study

6.6.1.1 Numbers and distribution of health workers and the factors influencing them

The number of Kenyan doctors and nurses within the country is estimated at somewhere between 3855–4506 and 26,267–37,112 respectively [4]. Approximately 500 nurses per year were estimated to be graduating with diplomas and 150/year with BSN degrees. The number of doctors produced each year was estimated as 350.

It was widely recognized that there was considerable unemployment among nurses and a figure of 7000 unemployed nurses was cited by some but could not be verified, but the presence of extensive unemployment was confirmed by the experience of the emergency hire programme (see below).

Public sector employment of both doctors and nurses had recently expanded with the public sector reported to have increased its recruitment of doctors and nurses last year by 300 and 3000 respectively.

The emergency hire programme was funded by several major external sources and the Government of Kenya, and implemented by the Capacity Project and recruited 830 nurses and other health professionals to work in 193 sites, 26 of which were able to open as a result of this initiative. It received approximately 7000 applications for these posts, funded only at allowable public sector rates (albeit with maximum allowances).

There was unequal distribution of the labour force between urban and rural and especially 'hard-to-reach' parts of the country. Within the public sector, deployment procedures appeared to be a source of the problem. Health workers were reported able to renegotiate their posting using various strategies, something that resulted in over-staffing in most urban Hospitals particularly those in Nairobi and Mombasa and under-staffing nearly everywhere else.

The situation had reportedly deteriorated further as a result of changing relative reimbursement packages between the faith based organization (FBO) sector and the public sector, with the latter paying significantly higher wages. The FBO sector dominates provision in the most hard-to-reach parts of the county.

According to one source, the FBO sector's total reimbursement package (worth approximately K.Sh. 12,000) was in 2007 worth only about one-half of that in the public sector (worth approximately K.Sh. 27,000). It was also reported that nurses in the FBO sector could fail to receive their wages if receipts at the relevant health facility were insufficient.

It had become very difficult for the FBO sector to recruit nurses under these terms, even from the pool of unemployed nurses. A representative of Christian

Health Association of Kenya (CHAK) mentioned a hospital that had advertised extensively and failed to recruit, and was currently trying (but apparently failing) to negotiate with the Nursing Council of Kenya (NCK), the entry of a Tanzanian nurse.

A Ministry of Health subvention paid to FBOs, estimated to have subsidized to the extent of 25% was removed in the late 1990s. After a period of no support, the Ministry of Health started to second some staff to FBOs, but it often proved difficult to retain these secondees who were able to negotiate redeployment.

Two large Kenya Ecumenical Council (KEC) hospitals closed during 2006–7. While difficulties of recruitment contributed, the main cause of closure appeared to be financial difficulties. This further worsened human resource distribution and removed services from some large areas of the country.

The Emergency Hire Programme experience suggests that it is possible to staff hard to reach areas at reasonable reimbursement rates. The contracts offered were fixed term (3 years) with no possibilities of redeployment. Sixty of the recruits were received by FBOs. The Ministry of Health plans to integrate the emergency hired nurses into the public health workforce at the end of the contracts, although this was not advertised.

6.6.1.2 Migration of doctors and nurses

The only internal source of data on doctor migration is the numbers seeking 'Certificates of Good Standing' from the Kenya Medical and Dental Association. These are required for doctors who are planning to practice outside the country or go abroad for postgraduate medical training. A register of these had only recently begun to be compiled in 2007, and showed that 28 doctors had sought these letters with an additional three in process in a four-month period. This rate is about 25% of the rate of training of doctors reported above. The total number of Kenyan born doctors practising outside Kenya is estimated at 3975, 56% of the total stock of doctors estimated. Of these, 2733 are estimated to be practising in the United Kingdom. These are probably over-estimates of Kenyan trained doctors practising outside because they include all those of Kenyan birth, including those who migrated as children or before basic training.

Obtaining a training post in another country is the usual vehicle by which doctors migrate—it was said to be relatively rare for a doctor to migrate directly to an overseas post other than a training post, or to set up an overseas private practice.

Figure 6.3 presents data compiled by the Nursing Council of Kenya on number of nurses whose qualifications were verified between January 1993

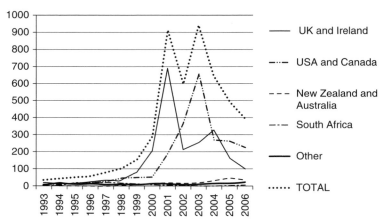

Fig. 6.3 Total number of nurses verified to apply for foreign registration from January 1993 to December 2006 [39].

and December 2006. Nurses require qualification verification as part of the registration process in a second country.

Figure 6.3 shows that verification numbers peaked in 2003 at 940, having first dipped from the 2001 level in 2002. This reflects a peak in the numbers seeking verification for exit to the United Kingdom in 2001, and a peak in the numbers seeking verification for exit to the United States in 2003. For both countries, numbers had fallen sharply since their peaks.

Better pay and conditions for doctors and to a lesser extent nurses were argued to provide some of the explanation. However, Reilly et al. [40] indicate that 50% of nurses wanted to migrate as late as 2004–5.

Greater difficulties in achieving access to the United Kingdom labour market dominated explanations. These included:

◆ Greater difficulties in obtaining visas. The categories of general nurse and general doctor had been removed from the list of occupations in short supply by the Home Office.

◆ More stringent 'adaptation' requirements and difficulties in securing placements. Until 2005, registration with the NMC required, apart from verified Kenyan qualifications, a period of United Kingdom-based 'supervised practice' or 'placement'. After September 2005 it required additionally completion of a class based course, an increased pass requirement in English language proficiency (increased further in February 2007). Placements were considered to have become almost impossible to identify.

◆ Increased total costs of the process, in part because of the difficulties addressed in the previous two bullet points.

Data did not allow analysis of the characteristics of nurses migrating. A common view was that those in the first wave of nurses who migrated were retirees, generating income to provide for a pension (in the public system the retirement age is 55). More recent emigrants were said to be younger—new graduates who were not absorbed into the public system. It was said that BSN graduates had found it difficult to be absorbed in a public system that had not adjusted to accommodate this higher level qualification. Some argued that the emigrants were the 'best' nurses—variously, because these were the ones with qualifications sought in the United Kingdom and elsewhere or because they were the more entrepreneurial 'risk takers'. One nurse described the perception that she was viewed by others as a failure because she had stayed.

However, migration did not appear to be the major factor driving health worker shortages that arose only in remoter, rural parts of Kenya. While some argued that public training resources were squandered in the process, it is not clear that they would not be equally squandered by the failure to absorb trained nurses into the labour force. There appeared to be a greater willingness on the part of the Ministry of Health to ensure all available doctors were absorbed into the labour force, but it is not clear that this would have been feasible if all Kenyan trained doctors had been available in Kenya, nor that this would be consistent with the direction advanced by the Health Sector Strategic Plan, 2007 (HSSP).

6.6.1.3 Human resources for health policy developments

The policy direction indicated by the HSSP was to emphasize strengthening the lowest levels ('level 1' and 'level 2') of the sector, which are the community and most basic facility levels. These levels require increased numbers of community health workers and nurses and clinical officers with the most basic qualifications. It was recognized that this conflicts with the professional aspirations of health workers, and that emphasizing this direction in personnel management may provide further impetus to migration.

6.6.1.4 Policy implications in Kenya

For high-income governments, particularly the United States and United Kingdom, many stakeholders considered that the most constructive intervention would be to develop government to government agreements over the exchange of health professionals. In 2007, there were agreements between the Government of Kenya and those of Sudan and Namibia of this type.

It was recognized that there may be differing comparative advantages in training of health professionals that current patterns of migration reflect. Basic training in Kenya may be lower cost at comparable quality, making it cost-efficient for the United Kingdom and United States to recruit nurses trained in Kenya. Similarly, pursuit of post graduate training opportunities in the United Kingdom and United States may suggest that the high-income countries have comparative advantage at that stage of the process. Foreign investment in basic nursing and other health professional training in Kenya would both recognize the benefits that the NHS gains from Kenyan public investment in training and directly benefit the NHS by adding further to the quality of training.

There are also measures that the Government of Kenya could take to support workforce balance. The code of regulation of civil servants explicitly rules out (reportedly) the return of civil servants to the public system at any higher grade than the one they left. This prevents recognition of education and experience gained overseas and confronts potential returnees with the prospect of working at the same level of those who were their juniors when they left. Some potential returnees are likely to be dissuaded by these provisions.

While Kenya loses many health professionals to international migration, it gains few. This appears to be as much by policy design as by market forces. For example, doctors from the Indian sub-continent who would like to practice in Kenya tend to be refused registration on the basis of their competence levels. The rationale for this appeared to be protectionism of the medical market for Kenyan practitioners.

6.6.2 Ghana case study

6.6.2.1 Numbers and distribution of health workers and the factors influencing them

Trends in training numbers for nurses and midwives (1999–2005), provided by the Nurses and Midwives' Council for Ghana are shown in Figure 6.4.

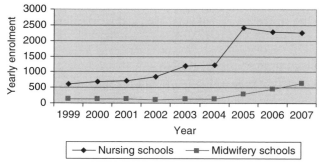

Fig. 6.4 Trends in training numbers: Nurses and Midwives, Ghana.
Source: data provided by Nurses and Midwives' Council for Ghana

These show that investment in training both categories has increased considerably over the nine-year period concerned, with growth in nursing numbers occurring earlier than growth in midwife numbers.

It is questionable whether quality was being maintained in the training schools. Anecdotal complaints included class sizes of 140 and more, inadequate increase in the number of tutors to cover the larger numbers of trainees and recruitment of under-qualified tutors, over-crowded practicals, leaving students volunteering at non-training institutions at weekends to gain experience, and failure to invest in the new infrastructure at a pace that reflects the growing student numbers.

The Ghana Health Services (GHS) estimated that there were 1446 doctors and 14,507 nurses in 2006. The Registrar, Pharmacy council estimated that there were 1600–1800 pharmacists. Numbers of unemployed nurses and doctors were considered to be insignificant. Both would be absorbed into the GHS if they met entry criteria. There were likely to be a few voluntarily unemployed, or a few who failed to meet criteria, for example because of years of non-practice. However, not all pharmacists were absorbed by the GHS and there was no automatic intake of new graduates as for nurses and doctors. Unabsorbed pharmacists were more likely to work in the private sector than be unemployed.

There was considerable regional variation in doctor and nurse density according to data supplied by the GHS. Northern Region had one doctor for every 85,957 people while Greater Accra had one doctor for every 5806 people. Nurses were less unevenly distributed. Western region was worst served with a population per nurse of 2368, and Northern, Brong-Ahafo, and Ashanti were nearly as poorly served with populations per nurse of 2126, 2036, and 2136 respectively. The ratio of population to health professional of the best to worse served region was 14.8 for doctors and 2.4 for nurses.

6.6.2.2 Migration of doctors and nurses

The Ministry of Health estimated total attrition in public, Christian Health Association of Ghana (CHAG) and military health facilities, suggesting that losses reduced between 2004 and 2006 in all categories, having shown an increasing trend between 2001 and 2004 in the cases of nurses/midwives, and medical officers. These data aggregate movement between facilities and loss to the system altogether. Causes of attrition in 2004–6 collated by the Chief Nursing Office were dominated by study leave. The category 'vacation of post' which is the usual one allocated for those migrating after 2004.

Darko et al. [41] reported a declining trend in rate of validation requests from nurses and midwives from a peak in 2003, with an overall 34.5%

reduction between 2003 and 2005. The Nursing and Midwives Council further reported that validation requests had fallen to 56 in 2006 from 686 in 2005. Many stakeholders agreed that migration was no longer prevalent, especially to the United Kingdom. Darko et al. [41] also reported the target destination of validation applications across the four years for which data are analysed. The dominant target destination was the United Kingdom (71%) followed by the United States (22%).

Two important explanations of these trends were advanced by respondents in Ghana: international labour market changes and Government of Ghana policy changes which have wider implications for HRH development (covered in the next section). Ghanaian stakeholders identified international labour market changes almost identically to Kenyan ones, so these will not be repeated.

6.6.2.3 **Human resources for health policy developments**

The Government of Ghana had put in place a number of policy measures designed to improve the HRH situation.

There had been significant developments over a number of years in the pay and conditions packages of doctors and other health professionals. At the end of the 1990s, doctors' lobbying and strike activity secured payment of the Additional Daily Hours Allowance that quickly extended to all doctors irrespective of their daily hours and had the effect of an approximate doubling of salary level. This allowance was then consolidated into the salary scale in 2005, as part of a rationalization and job evaluation process. Nurses and other health professionals also secured large pay increases as part of the same process.

There were questions about the sustainability of these rates of pay. The pay settlements may have been based on optimism that the National Health Insurance Fund which was at an early stage of implementation would generate sufficient funds, likely to be unrealistic.

The process of developing and implementing the new salary scales appeared to have encountered a number of difficulties with the effect that despite the sizes of these settlements, nurses in particular were dissatisfied with the new pay structure on the basis of its effect on changed differentials between nurses and doctors. It was expected that nurses would ultimately receive even larger settlements.

Since 2005, new procedures had made it more difficult to evade the provision of the bond by which nurses trained with public funds were required to work for five years for the Ministry of Health, or repay the cost of training. An updated, more accurate and much higher bond value had been calculated and was reported to be 200 million Ghanaian cedis, increased from two million. Additionally, there was a recent agreement between the Nursing and Midwifery

Council and the Ministry of Health/GHS that certificates of validation would not be issued without confirmation that the Bond had expired or been paid. This was credited as the factor underlying the falling migration rate [41]. A group of nurses interviewed confirmed the importance of this measure as a constraint to migration, although thought that some nurses were still able to evade the provision through personal contacts.

For doctors, similar measures to enforce a bond policy had not been taken. However, other measures had been put in place that constrained migration, according to a group of doctors interviewed. These included the extension of the period of house officership from one to two years and to include rotation through all four major specialties rather than a choice of two. Doctors should also have been directed to a rural posting for a period, although it seemed to have become increasingly easy to evade such a posting. It was pointed out by the group of doctors that these measures had the potential to backfire by making migration a more attractive option.

The Ghana College of Physicians and Surgeons was instituted in 2003 to expand provision of post graduate medical training. The College had received more applications than it had capacity to accept and was dealing with qualified candidates in batches, implying a growing waiting list for places. A greater emphasis on qualifications relative to experience in the recently revised pay scales was seen as partly responsible. Applying a higher qualification standard was under consideration. One issue in this development with the potential to aggravate workforce maldistribution was the almost exclusive accreditation of facilities in urban areas as post-graduate training centres.

Little progress had been made in tackling the maldistribution of health professionals across Ghanaian regions. The situation described above had changed little over the previous decade. However, two policies were in early stages of implementation that might tackle this more effectively:

- A new cadre of rural health worker had been created, with the capacity to support professional health staff operating in remoter areas. Some doubts were expressed about the feasibility of the plans. Most of those recruited had been younger women who might not be able to operate securely in isolation in these areas, which was consistent with a general view that these workers were difficult to retain.

- An attempt to better match individuals to the post to which they would be sent was planned by the Ministry of Health. There was in principle, a random system of allocation of graduates to posts within the services of the Ministry. It was planned to introduce a system of interviews so that individuals' preferences could play some part in the allocation. In the past it had been widely assumed that rural postings were universally unpopular and that random allocation was the only fair system. That view had been challenged.

6.6.2.4 Policy implications in Ghana

While there had been some attempts to implement bilateral agreements between the Ghana and United Kingdom health services in health professional exchange and training, these had floundered on the difficulties of securing the return of trainees supported to spend periods in the United Kingdom. Health Authorities involved in these were viewed as reneging on their commitments. There was as a result some scepticism about the potential for these sorts of arrangements.

It was suggested that the growing numbers of private nursing schools in Ghana could provide a suitable partner for international investment in Ghanaian training.

Pharmacists were perceived as marginalized and unrecognized in Government of Ghana policy making, and under-valued in the management of the district health system. Nurses cited problems of inconvenient accommodation, lack of equipment and low pay as factors affecting retention. Nurses had not yet received the pay increases expected. These issues highlight the inadequacy of improving remuneration as the sole plank of a policy that aims to increase health professionals' satisfaction with their work situations. Retention is likely to require further improvements to non-financial aspects of working conditions. Government of Ghana policy is likely to have played some part in the maintenance or even growth in health professional numbers in country over the period since 2000.

In general, there was a need for a stronger policy framework in relation to the expansion of training schools, the funding of pay agreements, and the addressing of health worker distribution.

6.7 Conclusions and global policy implications

Many factors influence the human resources for health situation in any given country: the 'push' and 'pull' factors that affect recruitment and retention; and the management and resource availability factors that affect motivation and performance. Only some of these are under the control of national Ministries of Health in the country affected, or are even factors under the control of national governments at all. However, those factors can be overlooked in an analysis that blames all human resources problems on external factors.

Low-income country governments could improve their situation by focusing on human resource management improvements at all levels of their health sector and offering political support to the project of task-shifting. The management of human resources is often confounded by political factors, such as the power of the medical profession which constrains task shifting, curbs on the migration of medical professionals, the provision of incentives to non medical health professionals and the allocation of management tasks to those with management skills. This is a problem contained within the national environment (even if a common one, internationally) but not one that can be considered under the control of national Ministries of Health or governments.

Nevertheless, external factors are important, and some of these can be influenced by governments in high-income countries. In relation to migration, such governments could offer compensation to the countries whose skilled professionals they are recruiting. Compensation for the cost of training would likely be a lower cost option than seeking to resolve imbalances in their local labour markets. It could help resolve the problem by allowing greater investment in training in source countries, yet it seems that this is a step such governments are reluctant to take. Acting through aid programmes, governments have new mechanisms illustrated by the Kenyan emergency hire programme and the Malawi Emergency Human Resources Programme by which aid programmes can support the remuneration of health personnel at their disposal. While these are relatively recently introduced and not yet well evaluated, there are some signs that they are starting to reduce the human resource crisis. Evidence of long-term impacts on sovereignty and sustainability will take longer to amass.

References

1 Speybroeck N, Kinfu Y, Dal Poz MR, Evans DB (2006). *Reassessing the relationship between human resources for health, intervention coverage and health outcomes* (Background paper prepared for The World Health Report, 2006). World Health Organization, Geneva. Available at: http://www.who.int/hrh/documents/reassessing_relationship.pdf.

2 The Rockefellor Foundation (2003). *Human Resources for Health and Development: a Joint Learning Initiative*. Available at: http://www.rockfound.org/library/03hrh.pdf (accessed 6 April 2007).

3 Bach S (2003). *International migration of health workers: labour and social issues* (Sectoral Activities Programme Working Paper). International Labour Office, Geneva. Available at: http://www.ilo.org/public/English/dialogue/sector/papers/health/wp209.pdf.

4 World Health Organization (2006). *The World Health Report 2006: Working Together for Health*. WHO, Geneva.

5 Dussault G, Franceschini MC (2006). Not enough there, too many here: understanding geographical imbalances in the distribution of the health workforce, *Human Resources for Health*, 4, 12. Available at: http://www.human-resources-health.com/content/4/1/12

6 Nigenda F, Machado H (2000). From state to market: the Nicaraguan labour market for health personnel. *Health Policy and Planning*, **15**(3), 312–18.

7 World Health Organization (2000). *World Health Report*. WHO, Geneva.

8 Chomitz K, Setiadi G, Azwar A (1998). What Do Doctors Want? In *Developing Strategies for Doctors to Serve in Indonesia's Rural and Remote Areas*. Policy Research Working Paper no. 1888. World Bank, Washington, DC.

9 Bangladesh Ministry of Health and Family Welfare (1997). *Human Resources Development in Health and Family Planning in Bangladesh: A Strategy for Change*. Human Resources Development Unit, Dhaka.

10 Machado M (ed) (1997). *Os Médicos no Brasil: um Retrato da Realidade*. Editora Fiocruz, Rio de Janeiro.

11 World Health Organization (1997). *Inter-country Consultation on Development of Human resources in Health in the African Region*. WHO Regional Office for Africa, Brazzaville.

12 Ghana Health Services. Available at: http://www.ghanahealthservice.org.

13 Bundrett PE, Levitt C (2000). Medical migration: who are the real losers. *Lancet*, **356**, 245–6.

14 Mensah K, Mackintosh M, Henry L (2005). *The 'skills drain' of health professionals from the developing world: a framework for policy formulation*. Medact, London. Available at http://www.medact.org/content/Skills%20drain/Mensah%20et%20al.%202005.pdf.

15 Pond B, McPake B (2006). The health migration crisis: the role of four Organisation for Economic Co-operation and Development countries. *Lancet*, **367**, 1448–55.

16 Aiken L, Buchan J, Sochalski J, Nichols B, Powell M (2004). Trends in international nurse migration. *Health Affairs*, **23**(3), 69–77.

17 Hagopian A, Thompson MJ, Fordyce M, Johnson KE, Hart LG (2004). The migration of physicians from sub-Saharan Africa to the United States of America: measures of the African brain drain. *Human Resources for Health*, **2**, 17.

18 The Guardian (2006). *Most new nurses still job hunting*. October 19th.

19 Marchal B, Kegels G (2003). Health workforce imbalances in times of globalisation: brain drain or professional mobility? *International Journal of Health Planning and Management*, **18**(supp 1), S89–S101.

20 Connell J, Stilwell B (2006). Merchants of medical care: recruiting agencies in the global health care chain. In Kuptsch C (ed) *Merchants of Labour*, pp.239–52. International Institute for Labour Studies, Geneva.

21 Buchan J (2005). Migration of health workers in Europe: policy problem or policy solution? In Dubois CA, McKee M, Nolte E (eds) *Human Resources for Health in Europe*, pp.41–62. WHO, Geneva. Available at http://www.euro.who.int/__data/assets/pdf_file/0006/98403/E87923.pdf

22 Labonté R, Packer C, Klassen N (2006). Managing health professional migration from sub-Saharan Africa to Canada: a stakeholder inquiry into policy options. *Human Resources for Health*, **4**, 22.

23 Mathauer I, Imhoff I (2006). Health worker motivation in Africa: the role of non-financial incentives and human resource management tools. *Human Resources for Health*, **4**, 24.

24 Penn-Kekana L, Blaauw D, Tint KS, Monareng D (2005). *Nursing staff dynamics and implications for maternal health provision in public health facilities in the context of HIV/AIDS*. Available at http://www.wits.ac.za/chp/docs/FR109_SA_Nursing_Staff.pdf.

25 Tilwell B, Zurn P, Connell J, Awases M (2005). *The migration of health workers: an overview*. WHO, Report to the World Health Assembly, Geneva.

26 Weiner R, Mitchell G, Price M (1998). Wits medical graduates: where are they now? *South African Journal of Science*, **94**, 59–63.

27 Available at: http://www.doh.gov.za/docs/discuss/2006/hrh_plan/exec_summary.pdf.

28 Huicho L, Scherpbier RW, Mwansa Nkowane A, Victora CG (2008). How much does quality of child care vary between health workers with differing durations of training? An observational multicountry study. *Lancet*, **372**, 910–16.

29 Pond B, McPake B (2006). The health migration crisis: the role of four Organisation for Economic Cooperation and Development countries. *Lancet*, **367**, 1448–55.

30 Kingma M (2005). *Nurses on the move: Migration and the global health care economy*. ILR Press, Ithaca, NY.

31 Maybud S, Wiskow C (2006). 'Care trade': The international brokering of health care professionals. In Kuptsch C (ed) *Merchants of Labour*, International Institute for Labour Studies, Geneva.

32 Bach S (2006). *International mobility of health professionals: brain drain or brain exchange?* UNU-WIDER, Research Paper No. 2006/82.

33 UK Department of Health (2004). *Code of practice for the international recruitment of healthcare professionals*. Available at: http://www.dh.gov.uk/assetRoot/04/09/77/34/04097734.pdf.

34 Willetts A, Martineau T (2004). *Ethical international recruitment of health professionals: will codes of practice protect developing country health systems?* Liverpool School of Tropical Medicine, Liverpool.

35 Ogowe A (2005). Brain drain: colossal loss of investment for developing countries. *The Courier ACP-EU 1996*, **159**, 59–60, cited in Eastwood JB, Conroy RE, Naicker S, West PA, Tutt RC, Plange-Rhule J. Loss of health professionals from sub-Saharan Africa: the pivotal role of the UK, *Lancet*, **365**, 1893–900.

36 UK Department of Health (2000). *The NHS Plan: a plan for investment. A plan for reform*. Available at: http://www.dh.gov.uk/assetRoot/04/05/57/83/04055783.pdf.

37 Arah OA (2006). The health worker migration crisis, letter. *Lancet*, **368**, 28.

38 *Country Case Study. Malawi's Emergency Human Resources Programme*. Available at: http://www.who.int/workforcealliance/knowledge/case_studies/Malawi.pdf.

39 Buchan J, McPake B, Rae G, Mensah K (2007). *The Impact of the Department of Health, England, Code of Practice on International Recruitment*. Report to Department of Health and Department for International Development, June 2007.

40 Reilly PL, Vindigni SM, Arudo J (2007). Developing a nursing database system in Kenya. *Health Services Research*, **42**(**32**), 1389–405.

41 Darko VM, Nyanteh F, Boni P (2006). Migration trends of Ghanaian nurses and midwives: impact of a recent policy implementation. *West African Journal of Nursing*, **17**(2), 178–82.

Chapter 7

Pharmaceuticals and the health sector

Prashant Yadav, Richard D. Smith, and Kara Hanson

7.1 Introduction

Pharmaceuticals, including vaccines, are used to prevent, treat, or cure a number of diseases and are often the expensive element within the health sector. The availability of affordable and effective drugs is, therefore, one of the most visible indicators of the quality of health services and the subject of intense debate in most developed and developing countries. Developing countries, especially, face a number of specific issues.

Pharmaceutical research and development (R&D) is carried out by a few large transnational companies in industrialized countries. The global pharmaceutical market is also highly concentrated with the top ten companies accounting for more than half of world sales. Over the last two decades, there has been a rapid growth in the generic pharmaceutical industry in India and China which manufactures both active ingredients and finished products. However, effective medicines for diseases of the developing world are lacking due to a variety of issues, but including the limited potential for return on this R&D. New mechanisms such as product development partnerships and pull incentives to promote development of pharmaceuticals for developing country needs have been put in place in the last decade.

In recent years increasing pressure on public budgets in industrialized high-income countries has put greater emphasis on pharmaceutical cost control in these large pharmaceutical markets. This has provided the impetus for pharmaceutical companies to shift their focus to finding bigger markets for their products in developing countries, especially middle-income countries. This shift in emphasis has coincided with the signing of the Trade Related Intellectual Property Rights (TRIPS) agreement by many developing countries.

Pharmaceutical markets within developing countries also differ widely from those in high-income countries. In developing countries, per capita spending on medicines is low but comes largely from out-of-pocket household expenditure. Drug shortages continue to undermine the performance of public sector clinics resulting in the growth of a larger private market for pharmaceuticals. Furthermore, national regulatory authorities of developing countries often do not have the capacity to handle numerous, complex product regulatory filings and this makes gaining regulatory approval for pharmaceuticals costly, complex, and lengthy.

This chapter consolidates existing knowledge around the role, structure, and improvement levers of pharmaceutical systems, and provides a review of issues facing the pharmaceutical component of health sectors in developing countries. It presents an overview of the approaches used to manage the development, production, distribution, and licensing of pharmaceutical products in developing country markets. The chapter first highlights the role of pharmaceuticals in the health sector, then the key issues affecting pharmaceutical product development. Next, the manufacturing and production of pharmaceuticals is outlined, followed by regulatory aspects, and the various options for financing the provision of pharmaceuticals. The chapter then turns to issues of distribution and access to pharmaceuticals, including trade and TRIPS aspects, before concluding.

7.2 Importance of pharmaceuticals in health sector expenditure

In recent years, health expenditure as a share of GDP has been increasing globally [1] with most countries witnessing a rise in the share of total healthcare expenditure going to pharmaceuticals. This increase in pharmaceutical expenditure is partly on account of the availability of new and more effective pharmaceuticals. However, increases in income, population aging, expansion in health insurance coverage, increases in physician-induced demand, and in some cases the rising administrative costs of running a pharmaceutical system also contribute to this increase. These trends are prompting governments and health policy makers to put a greater emphasis on understanding their pharmaceutical systems and policies.

While spending on pharmaceuticals represents a significant portion of the health expenditure in all countries, its level differs considerably between low- and middle-income countries and high-income countries. The proportion of health expenditure on pharmaceuticals is highest in middle-income countries (25%), and lowest in high-income countries (14%), even though the absolute level of expenditure is highest in high-income countries [2]. The average per capita pharmaceutical expenditure was US$396 in high-income countries compared to US$4.4 in low-income countries. Despite the low per capita absolute expenditure, pharmaceuticals are the largest item in household health

Table 7.1 Distribution of source of pharmaceutical expenditure, by income group (percentage of total expenditure on pharmaceuticals by source)

Income group	1990		2000	
	Private	**Public**	**Private**	**Public**
High-income	54.2	45.8	57.8	42.2
Middle-income	72.6	27.4	70.9	29.1
Low-income	71.4	28.6	71.6	28.4

Source: WHO (2004). *The World Medicines Situation.* WHO, Geneva.

expenditure the second largest line item in public health expenditure after healthcare personnel costs in most low- and middle-income countries. This is due to a large share of patients who buy drugs out-of-pocket and the extremely poor efficiency of the publicly run pharmaceutical provision systems.

Table 7.1 shows that high-income countries finance a larger percentage of pharmaceuticals from publicly funded sources than low- and middle-income countries, where a large share of pharmaceutical expenditure is borne directly by households, either in the form of direct out-of-pocket payments or contributions to insurance schemes.

Even within each income cluster the share of pharmaceutical expenditure on health varies considerably. Figure 7.1 shows 2007 data from the Organisation

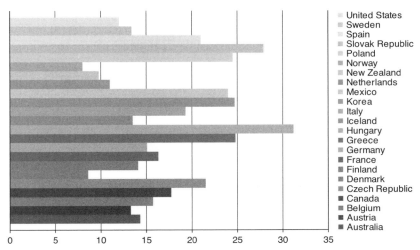

Fig. 7.1 Pharmaceutical expenditure as a percentage of total health expenditure in select OECD countries.
Source: OECD 2009.

for Economic Co-operation and Development (OECD) countries indicating high heterogeneity in pharmaceutical expenditure as a fraction of total health spending. Many of these countries do not differ significantly in their health outcomes, giving reason to believe that the organization of the pharmaceutical system and its efficiency are the drivers of observed difference in their pharmaceutical expenditures.

An obvious question arising from this considerable investment in pharmaceuticals is what health benefits arise from it. The relationship between total healthcare expenditure and gross domestic product (GDP) had been studied extensively, but studies of the effect of pharmaceutical expenditure on GDP or health status have been limited. French and Miller [3] examined the relationship between per capita pharmaceutical expenditures and life expectancy at different ages for a number of OECD countries. They found that pharmaceutical expenditure had a positive effect on remaining life expectancy at age 40 and at age 60. However, some of their results are not robust and it is not clear whether they are capturing the effect of life expectancy on pharmaceutical expenditure (older people tend to consume more drugs) or the effect of pharmaceutical expenditure on life expectancy. Interestingly, they also conclude that non-pharmaceutical health expenditure has no measurable effect on life expectancy, either at birth, or subsequently. Clemente et al. [4] trace the relationship between GDP and different subcomponents of health expenditure including pharmaceutical expenditure and show that pharmaceutical expenditure (among other subcomponents) is a significant predictor of per capita income. Other studies have found that higher pharmaceutical expenditures are associated with better health outcomes, but tend to have a focus towards high- or middle-income countries [5].

There are also multiple methodological issues and it is challenging to disentangle the contribution of new drugs from changes in disease management, changes in the distribution of healthcare, and other confounding factors [6]. Most studies agree that pharmaceutical expenditure improves health outcomes on average, but there is considerable heterogeneity in the benefits depending on the level of pharmaceutical expenditure. The relationship between pharmaceutical expenditures and health outcomes is non-increasing in nature i.e. successively higher pharmaceutical expenditures do not produce higher health outcome measures. Low- and middle-income countries are currently at low levels of pharmaceutical expenditure and thus the marginal gains there may be relatively higher as compared to high-income countries.

Pharmaceutical systems in countries of different income levels are organized using a wide array of structural and institutional forms. Usually, a heterogeneous set of stakeholders (including state and non-state institutions) are involved, each carrying out distinct roles of drug development, manufacturing, import, wholesaling, and retailing through complex (and often not well understood) relationship structures. It is imperative to clearly understand these complexities in order to design, operate, and run sustainable, effective, efficient, and equitable health sectors.

The following section provides an overview of the incentives (or lack of) for drug development, and new incentive structures that have been created to encourage the development of new drugs specifically focused upon the disease of the developing world.

7.3 Pharmaceutical research and development

Few other industries are as driven by R&D as the pharmaceutical industry. Increases in spending on R&D have been nearly matched by increases in revenue from drug sales, therefore industry's R&D intensity—the ratio of R&D spending to total sales revenue—remains higher than any other industry. The pharmaceutical industry also includes generic manufacturers who are an important player, especially in middle- and low-income markets. We focus in this section on innovative pharmaceutical companies, with a discussion on pharmaceutical manufacturing in the following section.

Pharmaceutical development is characterized by a lengthy development process with multiple risks and a high cost of development [7]. The most cited study on the cost of developing new drugs estimates the total cost of bringing a compound to market at US$802 million [8]. Basic research that improves fundamental understanding of biological processes is performed in academic research centers, universities, and companies. The output of this research is then utilized by pharmaceutical companies to create potential medicines which go through different phases of clinical trials before obtaining regulatory approval for commercial use. Large pharmaceutical companies are required by investors and management to achieve a high rate of return on these risky investments in product development. This leads to many potential drug candidates being terminated at fairly early stages in the development process where their perceived market potential is poor.

As a result of this economic risk–reward system, resource allocation for drug development is not correlated with disease burden, but rather with the market potential of a drug. Infectious and parasitic diseases of the developing world may generate a huge health burden, but because most of the people suffering from these diseases and their governments are poor, little is invested in developing treatments for such diseases [9,10]. Three diseases with the greatest burden are HIV/AIDS, malaria, and tuberculosis but until very recently there was little investment in development of drugs or vaccines for malaria or tuberculosis (HIV has a market in both developed and developing countries). Similarly, there are many other diseases of the developing world such as lymphatic filariasis, ascariasis, schistosomiasis for which drug development has been slow or non-existent.

The World Health Organization (WHO) classifies diseases as Type I, Type II, and Type III where Type I diseases know no geographic boundaries while Type II–III are predominantly or exclusively prevalent among populations of developing countries. Even within diseases of the developing world (Type II or Type III) or diseases with dual markets (Type I), research and development (R&D) efforts seem to have been targeted at small improvements to existing compounds instead of riskier and more drastic innovations. Not only are these small innovations less risky to develop, they may also achieve higher returns if they can be targeted at the inelastic segments of demand, such as those who are insured with minimal co-payments [11]. For diseases of the developing world with existing medicines, marginal innovations such as the development of easy to administer formulations to improve adherence, pediatric formulations, and enhancements to reduce adverse effects may have a significant impact on health outcomes without large or risky investments [12].

Several new approaches are now being used to address the lack of market and accelerate the development of drugs for neglected tropical diseases. The approaches to stimulate development of new products for neglected diseases are classified as 'push' and 'pull' [13]. Push approaches involve decreasing the cost of drug development by providing public or philanthropic funding along the development pathway. This decreases the cost of development borne by the developer and thus incentivizes product development even for those diseases which have a relatively small market. Pull approaches on the other hand either create a market for the product or create other return mechanisms such as prizes at the end of the development pathway.

7.3.1 Push mechanisms

The primary push mechanism is the Product Development Partnership (PDP), which is a non-profit organization that builds partnerships between the public, private, academic, and philanthropic sectors to catalyse the development of new drugs and vaccines for neglected diseases and underserved markets. PDPs receive donor monies for a specific product or therapeutic area and then part-finance the development of a few drug/vaccine candidates at academic or pharmaceutical company research centres [14]. Examples of PDPs include the Drugs for Neglected Diseases Initiative (DNDi), focusing on developing novel treatments for patients suffering from neglected diseases; FIND to develop and roll out new and affordable diagnostic tests for diseases of the developing world; the International AIDS Vaccine Initiative (IAVI) for the development of a HIV vaccine; Medicines for Malaria Venture (MMV) for developing new malaria drugs; and the Global

Alliance for TB (GATB) to develop new treatments for tuberculosis. Studies also show that PDPs achieve their objectives at a much lower cost than the commercial pharmaceutical approaches [8]. These costs may be lower due to the lower opportunity cost of capital for PDPs and in-kind time donations from academic and other partners which are not fully accounted for in the cost structure.

7.3.2 Pull mechanisms

There are several pull mechanisms that can help stimulate the development of new products for diseases in predominantly low-income markets. Advance Market Commitments (AMCs) are a market making mechanism under which a large group of donors guarantees to purchase a product for a developing country market at a pre-agreed price [15]. The target characteristics of the product are defined before the product is developed. The first AMC is currently being piloted for vaccines against pneumococcal disease with contributions from the United Kingdom, Italy, Russia, Canada, Norway, and the Gates Foundation. Being a relatively new mechanism, there are many open questions about AMCs, such as how to set pricing and volume levels and how to ensure that long-term guaranteed contractual commitments do not dilute research on second-generation products [16].

Orphan drug acts are a mechanism of providing R&D tax credits and enhanced market exclusivity to pharmaceutical companies that develop drugs to treat diseases which affect very few people. The United States and the European Union both have orphan drug legislation. Orphan drug status may provide some additional stimulus for commercial firms to develop drugs and vaccines for diseases of the developing world, but the effects are likely to be minor because potential revenues for treatments for acute infectious diseases, for which each patient needs only a short course of treatment, are likely to be smaller [17].

The priority review voucher is a scheme designed to promote the development of drugs for neglected diseases by large pharmaceutical companies through priority review of their regulatory approval applications for other products [18]. The voucher entitles the bearer to nominate a commercial drug for expedited review by the US Food and Drug Administration (FDA). Estimates show that such a priority review can shorten the time for FDA approval and review by up to 12 months. A pharmaceutical company with a potential blockbuster (US$1 billion in sales by year five) awaiting FDA review may gain over US$300 million in pre-tax revenues from such a voucher. Such vouchers can be sold on to another company for a market determined value. The FDA issued the first priority review voucher in 2007 to Novartis for the anti-malarial drug Coartem® and there are discussions about the introduction of a similar system for the European Medicines Agency.

7.3.3 Comparing push and pull mechanisms for neglected disease drug development

Although both push and pull approaches are gaining widespread acceptance, there is no clear theoretical or empirical evidence to understand which of the two approaches works better under what conditions. If the R&D investment decisions of a pharmaceutical firm are analysed based on its cost of capital and its marginal return on R&D investment, we see that the effectiveness of push interventions depends on the elasticity of the marginal return curve. Push incentives serve to lower the cost of capital thus if the marginal return curve is more elastic, a push incentive will be more effective. A pull incentive on the other hands works by shifting the marginal return curve outward. Thus, a combination of pull and push incentives may induce more investment than any of them used alone [13].

Principal agent models would suggest that pull mechanisms are superior when it is easy to specify the desired outcome, when agents are not capital constrained, and when the principal is risk-averse. In contrast, push mechanisms are expected to be superior when the desired outcome is easy to monitor and measure, and when the principal has a higher tolerance for risk [19]. Due to information asymmetries and non-verifiability of effort, it becomes very difficult for those who are financing push incentives to monitor the performance of the developers. It also makes such investments transaction cost heavy for the financier. In addition, financiers such as developed country governments (e.g. United Kingdom, Norway) who, due to taxpayer accountability have a lower appetite for product development risk, would prefer pull investments over push investments [19].

On the other hand, capital constraints and the differences in the cost of raising capital may result in push mechanisms being better suited to attract small innovators to develop products. Unlike large pharmaceutical companies, smaller biotech companies may not have the capital, or their cost of capital to take a product through the development pathway may be very high, compared with the value of a prize or market reward. The cost of capital for the financiers on the other hand may be very low and social welfare would be maximized if the donors helped the smaller innovators monetize their investment earlier in the process.

The developments in pharmaceutical markets in low- and middle-income countries also have the potential to remedy the problems caused by the lack of a market for drugs targeted at them. As pharmaceutical markets become more organized, with a clear role of a third-party payer, some of the market risks faced by developers for drugs for neglected tropical diseases will be reduced and this should accelerate drug development for neglected diseases.

Also, the willingness of pharmaceutical companies to work on drugs for poor countries is increasing, motivated in part by the greater concern for social responsibility and of honouring their 'social contract'. Many large pharmaceutical companies now have dedicated research centres for disease of the developing world and some are sharing their intellectual property in patent pooling arrangements to facilitate better research in this area [20].

7.4 Manufacturing/production

Pharmaceutical manufacturing is divided into two major stages: the production of the active pharmaceutical ingredient (API) and formulation i.e. the conversion of the APIs into products suitable for administration (pills, tablets, injections, syrups, etc.). Drug formulation and active ingredients involve very different manufacturing processes and technical capabilities. Active ingredients are manufactured by chemical synthesis, extraction, fermentation or by recovery from natural sources. Until recently the most common form of API manufacturing was chemical synthesis but the growth of biological products has led to an increase in cell culture and other biotechnology based manufacturing for this step. In drug formulation, the active pharmaceutical ingredient is combined with other active or inactive ingredients (excipients) in a physical transformation process involving unit operations such as granulation, drying, blending, grinding, and tabletting [21,22].

All aspects of pharmaceutical production are governed by Good Manufacturing Practices (GMP), which specify the facilities and processes to use for the manufacture, processing, or packaging of a drug to ensure that the drug meets the requirements of safety and has the identity, strength, purity and quality characteristics it is intended to possess [23]. GMP ensure that products are consistently produced and controlled to the quality standards appropriate to their intended use and as required under their regulatory approval. GMP only controls the risks in pharmaceutical production such as those arising from batch quality inconsistency, contamination, incorrect labelling, and lack of personal hygiene etc. GMP, however, should not be confused with regulatory approval of a pharmaceutical product which requires establishing safety, efficacy, and a robust method of manufacturing for the product.

The manufacture of APIs for a large number of pharmaceutical products now occurs in India and China as the API manufacturers there enjoy a cost advantage over their counterparts in Europe and North America, due to lower energy, labour, and environmental compliance costs. The high gross margins enjoyed by patented products have implied that formulation tends to be carried out in hubs that provide tax advantage. Ireland and Puerto Rico have been important hubs for the location of formulation plants owned by big pharmaceutical companies. Most large pharmaceutical companies operate production facilities across a very broad geographical base. This broad base allows them to leverage the varying taxation structures across countries and regions and produce products in the regions which allow the company to optimize their tax outflows [24].

The structure of the pharmaceutical industry today is such that a large proportion of the basic and advanced intermediate products are manufactured in China for producers of APIs based in Southern Europe and India. Increasing amounts of finished products for regulated markets are now also manufactured in India, either by Indian generic companies or by contract manufacturers for large pharmaceutical companies. China has so far not been a significant player in manufacturing finished products for regulated markets. For pharmaceutical products such as anti-retrovirals and anti-malarials with a pre-dominant market in sub-Saharan Africa, many small African manufacturers have emerged, most of them without GMP certification. Many low-income and least developed countries (LDC) are keen to pursue industrial policies that promote a domestic pharmaceutical industry and the issue of local manufacturing of drugs has become an important debate in pharmaceutical policy [25]. However, investments in local pharmaceutical production will be efficient only if quality-assured pharmaceuticals can be produced more cheaply locally than they can be imported on the open market.

7.5 Regulation

The pharmaceutical industry is distinct from any other industry in the careful regulatory attention it needs to assure that the products meet acceptable standards of quality, safety, and efficacy. The role of the pharmaceutical regulatory system involves assessing safety and efficacy before authorizing the use of a new product, ensuring adherence to GMP and other quality compliance standards, and post-marketing surveillance.

In developed countries considerable administrative and technical effort is directed to ensuring the quality of medicines allowed to be dispensed to patients. All pharmaceutical products available for use in a country are regulated by the national regulatory authority of that country and, in some cases, also regulated at the international level. Products that are marketed globally require the manufacturer to comply with regulatory requirements in the country of origin as well as the requirements of each country where the product is sold. The International Conference on Harmonization of Technical Requirements for Regulation of Pharmaceuticals for Human Use (ICH) coordinates drug regulation between Japan, the United States, and the European Union to reduce duplication. Similarly, countries in the European Union have created a centralized procedure for drug regulatory approvals through the European Medicines Evaluation Agency (EMEA) [26].

For developing countries there is no unified or harmonized approach to product registration and approval. Each country's national regulatory authority has its own standards and regulatory requirements, adding multiple layers of complexity for their relatively small market sizes. WHO has created a drug prequalification system to provide a global regulatory process that transcends national borders and to have unified standards of acceptable quality, safety, and efficacy [27]. A simplified global regulatory process should provide a simplified, systematic, and disciplined system that would reduce costs and speed up market access for new products.

7.6 Financing

Ultimately all funding for healthcare comes from households and corporations (either directly or indirectly), as noted in Chapter 4, and pharmaceutical funding is channelled through the same set of public and private intermediaries as funds for other health sector activities. While the issues of financing pharmaceuticals cannot be separated from the strategy for overall financing of the sector, there are a number of specific challenges with pharmaceutical financing.

One particular issue is the predominance—up to 90%—in developing countries of out-of-pocket spending on pharmaceuticals [2]. Such payments may expose households to the risk of catastrophic health payments. However, this high level of spending often produces limited health benefit due to poor prescribing, high prices, low quality of products, and inappropriate use. Improving the affordability of medicines is thus intrinsically linked to broader issues of pharmaceutical supply, dispensing and pricing. Out-of-pocket payments may take the form of purchases from private outlets (pharmacies, drug shops, dispensing health facilities, or market vendors) because they are more convenient or may be perceived to be less expensive than public facilities, or there may be charges imposed at public outlets, in the form of official user fees or informal 'under-the-table' payments to facility staff.

The burden of out-of-pocket spending on pharmaceuticals is exacerbated by poor availability and high prices, in both the public and private sectors. A review of 45 national and sub-national medicine price and availability surveys found that public sector availability of a basket of 15 essential medicines was only 38% (ranging between 29% in the WHO African region to 54% in the American region), while in all regions private sector availability was higher, at 64% on average. An important implication of poor public sector availability is that patients are frequently required to purchase needed drugs from private outlets where prices tend to be higher (ranging from 9.6 times to more than 25 times the international reference price in the private sector, compared with 3.2–11.95 times in the public sector). Medicine affordability was assessed by expressing the cost of a full course of treatment (for an acute illness) or a month's worth of medicines (for a chronic condition) in terms of the number of days' wages of the lowest paid government worker. These figures reveal the substantial burden on household budgets of financing medicine purchases. For instance, a month's course of medicines purchased privately to treat ulcer cost more than three days' wages in Africa, the Eastern Mediterranean and Europe [28].

Shifting pharmaceutical spending towards pooled financing sources, including public budgets, external financing sources, and social, private, or community-based health insurance, is therefore essential for increasing the affordability of medicines. Pooled funding both reduces the burden on households of paying for drugs at the time of illness, and generates the possibility of pooled procurement systems which should reduce costs and improve supply. The key pooled financing mechanisms, and some of their main challenges in relation to pharmaceutical financing, are described below.

Public spending on pharmaceuticals is financed from general revenues, and governments use their health budgets for purchasing drugs which are distributed through the health sector. Decentralization of public sector budgets has created new challenges for coordination and also for efficient procurement. For example, a recent study of the Tanzanian public sector supply system indicated the increasing fragmentation of medicines supply as districts use their budgets to procure medicines locally as well as from the central medical stores [29].

In recent years, the availability of external funding for major disease control initiatives in developing countries has expanded dramatically. These facilities include the Global Fund to Fight AIDS, Tuberculosis and Malaria, which includes commodity support in their regular grants; the GAVI Alliance, which finances purchases of vaccines for childhood immunization programmes, and UNITAID which seeks to improve access to treatment for AIDS, tuberculosis and malaria by leveraging price reductions for diagnostics and treatment. While these additional resources for pharmaceuticals are much needed, two challenges which are posed by these new funds are: 1) fragmentation and verticalization of funding supply arrangements, and 2) concerns about predictability of external funding and the implications for sustainability (see Chapter 9 for more details).

All of these mechanisms allow for a degree of pooling of risk among the sick and the healthy; in addition, social insurance arrangements allow for income-based cross-subsidies. Ensuring appropriate coverage of pharmaceuticals within these plans, particularly for newer and more expensive products, may be a challenge. Co-payments are often charged for pharmaceuticals, partly as a mechanism to reduce moral hazard on the part of prescribers and patients. The impact of such co-payments on controlling these behaviours must be weighed against the potential risks to access if there are inadequate exemptions for those who cannot afford to pay the charges. The experience with community-based insurance schemes has been highly mixed, with very few such schemes achieving high and sustained levels of coverage, and very little evidence about the extent of financial protection they provide [30].

Drug revolving funds (DRF) are a specific mechanism for pharmaceutical financing, in which a fund is set up in each community with an initial capital investment and thereafter drug supplies are replenished with the monies collected from the sales of drugs. Experiences from a variety of countries suggest that often the monies recovered are insufficient to replenish the pharmaceutical supplies and the fund soon requires recapitalization. Failure to collect payments, delays in cash flow velocity and price increases due to inflation or exchange rate fluctuations have been the most common reasons for the failure of DRFs. A prerequisite for a DRF to succeed is careful financial planning and a well managed cash to cash cycle which often require training and skills that are not available at the rural clinics [31].

7.7 Distribution and access

Since retail pharmacies cannot keep a large number of medicines in different pack sizes in stock, they rely on wholesalers and distributors, instead of buying directly from the pharmaceutical manufacturers. This leads to the existence of multiple third parties between the manufacturer and the dispensing pharmacists. The number of channel intermediaries involved, their ownerships and governance structure (publicly owned, privately owned or public–private partnerships) and the roles they play vary considerably from one country to another.

In most developed countries, there are a few privately owned national wholesalers who carry the full range of pharmaceutical products from multiple manufacturers in stock and distribute to clinics, hospitals and pharmacies. Such wholesalers make deliveries to retail pharmacies several times a day.

In most low- and middle-income countries, especially in sub-Saharan Africa, pharmaceutical distribution is entirely government run. The government procures drugs and distributes them to health clinics using a publicly run central medical store (CMS) and a government owned transport fleet. The procurement of pharmaceuticals by the government is a complex process and in some instances it can take up to 24 months to complete. Delays in planned funding, accompanied by delays encountered throughout the procurement process, contribute to delayed deliveries of drugs at the CMSs and the eventual stock outs of medicines. Procurement lines work slightly better for drugs for HIV/ AIDS, malaria, tuberculosis, and vaccines due to the tightly controlled architecture of financing. Additionally, in the public sector run pharmaceutical provision system, procurement and distribution are often organized as separate functions decoupled from each other with limited and infrequent flow of information between them. This decoupling of procurement from distribution leads to a greater need for safety stock in the system. Funding and resource constraints, however, prevent holding adequate quantities of safety stock, leading to frequent stock outs. In such a model, the managers of government-owned CMSs confront severe challenges in improving operational performance. They often have difficulty hiring people with business experience and skills because of poor wages and incentive systems in the public sector and often also lack the ability to remove incompetent workers [32]. Very few developing country governments (and global health policy makers) have begun to accept that pharmaceutical distribution is not necessarily a public sector role [32].

Distribution models such as decentralized medical stores, quasi-private or private drug distribution systems offer several advantages over fully public distribution systems but are rarely implemented. A few countries (e.g. Zambia, Kenya, Tanzania) have established para-statal drug distribution entities and have contracted out the operational management of such entities to private third party companies (e.g. Zambia, Botswana). Some countries such as Ghana have decentralized their distribution by allowing districts to purchase drugs and supplies from private sector suppliers, creating competition for the publicly run central medical store. Admittedly, many of these models have not yielded their promised successes, but implementation weaknesses should not be seen as weaknesses in the distribution model itself.

Within publicly owned and operated drug distribution systems, a large number of countries have a three-tiered distribution system with product flowing from the CMS to district or regional stores and then to the clinics. The most challenging part of such distribution systems (often called 'last mile logistics') is making deliveries to small clinics and health centres that are remote and have poor road access. In such instances, the clinic and health centre staff themselves travel to the district or regional medical store to receive their drug supplies using their own means of transport such as cars, motorcycles, etc., in the process taking extremely crucial healthcare worker time. When there is a system to distribute from the districts to the clinics, there is often a shortage of staff at the health centres that are trained to carry out the tasks of stock keeping, ordering, and requisitioning.

Despite the large investments in publicly run CMSs, the availability of medicines remains very poor in public health facilities [28]. Increasingly, the private sector plays an important role in the provision of medicines to large segments of the population in developing countries [33]. Although availability of medicines is usually not a bottleneck in the private sector, except for in remote areas, affordability remains poor due to high prices [28]. Channel mark-ups, tariffs, and duties can more than double the manufacturer's price, as illustrated in Table 7.2.

Table 7.2 Components of non-manufacturer costs in retail price of medicines in developing countries

	Sri Lanka	Kenya	Tanzania	South Africa	Brazil	Armenia	Kosovo	Nepal	Mauritius
Import tariff	0%	0%	10%		12%	0%	1%	4%	5%
Port charges	4%	8%	1%				4%		
Clearance and freight		1%	2%					2%	5%
Pre-shipment inspection		3%	1%						
Pharmacy board fee			2%						
Importer's margins	25%						15%	10%	
VAT				14%	18%	20%	0%		
Central govt tax									
State govt tax					6%				
Wholesaler	9%	15%	0%	21%	7%	25%	15%	10%	14%
Retail	16%	20%	50%	50%	22%	25%	25%	16%	27%
Total mark-up	64%	54%	74%	74%	82%	88%	74%	48%	59%

Source: adapted from [42].

In the private sector, the distribution from the manufacturer to the retail pharmacies or drug shops is carried out by the private wholesalers who distribute several times a week to retail pharmacies and hospital in large urban centres. However, the owners of private drug shops from rural areas in most cases have travel to the urban areas where the wholesaler is located to pick up their stock. This leads to poor availability in remote drug shops.

7.8 Trade and TRIPS

Pharmaceuticals are the single most important health-related product traded, comprising some 55% of all health-related trade by value (the share of the next most significant health-related goods traded, small devices and equipment, is 19%). In 2006 the global pharmaceutical market was valued at US$650 billion, of which the generic market contributed less than 10% (US$60 billion) [34]. As indicated earlier, the market is highly concentrated, with North America, Europe, and Japan accounting for around 75% of sales (by value), as indicated in Table 7.3.

Overall, high-income countries produce and export high value patented pharmaceuticals, and low- and middle-income countries import these products; although some produce and export low value generic products, such as India, as illustrated in Table 7.4. This leads to many developing countries experiencing a trade deficit in modern medicines, which often fuels an overall health sector deficit. Interestingly, however, is that even amongst high-income countries there are considerable trade deficits in pharmaceuticals, given their overall levels of consumption, as illustrated in Table 7.5.

Given the substantial investment made in pharmaceuticals, and this pattern of global trade, it is therefore not surprising that trade in pharmaceuticals has been the subject of intensive international dialogue. The debate began in earnest in the late 1970s when, on one side, multinational pharmaceutical producers based in the developed countries expressed growing concern over alleged 'misappropriation' of their patented technology by enterprises based in developing countries. At the same time, developing countries expressed deepening concern over the imbalance between technological capacity and ownership of technology between developed and developing countries. This dialogue played out in a series of negotiations at UNCTAD, WIPO, and ultimately at the GATT during the Uruguay Round of trade negotiations which culminated in 1993, and resulted in entry into force of the World Trade Organization's Agreement on TRIPS in 1995.

The TRIPs Agreement established global minimum standards for the protection of intellectual property, including a minimum of 20-year patent

Table 7.3 Top world pharmaceutical corporations, 2006

Company	Country	Sales (£M)	Market share (%)
Pfizer	USA	24,229	7.6
GlaxoSmithKline	UK	19,419	6.1
Novartis	SWI	16,596	5.2
Sanofi Aventis	FRA	16,337	5.1
Johnson & Johnson	USA	14,345	4.5
Astrazeneca	UK	14,056	4.4
Merck & Co	USA	13,150	4.1
Roche	SWI	12,328	3.9
Abbott	USA	9287	2.9
Amgen	USA	8494	2.7
Top 10		**148,244**	**46.4**
Wyeth	USA	7877	2.5
Lilly	USA	7737	2.4
Bayer	GER	6563	2.1
Bristol-Myers Squibb	USA	6476	2.0
Boehringer Ingelheim	GER	5903	1.9
Takeda	JAP	5271	1.7
Teva	ISR	4911	1.5
Schering-Plough	USA	4572	1.4
Daiichi Sankyo	JAP	2972	0.9
Novo Nordisk	DEN	2957	0.9
Top 20		**197,013**	**63.7**

M, million.
Reprinted from The Lancet , 373, Smith RD, Correa C, Oh C, Trade, TRIPS, and pharmaceuticals, 684–691, (2009), with permission from Elsevier..

protection on pharmaceuticals. Compliance was postponed until 2005 for developing countries and 2016 for least developed countries. TRIPS was seen to be an important step as patents have been the mainstay of policy to ensure investment in pharmaceutical research and development, acting as guarantor of monopoly rents. However, increasing globalization of the pharmaceutical industry, the complexity of dealing with many different national IPR systems,

Table 7.4 Indian pharmaceuticals and health care sector 2007

Generic market (US$B)	3.3
Generic market as proportion of total market	30
Exports (US$M)	1900
Imports (US$M)	710
Market share: imports (%)	35
Market share: domestic output (%)	65
Health expenditure (US$B)	44
Hospital sector (US$M)	16,400

B, billion; M, million.
Reprinted from The Lancet , 373, Smith RD, Correa C, Oh C, Trade, TRIPS, and pharmaceuticals, 684–691, (2009), with permission from Elsevier.

Table 7.5 World trade in pharmaceuticals, 2004

Country	Exports (£M)	Imports (£M)	Balance (£M)
Switzerland	12,052	6491	5561
France	12,302	8012	4290
Germany	19,616	15,349	4267
UK	12,354	8642	3712
Sweden	4082	1503	2579
Netherlands	6533	6094	439
Italy	6074	6690	−616
Australia	1141	2717	−1576
Spain	2716	4831	−2115
Japan	1677	3829	−2152
Canada	1815	4034	−2219
USA	11,989	19,099	−7109

M, million.
Reprinted from The Lancet , 373, Smith RD, Correa C, Oh C, Trade, TRIPS, and pharmaceuticals, 684–691, (2009), with permission from Elsevier.

and the absence of patent protection for pharmaceuticals in a large part of the world, led developed countries to push for the adoption of the TRIPS Agreement, which obligates WTO members to recognize pharmaceutical product patents, under the threat of trade sanctions.

There is a clear conflict between TRIPs and public health; by their nature, the monopoly rents afforded by patents are reflected in the final product's pricing, acting as a barrier to affordability. The early experience of developing countries with implementation of the TRIPS Agreement in this respect was problematic, and the TRIPS Agreement was quickly perceived as an obstacle to addressing public health problems. The WTO reacted to this, recognizing the importance of allowing governments to pursue flexible policies with respect to the protection of public health, by adopting in November 2001 the Doha Declaration on the TRIPS Agreement and Public Health. This was followed in August 2003 by adoption of a waiver authorizing exports of pharmaceutical products under compulsory license, and in December 2005 by adoption of a Protocol of Amendment to the TRIPS Agreement that would formally transform the waiver into a part of the TRIPS Agreement. Despite these positive steps, the political situation with respect to access to medicines has remained difficult, as compulsory licences issued by Brazil and Thailand in recent years have come under pressure from industry and supporting governments [35]. Meanwhile, concern has moved on from TRIPS to TRIPS-plus.

TRIPS-plus refers to unilateral or bilateral trade negotiations where standards beyond TRIPS are incorporated in exchange for trade concessions, particularly the promise of free access to markets for agricultural goods. Free trade agreements (FTAs), signed by the United States and European Union especially with a growing number of developing countries, have constituted one the main routes for TRIPS-plus standards [36]. For instance, both China and Argentina are on the 'Priority Watch List' of Special Section 301 of the US Trade Act [37] to apply pressure to introduce TRIPS-plus standards. Australia introduced data exclusivity as a result of a complaint by the United States [38]. There is also more diffuse political pressure, with some countries willing to accept TRIPS-plus measures in the hope of creating a more favourable 'climate' for foreign direct investment [39,40].

Patents have become, with the adoption of TRIPS, a key element in trade agreements, where higher protection for pharmaceutical patents is increasingly traded against potential access to developed country markets. The driving force behind changes in the international system, and consequent prices paid for pharmaceuticals, is hence not health improvement, but the need to pay for trade concessions. The immediate effect of this is to erect price (and other) barriers to access to medicines, although there seems no clear evidence that the costs incurred by the health systems will be compensated by the often-volatile trade advantages obtained in exchange.

TRIPS provides countries with options to overcome patent barriers for medicines with large public health needs. Countries are failing to make full use of flexibilities built in to TRIPS to overcome patent barriers, such as compulsory licences and parallel imports. Much of this may be due to a lack of domestic resources and capacity to exploit international trade provisions, but inequalities in power and influence between countries leave many vulnerable to pressure in order to protect broader trade and economic interests. Nonetheless, there are also widespread misunderstandings, such as the misconception that countries have to declare a national emergency before invoking a compulsory licence, and there are clear gains to be made from addressing these misunderstandings and misperceptions, together with greater support for development of legal and technical expertise to incorporate and implement TRIPS flexibilities in national policy. There may also be value in countries developing a South–South framework for collectively undertaking to implement TRIPS flexibilities, doing so as regional economic blocs [41].

In addition to the impact of TRIPS and TRIPS-plus, one also needs to be aware of other aspects of global pharmaceutical trade that define the availability of and access to pharmaceuticals. Critical among is recognition that the production, distribution, and trade of pharmaceuticals is subject to government regulatory control at a number of levels. Countries maintain substantially different regulatory standards to assure the safety and efficacy of the pharmaceutical supply chain. There are good reasons why governments adopt different standards; for example, to take account of differences in climate and geography. However, in some cases differential regulation may unnecessarily hinder the cross-border movement of pharmaceuticals, particularly among regions which share public health interests and trade policy objectives. Further, it has to be recognized that the ultimate objective of government policy with respect to pharmaceutical trade is not necessarily to promote and protect public health, as the pharmaceutical industry may be an important part of the national economy, providing employment and affecting the balance of trade. Governments may therefore choose to promote the development and maintenance of a strong local pharmaceutical industry as a part of national economic development policy.

7.9 Conclusions

Pharmaceuticals are an important component of a well-functioning health sector; and the different steps in the pharmaceutical supply system (ranging from upstream discovery through to distribution and supply of medicines) are substantially outside the control of national health sector authorities. Pharmaceutical provision systems in countries with different income groups are organized using a wide array of structural and institutional forms. Usually, a heterogeneous set of stakeholders (including state and non-state institutions) are involved, each carrying out distinct roles of drug development, manufacturing, import, wholesaling, and retailing through a complex (and often not well-understood) set of relationships.

Expansions in global trade especially, including the increasing concentration of the pharmaceutical industry, and the expansion of international legislation affecting patenting, not to mention the profile of patents in other free-trade agreements, is a critical area that the health sector has little control over; certainly in comparison with other areas. This wider aspect of the influence of increased globalization and trade in health-related goods and services is a topic that is the focus of Chapter 8.

At both the national and international levels, aspects related to pharmaceutical development, distribution and financing are areas that rely upon the negotiation abilities of those involved in the health sector to secure sufficient supplies to meet the needs of their populations' health. The critical nature of capacity in negotiation skills is the subject of Chapter 12.

References

1 WHO (2009). *World Health Statistics 2009*. WHO, Geneva.

2 WHO (2004). *Equitable access to essential medicines: a framework for action* (WHO Policy Perspectives on Medicines No 8). WHO, Geneva. Available at: http://whqlibdoc. who.int/hq/2004/WHO_EDM_2004.4.pdf (accessed 15 September 2010).

3 Frech, H., Miller R (1997). *The productivity of health care and pharmaceuticals: An international comparison. Working Paper in Economics*. University of California, Santa Barbara, CA.

4 Clemente J, Marcuello C, Montanes A, Pueyo F (2004). On the international stability of health care expenditure functions: are government and private functions similar? *Journal of Health Economics*, **23**(3), 589–613.

5 Crémieux, M-CM, Ouellette P, Petit P, Zelder M, Potvin K (2004). Public and private pharmaceutical spending as determinants of health outcomes in Canada. *Health Economics*, **14**, 107–16.

6 Grootendorst P, Piérard E, Shim M (2007). *The life expectancy gains from pharmaceutical drugs: a critical appraisal of the literature*. (Social and Economic Dimensions of an Aging Population Research Papers 221). McMaster University, Ontario.

7 Hansen RW (1979). The pharmaceutical development process: estimates of current development costs and times and the effects of regulatory changes. In Chien RI (ed) *Issues in Pharmaceutical Economics*, pp.151–87. Lexington Books, Lexington, MA.

8 DiMasi JA, Hansen RW, Grabowski HG (2003). The price of innovation: new estimates of drug development costs. *Journal of Health Economics*, **22**, 151–85.

9 WHO Commission on Macroeconomics and Health (2001). *WHO Commission on Macroeconomics and Health. Macroeconomics and Health: Investing in Health for Economic Development. Report of the Commission on Macroeconomics and Health.* WHO, Geneva.

10 Moran M, Guzman J, Ropars AL, Illmer A (2010). The role of product development partnerships in research and development for neglected diseases. *International Health*, **2**(**2**), 114–22.

11 Ganuza JJ, Llobet G, Domínguez B (2009). R&D in the pharmaceutical industry: A world of small innovations. *Management Science*, **55**(**4**), 539–51.

12 Nahata Milap C (1999). Lack of pediatric drug formulations. *Pediatrics*, **104**(3, Suppl), 607–9.

13 Sloan F, Hsieh CR (2008). Effects of incentives on pharmaceutical innovation. In Sloan F, Hirschel K (eds) *Incentives and Choice in Health Care*, pp.227–62. MIT Press, Cambridge, MA.

14 Widdus R, White K (2004). *Combating Diseases Associated with Poverty Financing Strategies for Product Development and the Potential Role of Public-Private Partnerships.* Initiative on Public-Private Partnerships for Health, Global Forum for Health Research, Geneva.

15 Kremer M, Barder O, Levine R (2005). *Making Markets for Vaccines: Ideas to Action.* Center for Global Development, Washington, DC.

16 Usher AD (2009). Dispute over pneumococcal vaccine initiative. *Lancet* 2009; **374**, 1879–80.

17 Adel M, Danzon PM, Barton JH, *et al.* (2006). Product development priorities. *Disease Control Priorities in Developing Countries*, 2nd edn. World Bank/Oxford University Press, New York

18 Ridley DB, Grabowski HG, Moe JL (2006). Developing drugs for developing countries. *Health Affairs*, **25**(**2**), 313–24.

19 Grace C, Kyle M (2009). Comparative advantages of push and pull incentives for technology development: lessons for neglected diseases. *Global Forum Update on Research for Health*, **6**.

20 Balch O (2009). How GSK's access to medicine plans will shake up big pharma. *Treatment News*, Wednesday, 1 April 2009.

21 Bennett B, Cole G (2003). *Pharmaceutical Production – An Engineers Guide.* Institution of Chemical Engineers, Rugby.

22 Allen LV, Popovich NG, Ansel HC (2005). *Pharmaceutical Dosage Forms and Drug Delivery Systems*, 8th edn. Lippincott Williams & Wilkins, London.

23 WHO (2007). *Quality assurance of pharmaceuticals: a compendium of guidelines and related materials. Vol. 2, Good manufacturing practices and inspection*, 2nd edn. World Health Organization, Geneva.

24 Mukherjee G, Yadav P (2005). Best practices in pharmaceutical supply chains. Master's Thesis, MIT-Zaragoza.

25 Anderson T (2010). Tide turns for drug manufacturing in Africa. *Lancet*, **375**, 1597–8.

26 Pignatti E, Boone H, Moulon I (2004). Overview of the European Regulatory Approval System. *Journal of Ambulatory Care Management*, **27**, 89–97.

27 WHO (2010). *The WHO Prequalification Project.* WHO, Geneva. Available at: http://mednet3.who.int/prequal/.

28 Cameron A, Ewen M, Ross-Degnan D, Ball D, Laing R (2009). Medicine prices, availability, and affordability in 36 developing and middle-income countries: a secondary analysis. *Lancet*, **373**, 240–9.

29 Management Sciences for Health (2010). *MDS-3: Managing Access to Medicines and other Health Technologies*. MSH, Arlington, VA.

30 Palmer N, Mueller DH, Gilson L, Mills A, Haines A (2004). Health financing to promote access in low income settings – how much do we know? *Lancet*, **364**, 1365–70.

31 Cross PN, Huff MA, Quick JD, Bates JA (1986). Revolving drug funds: Conducting business in the public sector. *Social Science and Medicine*, **22**(3), 335–43.

32 Yadav P (2010). In-country supply chains. *Global Health*, **5**, 18–20.

33 Goodman C (2004). An Economic Analysis of the Retail Market for Fever and Malaria Treatment in Rural Tanzania. PhD Thesis, London School of Hygiene and Tropical Medicine, London.

34 PIRIBO (2007). *Pharmaceutical Market Trends, 2007–2011: Key market forecasts and growth opportunities*, 2nd edn. URCH Publishing, London.

35 Dukes G (2006). *The law and ethics of the pharmaceutical industry*. Elsevier, Amsterdam.

36 Correa CM (2006). Implications of bilateral free trade agreements on access to medicines. *Bulletin of the World Health Organization*, **84**, 399–404.

37 Office of the United States Trades Representative (2007). *2007 Special 301 Report*. USTR, Washington, DC.

38 Priapantja P (2000). Trade Secret: How does this apply to drug registration data? Paper presented at ASEAN Workshop on the TRIPS Agreement and its Impact on Pharmaceuticals. Department of Health and World Health Organization, May 2–4.

39 Commission on Intellectual Property Rights (2002). *Integrating intellectual property rights and development policy*. Available at www.iprcommission.org.

40 Fink C, Reichenmiller P (2005). *Tightening TRIPS: The Intellectual Property Provisions of Recent US Free Trade Agreements* (Trade Note 20). World Bank, Geneva.

41 Musungu SF, Villanueva S, Blasetti R (2004). *Utilizing TRIPS Flexibilities for Public Health Protection Through South-South Regional Frameworks*. South Perspectives Report, South Centre, Geneva.

42 Levison L, Laing R (2003). The hidden costs of essential medicines. *Essential Drugs Monitor*, **33**, 20–1.

Health and systems in the wider context

Chapter 8

The health system and international trade

Richard D. Smith

8.1. Introduction

Over one million people travel to Asia each year to receive healthcare, contributing some US$2 billion to the region's economy. Over 50% of doctors trained in Ghana emigrate. Cuba is a regional hub for teleradiology services. Private companies from India, Singapore, and elsewhere invested more than US$1 billion last year in establishing hospitals or other ventures abroad [1,2]. The SARS (sudden acute respiratory syndrome) outbreak of 2003 resulted in a loss of some US$100 billion to global GDP and a potential pandemic influenza outbreak could create far greater economic as well a health losses [3,4]. The current global financial crisis and recession will reduce health and the affordability of healthcare. Global food price rises have increased malnutrition, yet at the same time record levels of type II diabetes are witnessed in developed and developing countries alike.

The expansion of countries opening up their frontiers and liberalizing their international trade is one of the key challenges facing health policy-makers in the 21st century [5–7]. Health systems and sectors are affected by trade liberalization in a number of direct and indirect ways; healthcare activities, products, and services can themselves be traded, health systems are impacted by changes in exchange rates, the health profile of a country is affected by global impacts on communicable and non-communicable disease, and there are a range of aspects of trade policy that impact upon health system flexibility [8]. This trade liberalization has both beneficial and detrimental effects for the health systems of the countries engaging in it. The challenge facing national governments is to capitalize on the positive effects and regulate their healthcare market appropriately to avoid the negative ones. To achieve this will place a premium on all those engaged in health to understand the importance of trade and to engage with their counterparts involved in trade and trade policy.

This chapter provides an introduction to the scope of the issues facing health systems concerning international trade. The next section provides an overview of the key linkages between trade and health, which is followed by an overview of international trade agreements, current trends in health services trade. The chapter concludes by examining the policies and processes required for health system strengthening.

8.2 Scope of influence of international trade on health systems

Increased trade in goods, services, people, and capital—whether directly health-related or not—will affect health through a number of channels, including the cross-border flow of infectious disease, advertising of unhealthy lifestyles, health professional migration, and so forth. Health, the health system, and health sector, will be affected by changes in general trade liberalization, international legislation, and international institutions, as well as those specific to health, and will in return impact on national economies [9] (the historical development of linkages between trade and health more generally can be found elsewhere [10]). In order to begin to develop an understanding of the implications for health and health systems of increased international trade, it is helpful to first systematically frame them and the linkages between them; as illustrated in Figure 1.2 in Chapter 1 [11].

Figure 1.2 summarizes the main proximal and distal determinants and linkages between trade and health. The lower half of the figure represents the individual country under consideration, and the upper half the aspects of international trade expansion and liberalization that impact upon the country, with the three arrows between them indicating the major linkages. This is a deliberately simplified picture to provide a concise and understandable frame of reference; a more comprehensive exposition is provided elsewhere [12].

Taking the lower half of the figure first, the standard influences on health are illustrated: risk factors, representing genetic predisposition to disease, environmental influences on health, infectious disease and other factors; household economy, representing factors associated with human capital and the investment in health by individuals/households; health sector, representing the impact of goods and services consumed principally to improve health status; and the national economy, representing the meta-influences of government structures and general economic well-being. The range of inter-linkages between these factors is also illustrated.

In the upper half, the influences of factors outside the national economy, or national 'control', are illustrated. For example, there are a wide variety of international influences directly upon risk factors for health, including: an increased exposure to infectious disease through the rapid cross border transmission of communicable diseases; increased marketing of unhealthy products and behaviours; and increased environmental degradation as a result of increased industrialization. Many of these factors may be considered externalities and have, to a greater or lesser extent, public good attributes. These global externality and public good aspects of, and impacts on, health are not considered further here, but are covered in detail elsewhere [13–16]. Trade will also affect health through influences upon the national economy. There is an extensive literature concerning the relationship between health and wealth, and to the extent that trade influences economic growth, and the distribution of positive and negative aspects of this growth, it will also influence health (e.g. changes in consumption of various goods beneficial or detrimental to health) [17,18]. Finally, trade will affect health through the direct provision and distribution of health related goods, services, and people, such as access to pharmaceutical products, health-related knowledge and technology (for example, new genomic developments), and the movement of patients and professionals [9]. Also in this upper half of the figure, we see the importance of international trade agreements in the cycle; as outlined in the next section of this chapter.

In terms of linkages between these influences, the solid black arrows indicate those between elements at the global or national level, which have been the subject of other literature. Many of these have been explored in other chapters, and the concern here is rather with the shaded black lines, which indicate the need to consider three specific forms of linkages between the global trade environment and the domestic circumstance. First, trade will bring associated changes in risk factors for disease. These will include both communicable diseases, as people and goods which are associated with such diseases (e.g. poultry and bird flu; cows and BSE (bovine spongiform encephalopathy)) cross borders, and non-communicable diseases, as changes in the patterns of food consumption for instance are influenced by changes in income and industry advertising. Second, trade will impact upon the domestic economy through changes in income and the distribution of that income, as well as influencing the levels of tax receipts and form of tax receipts (e.g. reduced import taxes). This will influence the household economy and also the abilities of government to be engaged in public finance and/or provision of healthcare. Finally, trade may be directly in health-related goods and services, such as pharmaceuticals and associated technologies, healthcare workers, patients, and so forth. Clearly the import and export of these will generate a variety of risks and opportunities for the health sector, and thus impact upon the breadth and depth of healthcare provision, and it is these linkages that are the focus of the rest of this chapter.

8.3 International trade agreements and health systems

Trade agreements have implications for health, the health system, and the health sector, whether multi-lateral or bilateral, or linked to the World Trade

Organization (WTO) or more regional trading systems, such as the European Community (EC), Association of Southeast Asian Nations (ASEAN), Southern Africa Development Community (SADC), or North American Free Trade Agreement (NAFTA) [19]. For instance, the Agreement on Trade-Related Intellectual Property Rights (TRIPS) adopted by the members of WTO in 1995 mandates patent protection for pharmaceutical drugs which has the potential impact of increasing the prices of drugs and therefore reducing their accessibility (as discussed in Chapter 7). In terms of non-WTO trade agreements, ASEAN has been promoting the development of agreements covering the migration of healthcare workers, and there are many concerns about recent bi-lateral trade treaties—especially between the United States and Europe with various developing countries—that include provisions going beyond WTO rules and offering even greater protection for instance to pharmaceutical patents [20]. In this section key aspects related to various trade agreements are reviewed with respect to their impact on health systems.

8.3.1 World Trade Organization agreements

In an effort to regularize an increasingly complicated system of international trade, the WTO was created in 1995, as the successor of the General Agreement on Tariffs and Trade (GATT), which was created in 1947. The WTO is a global agency that sets the rules for international trade (including trade in services, goods and intellectual property). In July 2008, 153 countries were members of the WTO. The aim of the WTO is to stimulate economic activity and promote economic development, through progressive trade liberalization. Its philosophical basis is that liberalization will encourage a global increase in efficiency, through the traditional economic arguments relating to comparative advantage, ensuring consumers continued product availability and reducing the economic power of individual economic operators [21]. It seeks to achieve this through creating a credible, reliable, and binding system of international trade rules to ensure transparency, consistency, and predictability in international economic policies [22]. In order to achieve this, the WTO negotiates and implements new trade agreements, serves as a platform for trade negotiations, settles trade disputes, reviews national trade policies, assists developing countries and cooperates with other international organizations (see Box 8.1 for an outline of key functions of WTO). The benefit of WTO in stimulating increased world trade is in securing stability and predictability through their legally enforceable and indefinitely binding nature, although this binding nature has, however, raised concerns [23,24].

The WTO Dispute Settlement Body has enunciated a set of principles that underscore the WTO's recognition of the importance of health as a political

Box 8.1 Key functions of the WTO

♦ Provision of a forum for negotiations between WTO members about their multilateral trade relations in matters dealt with under WTO agreements.
♦ Administration of multilateral trade agreements.
♦ Promotion of the transparency of WTO members' trade policies and actions regarding the implementation of WTO obligations, through regular monitoring and surveillance.
♦ Provision of a process for WTO members to mediate and settle trade disputes.
♦ Working in cooperation with relevant international organizations to achieve greater coherence in global economic policy making.

and social objective. In various cases, the WTO Dispute Settlement Body ruled that: 1) the protection of health is a national objective of vital importance; 2) WTO members are free to select the level of health protection they believe appropriate for their populations; 3) health effects should be included in the case-by-case analysis of whether products or services are alike; and 4) in cases analysing measures to protect human health under the necessity test, the potential effectiveness of less trade-restrictive alternatives should receive strict scrutiny. In this respect, health has a much stronger profile in international trade law than the protection of human rights, which is not an objective trade treaties recognize as a legitimate reason for restricting trade. In short, in implementing trade treaties, national policy makers and legislators have a foundation in the treaties on which to build coherency between trade and health.

The WTO has drafted several agreements in which health systems are involved. These include the General Agreement on Trade in Services (GATS), the agreement on Technical Barriers to Trade (TBT) (which require that technical product regulations and standards be applied in a non-discriminatory manner, be harmonized where possible on the basis of recognized international standards, and be the least trade-restrictive measures possible to achieve the level of health protection sought), the agreement on Sanitary and Phytosanitary measures (SPS) (national measures that aim to reduce hazards to animal, plant, and human health, including food safety regulations), and the agreement on Trade Related aspects of Intellectual Property Rights (TRIPS). In terms of health systems, there are two WTO trade agreements that are of primary interest: GATS and TRIPS. TRIPS has been discussed in detail in Chapter 7, and thus the remainder of this chapter focuses on GATS.

8.3.1.1 The General Agreement on Trade in Services

GATS is the WTO agreement that affects health systems most directly. It establishes the rules for trade in services (including health services), which are covered under four modes of service delivery, as outlined in Box 8.2.

GATS, like all other WTO agreements, is binding to all member countries who sign it. There are some obligations and exemptions associated with the GATS agreement. One such obligation is the 'most favoured nation' principle, where WTO members who adopt GATS agree to treat service suppliers from all countries equally. Furthermore, they must treat foreign health service providers in the same way as national ones. However, as with trade in goods, this principle does not appear to cause difficulty for robust public health measures. Exemptions include services provided by the government, which are not covered by GATS. Member countries have the right to restrict trade in services if they find that it poses a threat to human health. Although GATS is legally binding, countries have the opportunity to pull out after three years of officially adopting the agreement. However, they may have to compensate trading partners [25].

GATS permits WTO members to design the scope of their market access and national treatment commitments, should they decide to make such commitments. From the national implementation perspective, the specific commitments are more important than the general obligations because GATS makes modification of specific commitments difficult to achieve. To date, not many WTO members have made significant specific commitments in areas directly related to health services, and some have stated that they will not entertain any

Box 8.2 GATS four modes of supply of services

1. Mode 1: *Cross Border Supply of Services*. This mode regulates the remote provision of health services, such as diagnostics and radiology, from one country to another.

2. Mode 2: *Consumption of Services Abroad*. This mode covers 'health tourism', the movement of people across borders to receive medical services.

3. Mode 3: *Commercial Presence*. Mode 3 involves foreign direct investment from one country to another. In the health sector this usually involves setting up private hospitals and the presence of foreign insurance companies.

4. Mode 4: *Presence of Natural Persons*. This mode covers the movement of people from one country to another. In the case of health services, this would involve healthcare workers.

requests to liberalize trade in health services during the current Doha Development Round [26].

It is very difficult to measure the effects of GATS on health sectors. This is due to a lack of data, but also because it is difficult to isolate the influence of GATS amongst all the other factors that affect health systems and sectors simultaneously. All GATS modes have the potential to benefit health; however, there are concerns that these benefits maybe concentrated amongst the wealthy, increasing inequities within the health sector [9]. In this respect there are three specific aspects of importance [27]:

1 GATS applies to services provided in competition, thus excluding services provided in the 'exercise of government authority'. Whilst health services not supplied competitively fall outside GATS, if there is a combination of public and private providers then the public providers are covered by GATS. This is significant, as many health sector reform programmes have introduced some element of commercialization.

2 Sectors which are opened may contain qualifications, such as limitations to foreign equity investment, size limitations on facilities or exclusion from subsidy. However, GATS requires as an absolute general obligation that members extend to all other members the best treatment that they give to their most favoured trading partner (the most favoured nation (MFN) obligation in Article II).

3 GATS does not affect member rights concerning market regulation for social policy purposes, such as universal access to care, but it could affect what type of regulations are allowed. For example, the 'necessity test' allows governments to deal with economic and social problems as they wish, provided that the measures/regulations are not more trade restrictive or burdensome than necessary—obviously much depends here on how 'necessary' is defined.

In general, the number of sectors committed is positively related to the level of economic development, although there are anomalies with respect to the health sector. Here commitments are lower than any other sector except education, yet far more developing than developed countries have made commitments in health (information on GATS negotiations is available at http://gats-info.eu.int/, and up-to-date information on levels of levels of commitments can be found at http://tsdb.wto.org/) [28–30]. The low overall level of commitments is suggested as being for a number of reasons: many countries simply ratified already existing trade arrangements, which in health are historically low; health is seen by pace setters for trade—the United States and European Union (EU)—as of less comparative economic value (compared with telecommunications or financial services, for example); and for most countries health is an area of significant government involvement [31].

However, levels of activity and policy engagement in health-related services trade is growing under the combined influence of rising incomes in developed and developing countries, demographic change, particularly population ageing in developed countries and the ensuing pressures to contain health budgets, technological applications that facilitate the remote supply of an increasing range of health-related services, including to isolated populations in developing countries, continued liberalization of investment in services, and growing demand for skilled medical personnel and their cross-border mobility. A growing number of developing countries, particularly middle- and higher-income countries, today regard health services, especially those that can be combined with tourism-related activities, as a potentially significant source of foreign exchange earnings, foreign investment, and skills upgrading, devoting significant policy attention to building health-related export clusters, with some having developed targeted investment promotion strategies. Current, and especially future, rounds of negotiations may well yield much greater levels of commitments as these barriers are overcome, although there is emerging con-sensus that the balance of importance is moving away from GATS in towards more regional and bi-lateral agreements, as discussed in the next section.

8.3.2 Regional and bilateral trade agreements

Countries have different motivations for negotiating regional or bi-lateral trade agreements [32]. Often *liberalization is more easily negotiated at the regional level*, as it involves countries with geographical proximity, cultural ties, and similar levels of economic development. They also often involve a more limited number of participants and thus allow for greater reciprocity, as well as often being undertaken for *reasons other than purely economic ones*, such as strategic, cultural, and political reasons [33].

However, these recent developments in international trade are making the situation for health sectors more complex and less transparent. In addition to the trade negotiations taking place, albeit without much progress, in the WTO's Doha Development Round, many countries are pursuing regional and bilateral trade agreements, many of which include more aggressive provisions on liber-alizing health-related trade in goods and services and on protecting intellectual property rights than the equivalent WTO agreements. This is significant, as try-ing to adopt a health systems approach to the implications of trade agreements becomes more difficult as the number and type of agreements multiplies as, generally speaking, most health sectors, especially developing countries, do not have the capacity to participate and monitor all this activity in international trade. From the trade negotiator's perspective, consideration of health issues consistently across numerous negotiations and agreements might seem too burdensome given the perceived political and economic exigencies of getting agreements finalized [34].

There are some 250 regional and bilateral trade agreements, making up 30% of world trade [35]. These typically take place between developed countries and low- and middle-income countries, and have great implications for governance generally, and health systems more specifically. Regional and bilateral trade agreements pose the danger of benefiting developed countries and being detrimental to poorer countries. This is because they create the potential for trade diversion, as the most favoured nation principle does not apply in this sort of agreement. Furthermore, low- and middle-income countries have less negotiating power than developed countries, which may use this imbalance to exert pressure on them. As countries engaging in regional and bilateral trade agreements normally also take part in WTO agreements, their capacity to negotiate may be overstretched. Often, poorer countries engage in regional and bilateral agreements in the hope of securing their goods access to the market, without taking into account the impact of engaging in such agreements could have on their health systems [36].

Regional trade agreements (RTAs) tend to follow either a negative or a positive list approach. In the negative list approach, all RTA obligations apply across all sectors, and countries list those sectors and modes of supply which they wish to be excluded from the general obligations; sometimes, remaining restrictions are subject to negotiated elimination, sometimes combined with the so-called 'ratchet mechanism', which automatically binds unilateral liberalization of new services under the agreement [37]. The positive list approach, in turn, allows countries to list those sectors and modes of supply in which they would like to commit to liberalization. In theory, both approaches can provide the same level of liberalization. The positive list approach, however, provides greater flexibility in designing the scope and pace of liberalization commitments and it is considered to be the preferred choice for DCs, particularly when it comes to North-South but also South-South liberalization [38]. The positive list approach was adopted in EU–Chile, ASEAN, MERCOSUR (Mercado Común del Sur [Southern Common Market]), CACM (Central American Common Market), Japan–Singapore and United States–Jordan. The negative list approach was adopted in NAFTA-type RTAs, as well as CAN (Comunidad Andina [Andean Community]), and CARICOM (Caribbean Community and Common Market). In recent discussions on whether or not to cover services in Economic Partnership Agreements (EPAs), the choice between positive and negative listing has also received great attention. The health systems implications of international trade agreements must be taken into consideration by those engaging in the agreements in order to minimize the potential risks and maximize the benefits that may arise from such engagements.

8.4 Current trends in health-related services trade

This section provides an overview of aspects related to trade in health services, following the GATS classification [26,39].

8.4.1 E-health and telemedicine

Globalization has in part been made possible due to improvements in information and communication technology [40]. These improvements have also contributed to the remote provision of health services from one country to another, known as 'e-health' Examples of services provided include diagnostics, radiology, laboratory testing, remote surgery, and teleconsultation. Data in this area are limited, but the estimates of the global market on cross border supply of health services are between US$1 billion and US$1 trillion.

Such remote supply of health services has a great impact both on the health sector of the country contracting the services and those supplying them. The countries contracting the services will improve the efficiency and the flexibility of their health sector. This is because services could be carried out during the night if they are contracted to countries where there is a considerable time difference. More importantly, this has the potential to alleviate some of the staff shortages that some diagnostic services face. As some of these services are contracted to countries where salaries are lower, such as India, there is also potential for cost-saving from hiring out services like radiology. This type of trade can also increase the capacity of the country delivering the services. The health sector of these countries will benefit from increased profits and higher employment. There are concerns, however, that these services, and the higher salaries associated with them, may drive medical staff away from domestic services. There are further concerns about the quality of the services provided and the recognition of foreign degrees, as well as legal, malpractice and liability issues. Box 8.3 provides an illustrative case study of e-health trade.

8.4.2 Consumption abroad

Another type of trade in health services arises from the consumption of health services abroad. This is also known as 'health tourism' and it entails people choosing to go to another country to obtain heath care. This attracts approximately four million patients each year, with the global market being estimated to be US$40–60 billion [41]. These figures are likely to increase in the coming years. Consumers choose to travel abroad either because some services are not

Box 8.3 Offshore medical transcription (MT) services in the Philippines

MT is the process of interpreting/encoding electronically the oral dictation of health professionals regarding patient assessment, therapeutic procedures, diagnosis etc. United States outsourcing is the main driver of the global MT business. Since the entry into force of the Health Insurance Portability and Accountancy Act (HIPAA) of 1996 (which provides guidelines for safeguarding patient medical data) the need for medical transcription in the United States has expanded rapidly, growing at 20% per year coupled with a 10% decline in the number of transcriptionists in the United States every year.

The first large MT company, Outsource Transcription Philippines Inc, started in the late 1990s. As the third-largest English speaking nation in the world, with a large workforce, 94% literacy rate, and a strategic location with an ideal 12-hour time difference, the Philippines possessed key inherent advantages as a 'first choice MT outsourcing destination' for the United States (Business World Philippines). Medical transcription is one of the five sub-sectors identified by the Philippines Department of Trade and Industry in its campaign to promote the country as a global hub for outsourced IT-enabled services (CITEM). Of the US$13billion spent on medical transcription in the US per year, US$2.3billion was spent on outsourcing services in 2004. This is expected to grow to US$4.2billion by 2008 (IDC/Business World Philippines). The Philippines government has lent strong support to the MT industry by implementing an important e-commerce law, proposing the Data Protection Bill (2006) and setting up the Information Technology and Electronic Commerce Council. The government has further lent support to develop and expand the IT infrastructure of the country. These efforts have borne fruit as MT outsourcing to the Philippines experienced a cumulative annual growth rate of 13% (2001–4), by far the fastest growing of the outsourcing sectors in the Philippines.

While demand is expected to stabilize in the medium to long-term, the Philippines' share at US$483mn is still quite small compared to the potential market size. However, this is expected to grow rapidly in the short term, given the anticipated surge in United States outsourcing as hospitals have yet to convert records into electronic formats as required by the Federal authority. Furthermore, the vast majority of companies exporting these services from the Philippines are ultimately owned by investors in the United States. Hence the expectation is that as the benefits of outsourcing are fully understood the Philippines will be well positioned to benefit from outsourcing of other aspects of health-related administrative operations. In the case of Philippines–United States outsourcing, privacy concerns have so far not inhibited services exports. Patient information is protected though service contracts between importing hospitals in the United States and exporting transcription companies in the Philippines.

available in their home country, or because these services are too expensive or of poor quality.

For the country of origin, this type of trade may free up some space and be able to reduce its waiting lists. It may also lose revenue from its health sector, as patients are purchasing the services elsewhere. Other drawbacks of this type of trade include lack of insurance portability (so only rich patients will be able to afford to receive treatment abroad), concern about standards of care, safety, and recognition of qualifications. The country providing the services would benefit from the extra employment and revenues this type of trade will generate; the money raised should ideally be spent on the country's own healthcare. However, there is concern about equity and the creation of a two-tier health system in which health tourists receive better quality of care than domestic patients. This may result from more resources being input into treating foreign patients, which generates higher revenues, than to national health services. A case study of such trade is provided in Box 8.4.

Box 8.4 Health and medical tourism: the case of Jordan

Due to the high quality of medical services provided, Arab patients started visiting Jordan for medical treatment as early as the 1970s. In the 1990s Jordan began to consciously promote its health services exports. In 1998, the Ministry of Health established an office at the Queen Alia Airport to facilitate the entry of foreign patients.

While Jordan has invested in upgrading and modernizing its public hospitals and medical schools, it is private sector hospitals that dominate the market for medical tourism. The private sector accounts for 54% of the hospitals in the country and 46% of available beds. Jordan's private hospitals are state-of-the-art and many have links with renowned hospitals and medical centres in Europe and North America.

The Jordanian experience highlights the importance of public–private collaboration. A special directorate, established by the government in partnership with the private sector lays out the vision and strategy for promoting medical tourism in Jordan. Revenue from medical tourism was estimated to have crossed the US$1bn mark in 2003. The vast majority of medical tourists in Jordan come from the Arab world, mainly from Yemen, Sudan, Bahrain, Syria, Libya, Palestine, Saudi Arabia, and others. The majority of patients seek treatment in cardiology, neurology, bone, and other internal diseases.

Medical tourism in Jordan further highlights the importance of bilateral relationships and protocols between sending and receiving countries. Like in the case of Cuba and a few Asian health services exporters, some of the patients coming to Jordan are sponsored by their national funds. For instance, a protocol was signed between Jordan and the Algerian Social Security Fund in 1996, with the terms of payment for treatment in Jordan linked to Algerian Social Security. Jordan also has medical cooperation protocols with several other countries, while private sector hospitals have their own one-to-one agreements with government and private clients in foreign countries.

While the Ministry of Health (MOH) plays a limited role in the trade policy setting, it is notable that the MOH is represented at the Jordan Investment Board and actively functions on the board on matters related to the health sector. Success in the promotion of medical tourism has prompted Jordan to create incentives for national and foreign privet investment in the health sector.

However, Jordan is facing stiff competition in the medical tourism sector from countries like the United Arab Emirates and in the future possibly from Lebanon. There is a large inflow of foreign patients into Lebanon, with a majority coming from Gulf countries. The American University of Beirut Medical Centre attracts a large share of foreign patients in Lebanon. The Lebanese Ministry of Health has established a joint commission to promote 'medical tourism' and an independent company was assigned executive function to promote medical tourism on behalf of participating hospitals. Although the commission has achieved some success, medical care in Lebanon is still expensive compared to Jordan.

8.4.3 Foreign investment

Trade liberalization also applies to capital trade. Foreign direct investment (FDI), especially from developed into developing countries, in 2007 amounted to US$500 billion, over half of which was investment in services [42]. Investment in health is much lower than in other services, but it is still a significant amount [43]. In terms of health, this type of investment usually involves technology transfer, such as setting up modern hospitals or health insurance management practices. The health sectors of developing countries greatly benefit from this type of investment, as it improves their healthcare infrastructure, and therefore their health services delivery [44]. However, there are concerns over the privatization of national healthcare and foreign control of health services. There are further concerns that private foreign hospitals will only be affordable to the wealthy population, and that their poorer counter parts will not see any benefits from such investments. As these facilities will pay more competitive salaries, there are also worries that they could pose an internal 'brain drain' from the public to the private sector, again affecting the poor most [45].

8.4.4 Trade in healthcare workers

Healthcare workers are the core of national health sectors. As discussed in detail in Chapter 6, as liberalization increases and migration becomes easier, the movement of people across borders also increases. This has diverse impacts on the health sectors of the home and the destination countries. The destination country benefits from having more healthcare workers to fill their vacancies. The migrants also benefit from better living and working conditions. The picture is very different for the countries of origin, however. Whilst they may benefit from the remittances sent by the migrating workers, their health sector suffer, both in the quality and the quantity of the services they provide [46]. There is a financial loss, as there are high costs associated with training healthcare workers, which are lost if these workers migrate. Additionally, the workload of the remaining health professionals is heavily increased. There are often many unfilled posts (in Malawi, for example, 65% of nursing posts are not filled [47]). This means there are fewer services available to the population, and as the healthcare staff are overworked, these services are often of worse quality. This affects the remote, rural areas and poor urban dwellers more profoundly, as they have a higher rate of migration, disproportionately affecting the healthcare of the poorer population [48].

8.5 Policies and processes for health system strengthening

How might those engaged in health policy ensure that economic integration, international trade, and trade agreements contribute to health sector strengthening and not health sector weakening?

This chapter has outlined the main ways in which trade liberalization can affect health sectors, both positively and negatively. Positively, an increase in trade may improve efficiency, save costs, transfer skills and technology, increase revenues, and increase quality. On the other hand, the risks associated with liberalization include the loss of trained healthcare workers, an increase in cost, and the creation of a two-tier system in the services domestic and international patients receive. Furthermore, there are concerns that opening up health markets may threaten equity, access, and quality of services for the poor, and that all the gains from trade will be concentrated amongst the most affluent. There is much debate on the *likely* effects of increased trade; however, the lack of systematic data hinders our ability to assess the true impact of the increase in trade.

The first aspect that requires attention to ensure health sector strengthening with respect to international trade is therefore to improve data and indicators. Important data that are needed include: the volume of trade in health services that is taking place, the benefits and losses as a result of this trade, and what is being done with the benefits arising from trade in health services. Efforts in this area have already started, as WHO, WTO, the World Bank, and United Nations Conference on Trade and Development (UNCTAD) are working together to assist countries in collecting and interpreting the data needed [49]. In addition, governments should also start collecting more data at the national level. Chanda and Smith [49] have developed a framework—summarized in Box 8.5—that governments can use to report, analyse, and monitor the impact of trade and its related agreements on health sectors. This framework is only set here as an example of the steps governments could follow to report on trade and health. However, better methods are needed to assess some of the indicators. For example, there are difficulties in assessing point 1c, openness to trade [50].

A second critical area concerns collaboration between trade and health officials at the global level, with more coordination between WTO and WHO, and at the national level, with more linkages between the ministries of finance, trade, foreign affairs, and health [51]. Historically trade and health operated as separate policy spheres, but developments such as those mentioned mean that these areas have developed an increasingly expanded agenda of issues. Although some issues have produced closer cooperation between the two sectors, others have exposed tensions between the goals of protecting health and promoting trade in goods, services, and investment capital. In this respect, the potential risk associated with trade and health is further increased with the added complication of conflicts, or misunderstandings, between the trade and health sectors, and thus further confusion in estimating the potential benefits and risks of trade liberalization for health. National Ministries of Trade (and perhaps finance and foreign affairs), in making trade commitments, do so often in isolation from health ministries, yet they have an impact on health, of which they have limited knowledge. Conversely, Ministries of Health typically have very limited knowledge in trade issues. A critical factor in trade and health is therefore to address this asymmetry of information, by enabling Ministries of Health to make informed and comprehensive presentations to Ministries of Trade concerning decisions to be taken with respect to trade and trade agreements [52].

Balancing trade and health policies requires cooperation through international and national institutional mechanisms. Comparing the mechanisms within the two realms reveals why trade has so far dominated this relationship [53].

Box 8.5 Framework for collecting data on the impact of trade in health services on health systems (adapted from [49])

The following steps represent a framework that national governments may adopt to evaluate the impact of trade on their health system.

1. Establish the country's general background on macroeconomic and trade environment. This requires determining the following:

   Country's macroeconomic status and stability

   Trade and balance of payments

   Degree of openness to trade and investment regime

   Overall policy objectives

2. State of domestic health system. This is done by collecting data on:

   a. Amount of investment in the healthcare sector

   b. Demand and supply conditions

   c. Balance between public and private provision of care

   d. Policy environment

   e. Infrastructure conditions

   f. Regulatory framework

   g. Human resource capabilities

   h. Labour market conditions in the health sector

3. Agreement (or particular mode within agreement) specific elements. This requires determining the following:

   a. Current state of trade and investment in the health sector

   b. Direction of policy

   c. Current status of international commitments and proposed liberalization by the agreement or mode in question

   d. Institutional capacity with regards to trade in health services

   e. Data sources and availability of information on the health sector.

International trade has a highly structured, formalized, and demanding governance system. By contrast, global health governance exhibits little structural coherence, a greater diversity of actors and approaches, and weaker legal obligations on states. WTO is the centre of authority for the governance of trade, as indicated by the large number of its member states and the substantive reach of its agreements [10]. This contrasts with the unstructured plurality of governance in global health [54].

The importance of technical assistance and capacity building initiatives was underscored in the Doha Ministerial Declaration when Ministers confirmed that 'technical cooperation and capacity building are core elements of the development dimension of the multilateral trading system'. Ministers also endorsed the New Strategy for WTO Technical Cooperation for Capacity Building, Growth and Integration and instructed the WTO Secretariat, in coordination with other relevant agencies, to support domestic efforts for mainstreaming trade into national plans for economic development and strategies for poverty reduction. At the Hong Kong Ministerial Conference in December 2005, Ministers not only reiterated the significance of technical assistance and capacity building, but also outlined concrete measures to enhance them through a revamping of the existing Integrated Framework for Least Developed Countries and a new initiative on Aid for Trade. The rationale for the Aid for Trade initiative and the Integrated Framework process stems from the desire to strengthen the capacities of developing and least developed countries to take advantage of more open markets and to harness the multilateral trading system in support of their economic growth and development. Given the emphasis that is presently placed on harmonization of technical assistance and a holistic view of development these initiatives, provide an opportunity for health officials, as well, to articulate their needs in respect of the trade and health sectors and also access financial assistance under the projects initiated or to be initiated there under.

Nonetheless, the main challenge is how to position health more centrally in trade policy, to optimize opportunities to benefit health and healthcare, while minimizing the risks posed. To do so requires taking the initiative in the presentation of health at trade fora at the national level. This is taken up in more depth in Chapter 12.

References

1 Smith RD (2006). Trade and public health: facing the challenges of globalization. *Journal of Epidemiology and Community Health*, **60**, 650–1.

2 Smith RD (2008). Globalization: the key challenge facing health economics in the 21st century. *Health Economics*, **17**, 1–3.

3 Keogh-Brown M, Smith RD (2008). The economic impact of SARS: how does the reality match the predictions. *Health Policy*, **88**, 110–20.

4 Smith RD, Keogh-Brown M, Barnett A, Tait J (2009). The economy-wide impact of pandemic influenza on the UK: a computable general equilibrium modelling experiment. *British Medical Journal*, **339**, b4571.

5 Yach D, Bettcher D (1998). The globalisation of public health I: threats and opportunities. *American Journal of Public Health*, **88**, 735–8.

6 Yach D, Bettcher D (1998). The globalisation of public health II: the convergence of self-interest and altruism. *American Journal of Public Health*, **88**, 738–41.

7 Woodward D (2005). The GATS and Trade in Health Services: Implications for health care in developing countries. *Review of International Political Economy*, **12**(3), 511–34.

8 Blouin C, Drager N, Smith RD (eds). *Building a national health strategy on trade and health: A guide for policy making*. WHO, Geneva (forthcoming).

9 World Health Organization and World Trade Organization (2002). *WTO agreements and public health*. Available at http://www.who.int/media/homepage/en/who_wto_e.pdf

10 Fidler DP, Drager N, Lee K (2009). Managing the pursuit of health and wealth: the key challenges. *Lancet*, **373**(9660), 325–31.

11 Smith RD (2006). Trade in health services: Current challenges and future prospects of globalisation. In Jones AM (ed) *Elgar Companion to Health Economics*, pp.164–75. Edward Elgar, Cheltenham.

12 Woodward D, Drager N, Beaglehole R and Lipson D (2001). Globalisation and health: a framework for analysis and action. *Bulletin of the World Health Organization*, **79**, 875–81.

13 Smith RD, Beaglehole R, Woodward D, Drager N (eds) (2003). *Global Public Goods for Health: a health economic and public health perspective*. Oxford University Press, Oxford.

14 Smith RD, Woodward D, Acharya A, Beaglehole R and Drager N (2004). Communicable Disease Control: a 'Global Public Good' perspective. *Health Policy and Planning*, **19**(5), 271–8. (Also reprinted in: Kirton J (ed) (2009). *Global Health*, pp.191–8. Ashgate, Aldershot.)

15 Smith RD, MacKellar L (2007). Global public goods and the global health agenda: Problems, priorities and potential. *Globalization and Health*, **3**, 9.

16 Smith RD (2009). Global health governance and global public goods. In Buse K, Hein W, Drager N (eds) *Making Sense of Global Health Governance - A policy perspective*, pp.122–36. Palgrave Macmillan, Basingstoke.

17 Sachs J (2001). *Macroeconomics and health: investing in health for economic development* (Report of the Commission on Macroeconomics and Health). World Health Organization, Geneva.

18 Blouin C, Chopra M, van der Hoeven R (2009). Trade and social determinants of health. *Lancet*, **373**, 502–7.

19 Krajewski M (2003). Public services and trade liberalization: mapping the legal framework. *Journal of International Economic Law*, **6**, 341–67.

20 Correa CM (2006). Implications of bilateral free trade agreements on access to medicines. *Bulletin of the World Health Organization*, **84**, 399–404.

21 Chanda R (2002). Trade in health services. *Bulletin of the World Health Organization*, **80**, 158–361.

22 Adlung R, Carzaniga A (2001). Health services under the General Agreement on Trade in Services. *Bulletin of the World Health Organization*, **79**, 352–64.

23 Price D, Pollock A (1999). How the World Trade Organization is shaping domestic policies in health care. *Lancet*, **354**, 1889–92.

24 Pollock A, Price D (2000). Rewriting the regulations: how the World Trade Organization could accelerate privatization in health care systems. *Lancet*, **356**, 1995–2000.

25 Smith RD, Blouin C, Drager N, Fidler DP (2007). Trade in health services and the GATS. In Mattoo A, Stern RM, Zanini G (eds) *A handbook of international trade in services*, pp.437–58. Oxford University Press, Oxford.

26 Smith RD, Chanda R, Tangcharoensathien V (2009). Trade in health-related services. *Lancet*, **373**, 593–601.

27 Nielson J (2005). Ten steps before making commitments in health services under the GATS. In Blouin C, Drager N, Smith RD (eds) *International Trade in Health Services and the GATS: Current Issues and Debates*, pp.101–40. World Bank, Washington, DC.

28 Lautier M (2005). *Les exportations de services de santé des pays en développement–Le cas tunisien*, Agence Française de Développement, Notes et Documents n°25.

29 Mackinstosh M, Koivusalo M (2006). Health systems and Commercialization: In search of good sense. In Mackintosh M, Koivusalo M (eds) *Commercialization of Health Care: Global and Local Dynamics and Policy Responses*, pp.3–21. Palgrave Macmillan.

30 Holden C (2005). Privatization and trade in health services: A review of the evidence, *International Journal of Health Services*, **35**(4), 675–89.

31 Adlung R, Carzaniga A (2005). Update on GATS negotiations. In Blouin C, Drager N, Smith RD (eds) *International Trade in Health Services and the GATS: Current Issues and Debates*, pp.83–100. World Bank, Washington.

32 Crawford X and Fiorentino X (2005). *The Changing Landscape of Regional Trade Agreements*. WTO Discussion Paper No. 8. WTO, New York.

33 UNCTAD (2007). *Trade in Services and Development Implications*, Note by the UNCTAD secretariat, TD/B/COM.1/85, 2 February 2007. UNCTAD, Geneva.

34 Roy M, Marchetti J, Lim H (2006). *Services Liberalization in the New Generation of Preferential Trade Agreements (PTAs): How Much Further than the GATS?* (WTO Staff Working Paper No. ERSD-2006-07). World Trade Organization Economic Research and Statistics Division, Geneva.

35 Oxfam (2007). *Signing Away the Future: How trade and investment agreements between rich and poor countries undermine development*. Briefing Paper, p.5. Oxfam, Oxford.

36 Fink C, Mattoo A (2004). Regional Agreements and Trade in Services: Policy Issues. *Journal of Economic Integration*, **19**(4), 742–79.

37 UNCTAD (2006). *Preserving Flexibility in IIAs: the Use of Reservations* (Series on International Investment Policies for Development). UNCTAD, New York.

38 UNCTAD (2007). *Trade in Services and Development Implications* (Note by the UNCTAD secretariat, TD/B/COM.1/85, 2 February 2007). UNCTAD, New York.

39 Blouin C, Gobrecht J, Lethridge J, Singh D, Smith R, Warner D (2006). Trade in health services under the four modes of supply: review of current trends and policy issues. In Blouin C, Drager N, Smith RD (eds) *International Trade in Health Services and the GATS: Current Issues and Debates*, pp.203–34. World Bank, Washington, DC.

40 Yach D (1998). Telecommunications for health–new opportunities for action. *Health Promotion International*, **13**, 339–47.

41 Datta P, Krishnan GS (2003). The Health Travellers. *BusinessWorld*, 22 December 2003. Available at: http://www.businessworldindia.com/issue/pharma.asp.

42 WHO-EMRO (2004). *Trade in health services: Case-Study on Jordan*. WHO-EMRO, Geneva.

43 Zhang Q, Felmingham B (2002). The role of FDI, exports and spillover effects in the regional development of China. *Journal of Development Studies*, **38**, 157–78.

44 Outreville JF (2007). Foreign direct investment in the health care sector and most-favoured locations in developing countries. *European Journal of Health Economics*, **8**, 305–12.

45 Smith RD (2004). Foreign direct investment and trade in health services: a review of the literature. *Social Science and Medicine,* **59**, 2313–23.

46 Connell J, Pascal Z, Stilwell B, Awases M, Braichet JM (2007). Sub-Saharan Africa: Beyond the health worker migration crisis? *Social Science & Medicine,* **64**, 1876–91.

47 Palmer D (2006). Tackling Malawi's human resources crisis. *Reproductive Health Matters,* **14**(27), 27–39.

48 Wibulpolprasert S, Pachanee C, Pitayarangsarit S, Hempisut P (2004). International service trade and its implications for human resources for health: a case study of Thailand. *Human Resources for Health,* **2**, 10.

49 Chanda R, Smith RD (2006). Trade in health services and GATS: A framework for policy makers. In Blouin C, Drager N, Smith RD (eds) *International Trade in Health Services and the GATS: Current Issues and Debates,* pp.245–304. World Bank, Washington, DC.

50 Smith RD (2006). Measuring the globalisation of health services: a possible index of openness of country health sectors to trade. *Health Economics, Policy and Law,* **1**, 323–42.

51 Blouin C (2007). Trade policy and health: from conflicting interests to policy coherence. *Bulletin of the World Health Organization,* **85**(3), 161–244.

52 Smith RD, Lee K (2009). Trade and health: an agenda for action. *Lancet,* **373**, 768–73.

53 Smith RD (2010). The role of economic power in influencing the development of global health governance. *Global Health Governance,* **III** (2).

54 Bartlett C, Kickbusch I, Coulombier D (2006). Cultural and governance influence on detection, identification, and monitoring of human disease. *Foresight Project on Infectious Diseases: preparing for the future.* Available at: http://www.foresight.gov.uk/InfectiousDiseases/d4_3.pdf (accessed 8 December 2008).

Chapter 9

The health system and external financing

Anna Vassall and Melisa Martínez-Álvarez

9.1 Introduction

Building stronger health systems and sectors in low-income countries will continue to require international finance for some time to come. However, despite the significant growth in development assistance for health in recent years, fundamental challenges remain; both to raise the finance required and to ensure funds are spent effectively. At the global and national level, new policies and aid instruments are being developed to improve aid effectiveness. These are being shaped in the context of an evolving health policy environment: the prioritization of interventions to achieve the Millennium Development Goals (MDGs); the wider involvement of the private sector; and the challenges of health service delivery in fragile states. This chapter examines the experiences, emerging evidence, and lessons learned that are influencing the way in which the international community funds health-related development in low- and middle-income countries.

External financing can take many forms. Official development assistance (ODA) is defined as flows to the Organisation of Economic Co-operation and Development, Development Assistance Committee (OECD-DAC) list of recipients; which are administered with the promotion of the economic development and welfare of developing countries as their main objective and are concessional in character. This includes loans with an equivalent grant element of 25% or more. Development assistance for health (DAH) is slightly broader than ODA and includes non-concessional loans and funds from private foundations and non-government organizations (NGOs) that contribute directly to the promotion of development and welfare in the health sector in developing countries. This chapter will concentrate on DAH.

The provision of development assistance to the health sector is complex, with no dominant group of actors, set of aims, or consistent approach. There are a wide variety of public and private institutions providing assistance, from both OECD and non-OECD countries. Moreover, development funds often do not flow directly from sources of finance (government treasuries, private contributions to NGOs) to the recipient. Instead they may flow through a variety of different channelling institutions such as bilateral aid agencies, multilateral institutions and development banks, or intermediary funds such as the Global Fund for Aids, Tuberculosis and Malaria (GFATM).

Furthermore, development assistance can support population health in a myriad of different ways. Funds can be provided with the direct aim of improving health services and/or sectors. Funds may also be given to interventions that have an indirect impact on health sectors, for example, improving governance, public finance systems, or community involvement in public services. Moreover, development assistance that supports economic well-being, addresses poverty, or areas such as transport policy may also impact the determinants of health. Conversely, funding to health sectors may also be used to support and complement broader development objectives such as good governance or ensuring security.

Funding can also be provided with a wide range of different objectives. First, development assistance may be given in support of specific health services or targets, or it may be used to support the whole health sector. It can also be provided directly to governments, para-statal institutions or NGOs. The processes of planning and prioritizing development assistance can range from being driven and determined by domestic governments, to projects being planned and designed from donor headquarters. Finally, implementation can be done directly by governments, by donors, or through third parties, such as private companies.

In the last two decades, this complex system of development financing has come under increased scrutiny. While progress has been made, a failure to reach MDG targets has meant that both donors and recipients have been forced to examine which funding arrangements and aid instruments work most effectively—and provide the best value for money. Concerns have been voiced around issues such as: the lack of country ownership, the fragmentation of aid (the division of aid into numerous small projects or investments), high administration costs, the transparent use of aid, targeting of aid to those who need it, the inefficient allocation of funds, and the crowding out of domestic financing to health sectors. Development assistance for health has been at the forefront of this debate, and whilst many concerns remain, consensus is now emerging on the key principles required to deliver DAH effectively. The main challenge in the coming years will be putting these principles into practice, not as a blueprint, but in a way that responds to the very different needs of each recipient country.

This chapter will outline the pattern of aid flows to low- and middle-income countries in recent years. It will then present and discuss concerns and evidence relating to aid effectiveness in the health sector, focusing on health sector development. Finally, it will outline the policy response and examine the way ahead.

9.2 **Patterns/trends in development assistance**

Before describing the main trends in development assistance in the past years, it is important to first understand the nature and limitations of the data available on DAH. There is presently no comprehensive system for tracking development assistance for health. The main source of data is the OECD-DAC. OECD-DAC provides two online databases, one listing aggregate commitments and disbursements and the other detailing projects for all OECD donors, several multilateral agencies, and a number of NGOs from OECD countries. This data is compiled from information provided by each donor, guided by a set of consistent reporting directives. While both the quantity and quality of the data reported to the OECD has been improving in recent years, some important gaps remain. These include: the under-reporting by several donors of disbursements, absence of some key multilaterals, limited reporting by the private sector, and the incompleteness of project descriptions and data fields [1,2]. Furthermore, the database does not include development assistance from non-OECD countries; a source of development finance that is playing an increasing role in health sector development in several countries [3].

The limited data on DAH restricts the extent to which aid effectiveness can be properly assessed. Although governments and donors regularly conduct evaluations using internal expenditure and effectiveness data, there is a growing realization that this approach is inadequate. In a context of multiple development assistance flows, effectiveness is increasingly defined in terms of contribution to the overall health sector development effort. A comprehensive assessment of all development assistance flows is therefore required, based on a picture of overall health sector expenditures and outcomes. More fundamentally, the need for timely, good quality and comprehensive DAH data goes beyond donor accountability; it is required by recipient countries to effectively lead, plan and implement health sector development.

Despite the data limitations, several substantive efforts have been made to provide insight into DAH flows in recent years. In 2009, an estimate was made of the DAH contribution to health expenditure in 42 low- and middle-income countries by the Taskforce on Innovative International Financing for Health Systems [4]. This showed that, on average, external resources accounted for

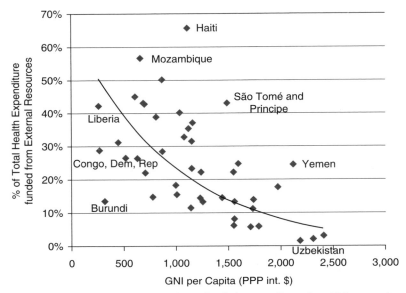

Fig. 9.1 Percentage of health expenditure funded externally against GNI per capita.

around 25% of total public and private health expenditure in the countries studied. In some countries, externally financed expenditures amounted to more than 50% of total health expenditures, illustrating a high level of external dependency of the health sector in many countries. Figure 9.1 plots these findings against GNI per capita, suggesting a negative association between the two. This illustrates the significant role of DAH for those countries that are likely to have weak health systems.

In 2009, the Institute for Health Metrics and Evaluation conducted an analysis of development assistance expenditures for health between 1990–2007; based on OECD-DAC data, supplemented with data from various multilaterals and United States-based NGOs [5]. The results showed a significant rise in development financing for health during the period. In 1990, total expenditures were estimated to be around US$5.59 billion globally, by 2007 this had risen to US$21.79 billion. This rate of growth was slow at first but then accelerated substantially post-2002. New funds like the GFATM and Global Alliance for Vaccines and Immunisation (GAVI) channelled increasing amounts of resources. The amount of funding provided through bilateral agencies also rose substantially. Several charitable foundations, such as the Bill and Melinda Gates Foundation increased the level of private sector contributions to the health sector.

For those DAH expenditures that could be allocated to a specific disease area, increases were observed in the funding for HIV/AIDS and more recently also for tuberculosis and malaria. This was in sharp contrast to the volume of funds that could be identified as broader health sector support; these remained stagnant and low, at under 10% of total DAH. Some had argued that the increasing funding to HIV/AIDS and other infectious diseases would attract more funding to the broader health sector. But it is now widely accepted that, at least up until 2007, no substantial increase in health systems development funding occurred [6].

Regionally, the relative share of resources allocated to sub-Saharan Africa increased from 9.7% in 1990 to 22.7% in 2007. Broadly, aid allocations were found to be linked to the burden of disease, although there were considerable variations between countries. At the beginning of the period studied development assistance was not correlated to per capita GDP, but by the end poorer countries began to receive increasing amounts of development assistance, compared to relatively richer ones. An increasing proportion of expenditure was managed by recipient countries, either by the provision of direct contributions to government budgets, or using integrated or joint management procedures; the most marked increase occurring since 2002 [5].

Several disease/health specific studies complement these findings. For example, a study tracing donor assistance to maternal, newborn and child health (MNCH) between 2003 and 2006 found a 60% increase in total funding for MNCH, but little change in the overall proportion of development assistance on health allocated to MNCH [7]. Another study comparing development assistance for reproductive health found that non-conflict countries received 50% more aid per capita for reproductive health than conflict-affected countries; highlighting that, although the broad trend is in favour of poorer countries, large variations in DAH remain between subsets of countries [8].

Data on development expenditures by non-OECD donors are scarce. The main source of data is the PLAID database, produced by Aid Data. A study comparing the patterns of aid from non-OECD donors using the PLAID database found that non-OECD donors tend to provide most aid to neighbouring countries and their poverty orientation tends to be weaker that OECD donors. However, they are no more likely to be present in countries with weak governance than OECD donors [3]. It should be noted that this database excludes some important new donors such as India and China. However, the Chinese Statistical Yearbook estimates that the total amount of aid (to all sectors) provided by China amounts to around US$2 billion per year, suggesting that they are among the smaller of international donors.

The trends cited above have substantial consequences. First, the balance between infectious diseases, reproductive health, other areas of health, and health sectors has significantly shifted, in favour of disease-focused financing.

Second, (often weak) health sectors have had to absorb unprecedented increases in DAH and scale-up several interventions at a speed not previously seen. Third, new actors are emerging, such as charitable foundations and non-OECD donors, who are now operating at the scale where they can influence international health sector policies, and interact with domestic governments in new ways. Finally, there have been some slow, but steady moves to focus DAH on poorer, often more fragile, countries. While few in the health sector would not welcome the large influx of funding in recent years, these factors have raised concerns about the impact of these flows on the development of sustainable health sectors.

9.3 Aid effectiveness and health development

Arriving at general conclusions about the impact of development assistance on health is problematic. There have been some notable improvements in health service indicators in recent years. Access to antiretroviral drugs, case detection for tuberculosis and the ownership of long-lasting insecticide treated bed-nets have all increased. However, attributing these improvements to increased DAH flows is complex. Even where sophisticated modelling methods are used, the empirical literature on impact of DAH on health sectors has yielded unclear and ambiguous results [9]. Even less is known about the specific relationship between DAH and health systems development. Although donors and recipient countries regularly produce unpublished internal evaluations of numerous projects and investments, there are little published data available that relate aid flow patterns to health system improvements. Nevertheless, there is a consensus emerging on how development assistance can be best provided for health systems strengthening, based on a variety of experiences and academic literature on overall ODA and the numerous unpublished evaluations of DAH conducted over the last two decades.

9.3.1 Underfunding of health sector development

Whilst the need for health sector investment is apparent, until recently there were few estimates of the level of expenditure required. The High Level Taskforce for Innovative International Financing for Health Systems was set up in 2008 in part with the aim of assessing the resource gaps in financing the health sectors of the poorest countries (the Taskforce also had other goals, see below). To do this, two approaches were used: the World Health Organization (WHO) normative approach and the marginal budgeting for bottlenecks (MBB) approach. Briefly, for the WHO normative approach, the amount of resources required to scale-up health sectors to a level deemed 'best practice' by experts and practitioners was estimated. The MBB approach consisted in identifying bottlenecks to scaling-up effective interventions and costing strategies to overcoming them. Both methods looked beyond the simple costing of services at the facility/local level, and systematically examined the broader investments required to enable the scale-up of basic health services. The results from the two approaches were broadly comparable. The extent of underfunding for health sectors was estimated to be US$10 billion per year [11]. Further, the Taskforce made some recommendations on how the extra funds should be allocated. Importantly, it was estimated that around 40% of funds should be invested in capital (human and physical), in order to increase absorption capacity. The remainder should be spent on recurrent costs (health workforce, drugs, and supplies) [11]. The Taskforce did not recommend a re-allocation of funds within the health sector, instead it concentrated its efforts on raising the additional funds required.

9.3.2 Absorption capacity

The second emerging issue concerns absorption capacity. This addresses the inter-relationship between macro-economic, fiscal and sector constraints, and the achievement of health service expansion. First, examining the macro-economic level, there is a risk that high levels of external aid flows may increase domestic demand, thus driving up the prices of local goods and create inflationary pressures. As a consequence exports may suffer, which may damage investment and growth prospects. This phenomenon is often referred to as 'Dutch disease', following a similar experience after the exploitation of natural gas in the Netherlands. DAH is hence constrained by the capacity of an economy to adjust to the increased domestic demand it generates. DAH investments in areas which require a high proportion of imported goods are likely to be less affected. Likewise, if DAH flows are transparent this effect may be mitigated with domestic economic management. Second, at the fiscal level, large inflows of funds affect the balance between government revenues and expenditures. DAH investments typically require complementary domestic resource use. For example, many donors are only willing to fund capital goods, such as training and equipment. These investments need to be complemented with long-term domestic funding for human resources and areas like repair and maintenance. The effective absorption of DAH funds is therefore constrained by medium term domestic revenues. Finally, the absorption of DAH can be impeded by constraints at the sector level. For example, limited human resource capacity poses the risk that increased DAH funding simply results in increase wages. Limited domestic management and administrative capacity can also restrict the speed at which DAH funds may be effectively absorbed.

Likewise, complementary infrastructure development may take time and limit the speed at which services can be expanded.

All of these factors have focused attention on how to mitigate or reduce absorption constraints. Transparent and predictable DAH flows are seen as essential for this effort. Planning DAH in the context of National Development Plans that deal with macro, fiscal, and sector levels in a cohesive way, are also seen as key.

9.3.3 Fragmentation of DAH

The way DAH is delivered also impacts its effectiveness. A key issue is the high level of fragmentation of aid provided to the health sector. Fragmentation refers to the division of DAH into numerous different projects or programmes, provided by a wide variety of different actors. There has been a substantial proliferation of donors active in the health sector in recent decades. The Taskforce on Innovative Financing for Health Systems observes that the health sector now suffers, more than most other sectors, from a fragmentation of donor support with different interests in and funding of specific activities and projects [4]. This viewpoint is supported by several OECD analyses [12], which observe higher levels of fragmentation in social sectors, most notably health and education. It is suggested that this, combined with the increase in social sector funding over the past years, has been responsible for an overall increase in the fragmentation of development assistance.

The presence of high numbers of donors in a country (or sector) is associated with aid ineffectiveness [13]. Fragmentation may be as much as symptom as a cause; country characteristics such as population size, poverty and democracy are likely to increase fragmentation [12] and at the same time are likely to impact aid effectiveness. However, a number of interactions can be identified that suggest that fragmentation may directly reduce the effectiveness of aid. First, high numbers of different projects result in high administrative and transactions costs [14]. Second, recipient governments may find it difficult to keep track of all assistance and prevent inefficient duplication. Moreover, effective domestic priority setting may be inhibited, as numerous different interests need to be balanced. Third, although each individual donor may be satisfied with their own project, fragmentation may become a barrier to those seeking to address broader fiduciary performance concerns [15]. Finally, fragmentation reduces the extent to which governments and donors can comprehensively plan health sector improvements resulting in patchwork investments.

Having said this, it should be noted that the other extreme of no fragmentation would also be a concern. Whilst having many small and disparate actors may not be efficient, having no diversity may also restrict innovation; and also confront domestic governments with an effective monopoly of DAH. Therefore a balance needs to be made, whereby aid flows are sufficiently uniform to enable broad system development, but at the same time allow for new actors and, provide governments with a degree of choice of finance for their health sector development efforts.

A related concern is the disconnection of DAH flows between those that are intended for a particular disease, such as HIV/AIDS, and those which are targeted at health sector development. While, at the implementation level, they are fundamentally intertwined, in recent years the management of DAH funding flows to each area has become fragmented—with the establishment of funds that have a specific disease focus. These came about primarily as a consequence of the need to respond to the global HIV/AIDS emergency. As such they were designed to leverage funding, achieve rapid results, with an emphasis on providing funding based on results (in terms of the rapid scale-up of interventions). Applications for funding from these organisations are commonly coordinated at the domestic level and funding can be channelled to a variety of private and public actors from within the health sector and beyond. As originally designed, engagement in government and public processes was minimal, arguably enhancing the speed of disbursement.

There is a long-standing debate between those who see these funds as effective and pragmatic financing vehicles for focused health service development, with positive externalities, and those who emphasize the distorting impact of vertical financing channels on sustainable and comprehensive health service and system development. Proponents on both sides of this debate primarily rely on anecdotal examples and case studies. A review of a wide range of case studies carried out in 2009 by the WHO Maximizing Positive Synergies Collaborative Group of the interaction of global health initiatives and country health sectors found substantive evidence gaps [16]. Nevertheless, it did identify some evidence that strengthening infectious disease programmes can have a positive impact on broader health systems development. Effects ranged from keeping health professionals, who may succumb to the diseases such as HIV/AIDS, alive, to improving health service staff skills. Disease focused funding can, on occasion, also improve wider health service delivery. A notable example is the case of Rwanda, where improvements in disease programmes have simultaneously increased the overall utilization of services [17]. Moreover, some funds, like GAVI and the GFATM, have been successful at leveraging funds for health system development. Finally, many of these funds make considerable effort to involve domestic institutions in their steerage and planning processes; often bringing new stakeholders into previously closed discussions [18].

Critics of global health funds argue that these programmes have pulled scarce domestic resources away from key health sector functions towards a more narrow short term focus. For example, highly qualified management staff may be attracted away from essential public service functions by the higher salaries provided by some of these funds [17]. Evidence of fund contributions to pre-service training or health worker production remains scarce, although there are some notable exceptions [16]. Arguably these funds have also 'crowded out' DAH that would have otherwise been available for health systems development, although this is hard to verify. Perhaps the most serious issue concerns the incentives that international vertical financing provides for the maintenance of vertical planning by domestic institutions. These may impede domestic priority setting, resulting in systemic resource imbalances and sector inefficiencies. For example, efforts to encourage decentralized district health service priority setting and planning can be hindered when vertical programmes operate under centrally driven planning processes—with independent finance. Critics point out that, although these funds make considerable effort to involve national actors in their planning processes, efforts to do the reverse—integrating themselves into national planning processes—appear to be weaker [16].

Whatever the perspective, in the last few years there has been a growing realization that, both the fragmentation between disease-orientated and health sector funding—and the imbalance of funding between these two areas—need to be simultaneously addressed if the MDGs are to be achieved and sustained. In part due to the increased focus on HIV/AIDS treatment, those advocating for infectious disease programmes are increasingly recognizing that the successful scale-up of interventions is dependent on the underlying health sector absorption capacities [4]. Likewise, those coming from a health system perspective are accepting that investments in health need to demonstrate real (and reasonably rapid) impacts on health service outputs and outcomes—particularly if funding is to be leveraged from sources that require results on these terms.

Addressing these mutual objectives requires intervention at the sectoral level and above. An example is the case of building the human resource capacity necessary for TB and HIV/AIDs treatment. Ensuring sufficient human resources for health does not simply depend on the short term employment and training of disease focused staff, but, more fundamentally, on a sustainable growth in capacity to provide long-term training and finance and, to allocate and manage human resources effectively [20]. In turn, this may require sustained public finance commitments, and possibly changes to employment law and/or civil service rules, requiring engagement at the macro-level. Nevertheless, despite the growing recognition of these issues agreement on the aid architec-ture—the structure of DAH institutions globally and at the country level required—is still a work in progress.

The last aspect of fragmentation that deserves some attention is the division between DAH provided to NGOs and that provided to public institutions. The complex debate surrounding the relative merits of developing capacity through NGOs and the public sector is not dealt with here. However, it should be noted that considerable concern has been raised in recent years about the conse-quences for fragmentation when relying on disparate and externally financed NGOs as vehicles for health service and sometimes system development. This issue is particularly acute in post-conflict environments.

9.3.4 Short-term and unpredictable financing

The negative consequences of fragmentation for health system development are compounded by the often short-term and unpredictable nature of DAH investments. Although data in this area is weak, volatility of DAH at the coun-try level is thought to be considerable. In contrast, health systems development is a long-term process that requires substantial initial outlay followed by sustained financial commitment. As long as there is uncertainty about growth in future financing, domestic governments are unlikely to favour substantial scale-up of their physical infrastructure and human resources. In both developing and developed countries alike, a reduction in services, staff or infrastructure can present a political challenge. Moreover, any subsequent contraction of health services can result in serious funding imbalances; where funding for areas that are challenging to reduce, such as health service staffing is maintained; but funding for other essential and recurrently funded areas like drugs or repair maintenance becomes severely constrained. As a consequence the scale-up of services that cannot be financially sustained is often avoided.

Sustained and predictable recurrent financing is therefore an essential pre-requisite of health sector expansion. This can be provided by development assistance, but requires long-term commitment—and disbursements that match them. Long-term DAH may also be used to leverage sustained domestic funding allocations to the health sector. The question of how to and whether governments can and do provide appropriate levels of health sector financing is extensive in itself and will not be addressed here. However, the engagement at the fiscal and sectoral level of all financing partners is required. Ideally, increased DAH would, at the very least, demand the maintenance of the level of domestic resourcing to the health sector, and at best encourage a commit-ment of additional domestic funding.

9.3.5 **Fungibility of DAH**

This raises the issue of the fungibility of DAH. That is, the extent to which domestic governments adjust their own spending to offset donor funding [21]. Before examining this issue further, it is important to first recognize the perspective from which this is seen as a concern. From a health sector perspective, the donor's aim is to ensure that every euro, dollar, or pound of DAH provided adds to the total funding available for the health sector. A failure to do this is seen as problematic. However, this presumes that the donor has judged the relative needs of different sectors correctly; that, if domestic health sector funding falls, this represents a reduction in the aggregate allocative efficiency of domestic expenditures. This may not be the case. Indeed, many development economists view reductions in domestic health funding by governments as a rational response to the high level of additional external health sector funds in recent decades [22]. Any concern over the issue of aid fungibility raised is argued to represent narrow sectoral interests and should not be central to debates around development assistance [23]. At the very least, the fungibility of DAH should be assessed and judged in the context of national spending priorities, rather than as a necessarily negative phenomenon.

Having said this, from a health sector development perspective, it is valid to ask whether the increases in DAH have resulted in an overall increase in financing for the health sector in the last decades. Unfortunately for those with health sector development aims, most the evidence to date suggests that health sector fungibility has been particularly acute [24,25].

An improvement of data on both domestic and development health expenditures has recently enabled increasingly accurate estimations of the extent of the fungibility in the health sector [26]. A panel regression analysis used to estimate the association between government domestic spending on health and DAH disbursements globally, conducted in 2010, showed that DAH had a negative impact on domestic government spending on health. The extent was profound, in that for every US$1 of DAH to government, government health expenditures were reduced by $0.43–1.14 [22]. However, these results need to be interpreted with some caution. Despite the improvements, neither data on DAH funds or domestic health expenditures can be seen as fully reliable [27].

When funds are earmarked to particular areas, fungibility may also occur within the health sector. For example, during the 1980s significant development assistance funds were provided for primary healthcare, and many governments responded by allocating higher proportions of the domestic budget to hospital care, worsening the apparent domestic neglect of the primary healthcare [21]. There is also some evidence of the crowding out of health system expenditures associated with increased development expenditure on HIV/AIDS [28]. Both examples however, illustrate the importance of taking a 'systems' approach when delivering DAH, to ensure that efforts to support one part of the health infrastructure are truly additional.

The degree of fungibility of DAH varies substantially between countries and circumstances, and more attention and research is required to fully understand the processes which promote or decrease it. Arguably, fungibility is directly linked to the short-term and unpredictable nature of DAH flows. It is not simply that governments are reluctant to expand health spending, but that short-term aid flows encourage governments to restrict expenditures. Governments use their own funds to create a buffer—a practice encouraged by the International Monetary Fund—saving them for times when development assistance declines or economic conditions worsen [29]. It is also suggested that fungibility is lower when DAH is channelled through NGOs [22], possibly reflecting the fact that governments find it hard to keep track of the magnitude of the funds channelled through NGOs and therefore are less likely to adjust their spending accordingly. However, responding to these influencing factors is unlikely to comprehensively address this issue. Ultimately, the only way to remove fungibility entirely may be to provide DAH in the context of overall budget support—where funding is provided on the basis of nationally agreed plans with appropriate sectoral allocations.

9.3.6 Weak governance and institutional capacity

Finally, aid effectiveness is substantially influenced by the ability of domestic institutions to effectively plan and channel DAH funds [30]. The domestic management of DAH—from planning investments to being responsible for procurement—has the potential to be more responsive to need—and legitimate—than the external management of these processes [27]. Good governance, whether by the public or private sector, is the key to the realization of this. Corruption and rent-seeking behaviour, particularly around the substantial contracting of infrastructure or other capital investments associated with development is a valid concern. Corruption is notoriously difficult to measure, but nevertheless there are a number of recent cases that highlight the potential danger of high levels of DAH leakage from the health sector in several countries. In addition, the fragmentation of aid is more likely in states with a high level of corruption, perhaps reflecting donors desire to directly control funds.

A tension exists between the demand on the donors to disburse commitments and achieve results within short time frames, and weak domestic ability to deliver these results. The path of least resistance may be sought, focusing on 'easy wins', rather than build the institutional capacity necessary to domestically manage funds for development. Donors may avoid the public sector in states with weak governance on the assumption that systemic corruption and poor management is less endemic in the private sector [27], thus side-stepping a more broadly focussed health system development approach.

9.3.7 Summary

In summary, while DAH has supported some notable successes—including the rapid mobilization of resources to respond to the global HIV/AIDs emergency—there is a growing recognition that health system development has been underprioritized and underfunded in recent years. In particular, it is increasingly being recognized that the achievement of the health related MDG's is not solely dependent on funds to improve health services, but also requires funding to address absorption capacity—at the macro, fiscal, and sectoral levels. The manner of aid delivery, in terms of high levels of fragmentation, the disease/systems disconnection, and short-term nature of funding are likely to have weakened the effectiveness of DAH, impeded health systems development, and failed to adequately address the domestic policy and governance issues required. Furthermore, there is a suggestion that—in part as a consequence of all these factors—increases in DAH may have been highly fungible; where funds provided with the intention to address health related MDGs, are not fully additive and in some case may have reduced the domestic finance available to sustainably fund the health sector. This section of the paper has already touched upon some of the solutions; the next section of this chapter examines these further and discusses the way forward.

9.4 The response—key issues and emerging evidence

In the last few years, the concerns outlined above have led to concerted international effort, both within the health sector and beyond. In 2005, numerous developed and developing countries signed Paris Declaration on Aid Effectiveness, aimed at improving ownership, harmonization, alignment, results, and mutual accountability. In 2008, a High Level Task Force on Innovative Financing for Health Systems was formed to identify new sources of sustainable financing for health systems development. Finally, a plethora of new financing and funding instruments are being promoted to improve the delivery of assistance at country level. This section briefly summarizes some of these efforts.

9.4.1 Reaching a consensus on aid effectiveness

There has been a long history of negotiations between donors on international policy on aid effectiveness. Several agreements have been signed, including the Monterrey Consensus on Financing for Development (2000), the Rome Declaration on Harmonization (2003), and the Marrakesh Memorandum on Managing for Results (2004). The most prominent was the Paris Declaration on Aid Effectiveness endorsed by over 100 countries and international agencies in 2005. The Paris Declaration is characterized as a set of five Partnership Commitments between the partner (recipient) countries and the donors.

9.4.1.1 Ownership

The principle of ownership recognizes the need for recipient countries to provide leadership over their development policies and strategies, and to coordinate development activities. Improved ownership is also recognized as essential for health systems development; to avoid fungibility and to provide support for the often difficult domestic policy decisions required to support health sector reform. When signing the Paris Declaration, recipient countries agreed to lead the development and implementation of their national development strategies, including national strategic health plans, through a consultative process; to make these results oriented and linked to a medium-term expenditure framework, and reflect them on their annual budgets; and to play a leading role in the coordination of aid at all levels.

9.4.1.2 Alignment

Strong country ownership facilitates the alignment of donors. Alignment requires donors to define their support in relation to partners' national development strategies, institutions, and procedures, rather than the converse. To achieve this, partners and donors committed to working together to use (and thereby strengthen) country systems, improve partners' development capacity, strengthen public financial management capacity and national procurement systems, and untie aid; thus avoiding the worse consequences of fragmentation. Alignment is expected to make aid consistent with partners' priorities and systems, reduce transaction costs, and improve developing countries management capacities and accountability [31]. If donors and partners keep to their commitments, it is hoped that it will lead to a 'virtuous circle', where partners strengthen their systems, which results in donors trusting and using them, which promotes the further strengthening of country systems [31]. Country ownership and alignment are interlinked, and can reinforce each other. If partners have ownership and leadership over their development programmes and strategies, they are more likely to get donors to align to them. Similarly, by aligning to country systems, donors provide incentives for partners to strengthen and reinforce these [31].

9.4.1.3 Harmonization

The aim of harmonization is for donors to act in a transparent and collectively effective manner; this is facilitated by aligning behind national development plans. When signing the Paris Declaration, donors committed themselves to implementing common management arrangements and simplifying procedures at all levels, including planning, funding, disbursement, monitoring, evaluating, and reporting. A key aspect is for donors to work together to avoid (or greatly reduce) duplicating projects and diagnostic reviews, and share lessons learnt. Ideally this coordination should be government led. Donors and domestic partners should work towards complementarity; aiming for an effective division of labour. In doing so, again the worse consequences of fragmentation can be avoided, enabling a coordinated approach to health systems development.

9.4.1.4 Managing for results

Managing for results means delivering aid focusing on results, and using information to improve decision-making. To achieve this, partner countries committed to establishing results-oriented reporting and assessment frameworks, based on national and sector priorities. Similarly donors committed to linking their programmes to results and aligning them with country performance frameworks. This will benefit health sectors by ensuring that only effective programmes are pursued, and that aid is allocated in an evidence-based manner.

9.4.1.5 Mutual accountability

The final commitment is mutual accountability, where donors and partners agreed that both would be accountable for development results. This would involve both donors and partners to be transparent, inclusive in their approach (including all development partners) and assess their mutual progress through country-level mechanisms.

These principles also apply to fragile states, although the commitments were slightly revised for these countries. In the case of harmonization, partner countries committed to work towards building institutions and governance structures, to develop simple planning tools in conjunction with donors, and to encourage the participation of a wide range of national actors in setting development priorities. At the same time, donors committed to harmonize all their activities, align as much as possible behind country systems, avoid undermining national institutions and use an optimal mix of aid instruments, in order to achieve the best results.

9.4.2 International financing for health systems and the international health partnership

Within the broad policy framework for ODA outlined above there have been several notable efforts to improve the specific effectiveness of DAH. The Taskforce on Innovative International Financing for Health Systems was established in September 2008 and chaired by the then United Kingdom Prime Minister Gordon Brown and the World Bank President Robert Zoellick; acknowledging at the highest level that that new and innovative ways of financing health systems needed to be identified to accelerate progress on the MDGs, as well as make better use of DAH. The aim of the Taskforce was to help strengthen health systems in the 49 poorest countries in the world, by 'filling national financing gaps to reach the health MDGs through mobilizing additional resources; increasing the financial efficiency of health financing; and enhancing the effective use of funds' [4]. The Taskforce was organized into two phases of work: the first one was undertaken by two working groups who were charged with producing a set of recommendations, and the second involved a group of 'champions' who advocated for the Taskforce recommendations.

In May 2009 the Taskforce launched its report, with ten recommendations. These included raising an additional US$10 billion per year to spend on health in low-income countries, by expanding the mandatory solidarity levy on airline tickets (UNITAID), exploring similar levies, and expanding on the use of International Financing Facility for Immunization (IFFIm). UNITAID was set up in 2006 to improve access to medicines and diagnostics for HIV/AIDS, malaria, and tuberculosis. Most of its income (82%) is raised through a levy on plane tickets, although some countries also make direct budgetary contributions. Its original aims are to make the supply of drugs more predictable and sustainable, to make drugs more affordable and available, of better quality and more adapted to patients' needs. UNITAID has been praised for raising funds in an efficient manner, with further positive developmental impacts (environmental). IFFIm raises money from the international capital markets and channels it through GAVI to improve immunization coverage and access to new vaccines. It has the advantages of being predictable (it is legally binding), providing significant up-front support and providing some funds to health systems strengthening (through the GAVI framework). However, there is a premium that IFFIm must pay (borrowing and transaction costs), which makes it more expensive than other forms of DAH.

Furthermore, the Taskforce examined the way in which these additional funds could be delivered in a way that avoided past concerns. In particular, it provided the outline of the application of the Paris declaration principles to health systems development, by recommending the strengthening of governments' performance and capacity to secure investment from non-state actors; ensuring the efficient allocation of funds; undertaking a review of all current technical assistance and focusing it on strengthening domestic institutional capacity. Whilst stopping short of advocating a singular health systems funder, it suggested the establishment of a joint health systems funding platform for the GFATM, GAVI, and the World Bank to manage the flow of resources to health sectors [11]. This platform would pool and coordinate funds from different international agencies at the country level, thus improving harmonization. It would channel funds (possibly using different mechanisms) based on a national health plan encouraging a joint approach to development.

In addition, several donors have signed up to an International Health Partnership (IHP). This was established to support this effort, with the aim of mobilizing resources around single country led health plans. Here again the focus is on coordination at the country level, the partnership now being piloted in several countries.

9.4.3 New funding instruments

The implementation of this new approach has required the development of new funding instruments. Historically DAH has been delivered through projects; defined as 'externally financed discrete interventions', which are independent of government systems and management [32]. However, project aid has attracted considerable criticism with only half of all projects estimated to have succeeded [33]. Project aid has allowed donors to work through a variety of implementing partners, avoid fiduciary risk, target resources and work where there are weak governments [34,35]. Despite this, some argue that sustainability has been weak [35], transaction costs high (due to the frequent reports and coordination meetings recipients must deliver and attend) [36,37], and there has been little country ownership with the undermining of local systems [32,36]. In summary, project aid has been recognized to be one of the key drivers of fragmentation and highly donor-driven [38], and therefore an inappropriate vehicle for comprehensive health systems development. As a result, increasing attention has focused on programme aid and more recently direct support for government budgets.

9.4.4 Programme aid, including multi-donor trust funds

In the last 20 years, programme aid has become increasingly common and now is the main aid instrument used by many of the global health funds. Programme aid provides multi-year support to achieve a broad set of objectives, often cofinanced by donors and recipients. It is considered more stable and predictable than project aid. It can be managed by governments or other implementers, often using donor procedures, moving some way towards alignment and country ownership. Programmes maintain a transparent link between financing and defined objectives, such as improving disease control or strengthening health sectors. In principle they can be used in a coordinated way to help the recipient country overcome systemic funding gaps [39] and can support broad sector objectives and harmonization. However, programme aid may still be highly fungible [39] and vulnerable to politically-triggered 'freezes', which can hinder its predictability [32].

Multi Donor Trust Funds (MDTFs) provide a mechanism for donors to pool their funds for programme support, furthering harmonization. They are managed using donor procedures, but can be implemented within government structures. They are often administered by the World Bank or the United Nations. They have the advantages of attracting resources from a range of donors, and can be tailored to meet specific needs (for instance the Health Result Innovation Trust Fund that focuses on strengthening health systems). Programmes can be results-based, and may strengthen links between health and finance ministries [40]. However, they have been criticized for having slow disbursement, due to the requirements of donor procedures and some argue they reduce accountability to financiers [35]. Nevertheless, they are currently one of the main instruments used to finance health sector development in post-conflict environments.

A more aligned approach is budget support that provides funds directly to government budgets. This has the potential to significantly reduce transactions costs and can take two forms: sector budget or general budget support. General budget support is provided directly into the recipient government's budget. It has little or no earmarking [35], but is linked to a national development plan. It is planned and managed using government processes and any link to a specific donor supported objective is broken. If negotiated carefully, there is a potential for more funds to be delivered to a specific sector than in the case of programme aid, as the risk of fungibility is removed. Negotiations can focus on overall allocations to the health sector, although may not deal with sector specific issues. Potential benefits may also include: strengthened government ownership, national decision-making processes and government accountability; better policy coherence and a more rational allocation of expenditure; reinforced government channels improved coordination and alignment; and more predictability of funding [32,35].

However, budget support is highly dependent on the quality of governance and policies of the recipient country. There are fiduciary concerns, including a risk that corruption may result in the money being misspent [9]. The application of budget support therefore requires substantial pre-conditions, which many governments find hard to meet. Only 6.4% of all ODA between 2000 and 2006 was spent on general budget support [42], although its popularity is growing [32]. This type of aid is particularly favoured by European countries, with DFID now providing general budget support to Uganda and Tanzania [34]. There is some concern however, from some in the health sector that budget support may not provide adequate attention for health sector issues, as negotiations tend to concentrate on macro-economic and public financing issues.

Sector budget support is budget support earmarked for a specific sector and is disbursed and accounted for using government systems, although additional sector reporting may be required [34]. Sector budget support may also deliver similar benefits to general budget support (lower transaction costs and alignment with national priorities) [42]. In addition, it can be used even if the policy and institutional frameworks are weak, provided that the sector-level structures are strong enough [35]. It can further be used as a pilot, before committing to general budget support [35]. Nearly 8% of all health ODA in the period 2002–2006 was spent on sector programmes [42]. Finally, it can avoid fungibility by attaching conditions ensuring that governments only receive support if domestic allocations to the sector are also maintained.

MDG contracts are a new funding mechanism used by the European Commission (EC). They are part of general budget support, but they place an emphasis on achieving MDG results, as well as addressing wider macro-economic and public finance issues. In this way they provide non-earmarked financing to governments, linked to both macro-economic and sector specific objectives. MDG contracts can bring in additional resources, as well as complementing other instruments and can be used to operate in difficult settings. However, given that these instruments are such a novel funding instrument, their impact has yet to be evaluated [43].

9.5 **The way forward**

At the global level many of the building blocks are now in place to encourage and enable sufficient, predictable and efficient flows of DAH to build health systems. Some substantive issues are still evolving, most notably the determination of the most appropriate aid architecture to raise and deliver 'health systems strengthening funds'. Key questions remain in relation to how any health systems platform should be led, organized, managed, and implemented at the country level. Moreover, although the importance of health system development and the broad principles of aid effectiveness have been agreed globally, enthusiasm between donors is varied. Several key donors and institutions remain bound by domestic laws that limit their ability to engage in some of the processes demanded. And, while many donors officially recognize the importance of aid effectiveness principles, the same cannot always be assumed of their political leaders, who may need to respond to the particular needs of their constituencies. There also remains considerable scepticism from some academic quarters and interest groups about any use of DAH financing beyond emergency health needs; given the limited evidence of the effectiveness of past efforts in health sector strengthening.

Having said this, the primary challenge facing most donors now surrounds the application of these aid effectiveness principles at the country level. Significant progress has been already been made in some areas. For instance, the Paris Declaration evaluation found that many donors have increased their alignment of high level policies with partners' national development plans, medium-term expenditure strategies and budgets [31]. Some countries have also made remarkable progress towards country ownership. For example, the Government of Vietnam successfully set out a policy framework to manage donor money. This was achieved through a broad consultative process (which included civil society and international partners), which meant it was widely owned and supported by the donors, which consequently facilitated donor alignment [20]. Similarly, progress has been made on domestic capacity development to manage DAH, most notably in improved financial management (although there have been mixed results on the reduction of parallel project implementation units). Pooled aid instruments such as MDTFs and implementation arrangements are being increasingly used in a wide variety of environments, particularly in post-conflict settings.

However, progress is uneven across countries and donors and concerns remain. In part this simply reflects the real personal, cultural and institutional change that these principles demand of donor employees, donors, and their financiers. These new approaches need to be implemented by individuals who have varying degrees of interest, understanding, and commitment to the substantial institutional changes demanded. The internal structure of donors often needs to be revised; sometimes reducing the role of donor staff with sector specific expertise. Signing up to an international agreement is rarely sufficient. It takes time and commitment to embark on a concerted effort to sell these principles within (often large and disparate) donor institutions.

Even where donors have succeeded, structures are in place and staff orientated, incentivized, and motivated by the aid effectiveness agenda, much skill and judgement is required to guide DAH delivery at the country level. There is no blueprint available—nor should there be. While much has been made of the positive experiences in countries like Tanzania and Vietnam, there are more mixed (and arguably more realistic) experiences of the application of aid effectiveness principles in more challenging environments. Donor coordination can be difficult, different interests do not always neatly coincide, and there is an inherent tension between achieving one's own goals and slowing down to accommodate the views of all. Country ownership is an admirable objective, but compromise is often required. Even embarking on the first step—the joint development of National Health Plan—can require careful navigation between donor expectations and requirements and domestic capacity to produce the plan. Organizing donor engagement with governments can also present dilemmas: for example, while it may be beneficial to include all donors in joint DAH planning, this may result in meetings where national representatives become rapidly outnumbered. Promoting the management of aid through joint procurement mechanisms sounds achievable, but may take years for those new to them to master. Public finance reform may take substantially longer. Moreover, although the aim of the Paris declaration was primarily to reduce transactions costs for recipients, much of this has to take place in a context where donors are trying to reduce their own transactions costs.

Finally, it should not be assumed that following and applying aid effectiveness principles are sufficient for health system development. At best, they merely provide an enabling environment for the effective financing of core health sector functions. Consistent domestic, donor and technical support is often required. Proponents of health systems development, on the one hand, may also need to make compromises in the broader context of macroeconomic growth and stability; and, on the other, accept that health sector strategic plans and expenditure frameworks may remain developed, structured, and focused along the lines of vertical health programme outcomes for some time to come. As financing for health system development increases, so too will the pressure to demonstrate overall health sector improvement. Success is not guaranteed, and failures may renew the case for more targeted and externally controlled forms of aid. Governments may still not be willing to absorb and complement the high level of funding required to build systems quickly, they simply may have other priorities. But in spite of all the obstacles, the alternative, of failing to tackle head-on these deep-seated development finance issues, will mean that the limited, short-term and patchwork development of health systems (and services) in low- and middle-income countries will remain with us for many years to come.

References

1 Ravishankar N, Gubbins P, Cooley RJ, *et al.* (2009). Financing of global health: tracking development assistance for health from 1990 to 2007. *Lancet*, **373**(9681), 2113–24.

2 Powell-Jackson T, Mills Mills A (2007). A review of health resource tracking in developing countries. *Health Policy and Planning*, **22**(6), 353–62.

3 Dreher A (2010). *Are 'New' Donors Different? Comparing the allocation of bilateral aid between Non-DAC and DAC donor countries.* Kiel Working Papers, Kiel Institute for the World Economy, Kiel.

4 Taskforce on Innovative Financing for Health Systems Working Group (2009) *Taskforce on Innovative Financing for Health Systems Working Group 1 Report.* Available at: www.internationalhealthpartnership.net.

5 Institute for Health Metrics and Evaluation (2009). *Financing Global Health 2009.* University of Washington, Seattle, WA.

6 Shiffman J, Berlan D, Hafner T (2009). Has aid for AIDS raised all health funding boats? *Journal of Acquired Immune Deficiency Syndromes* **52**(Suppl 1), S45–S48.

7 Greco G, Powell Jackson T, Borghi, J, Mills A (2008). Countdown to 2015: assessment of donor assistance to maternal, newborn, and child health between 2003 and 2006. *Lancet*, **371**, 1268–75.

8 Patel P, Roberts B, Guy S, Lee-Jones L, Conteh L (2009). Tracking official development assistance for reproductive health in conflict-affected countries. *PLoS Medicine*, **6**(6), e1000090.

9 Bourguignon F, Sundberg M (2007). Aid effectiveness – opening the black box. *American Economic Review,* **97**(2), 316–21.

10 World Bank/UNICEF/UNFPA/Partnership for Maternal, Newborn and Child Health (2009). *Health Systems for the Millennium Development Goals: Country Needs and Funding Gaps. Background Document for the Taskforce on Innovative International Financing for Health Systems, in Working Group 1: Constraints to Scaling Up and Costs.* United Nations, New York.

11 Taskforce on Innovative Financing for Health Systems (2009). *More money for health, and more health for the money.* www.internationalhealthpartnership.net

12 Frot E, Santiso J (2010). *Crushed aid: Fragmentation in sectoral aid.* OECD Development Centre, Paris.

13 Djankov S, Montalvo JG, Reynal-Querol M (2009). Aid with multiple personalities. *Journal of Comparative Economics*, **37**(2), 217–29.

14 Acharya A, Fuzzon de Lima AT, Moore M (2006). Proliferation and fragmentation: transaction costs and the value of aid. *Journal of Development Studies*, **42**(1), 1–21.

15 Pearson M (2008). *IHP+: Expanding predicable finance for health systems strengthening and delivering results.* HLSP, London.

16 WHO Maximising Positive Synergies Collaborative Group (2009). An assessment of interactions between global health initiatives and country health systems. *Lancet*, **373**, 2137–69.

17 Levine R (2009). Global HIV/AIDS funding and health systems: Searching for the win-win. *Journal of Acquired Immune Deficiency Syndromes*, **52**(Suppl 1), S3–S5.

18 Spicer N, Aleshkina J, Biesma R, *et al* (2010) National and subnational HIV/AIDS coordination: are global health intiatives closing the gap between intent and practice? *Global Health*, **6**, 3.

19 Pearson M. *Cambodia: does disease-targeted funding help or hinder the development of systems?*

20 World Health Organization (2006). *The World Health Report 2006 – Working together for health.* World Health Organization, Geneva.

21 Waddington C (2004). Does earmarked donor funding make it more or less likely that developing countries will allocate their resources towards programmes that yield the greatest health benefits? *Bulletin of the World Health Organization*, **82**(9), 703–6; discussion 706–8.

22 Lu C, Schneider MT, Gubbins P, Leach-Kemon K, Jamison D, Murray CJL (2010). Public financing of health in developing countries: a cross-national systematic analysis. *Lancet*, **376**(9741), 592–3.

23 Pettersson J (2007). Foreign sectoral aid fungibility, growth and poverty reduction. *Journal of International Development*, **19**(8), 1074–98.

24 Jones K (2005). Moving money: aid fungibility in Africa. *SAIS Review*, XXV(2), 167–80.

25 Lancaster C (1999). Aid Effectiveness in Africa: The unfinished agenda. *Journal of African Economics,* **8**(4), 487–503.

26 Farag M, Nandakumar AK, Wallack SS, Gaumer G, Hodgkin D (2009). Does funding from donors displace government spending for health in developing countries? *Health Affairs*, **28**(4), 1045–55.

27 Sridhar D, Woods N (2010). Are there simple conclusions on how to channel health funding? *Lancet*, **375**(9723), 1326–8.

28 Ooms G, Decoster K, Miti K, *et al.* (2010). Crowding out: are relations between international health aid and government health funding too complex to be captured in averages only? *Lancet*, **375**(9723), 1403–5.

29 Stuckler D, Basu S, and McKee M (2011). International Monetary Fund and aid displacement. *Int J Health Serv*, **41**(1), 67–76.

30 Lewis M (2006). *Tackling Healthcare Corruption and Governance Woes in Developing Countries.* Center for Global Development, Washington, DC. Available at: www.cgdev.org.

31 OECD (2009) *Aid Effectiveness: A Progress Report on Implementing the Paris Declaration.* OECD, Paris.

32 Marshall J, Ofei-Aboagye E (2004). *Donors and childhood poverty in sub Saharan Africa: Approaches and aid mechanisms in Ghana and Tanzania.* Childhood Poverty Research and Policy Centre, London.

33 Doucouliagos H, Paldam M (2008). Aid effectiveness on growth: a meta study. *European Journal of Political Economy*, **24**(1), 1–24.

34 Foster M, Leavy J (2001). *The Choice of Financial Aid Instruments.* Overseas Development Institute, London.

35 Leader N, Colenso P (2005). Aid instruments in fragile states. In *Poverty Reduction in Difficult Environments* (Working Paper 5). UK Department for International Development, London.

36 Quartey P (2005). Innovative ways of making aid effective in Ghana: tied aid versus direct budgetary support. *Journal of International Development*, **17**(8), 1077–92.

37 NORAD (2008). *Support Models for CSOs at Country Level*. Norwegian Agency for Development Cooperation, Oslo.

38 World Bank (2001). *Education and Health in Sub-Saharan Africa: A Review of Sector-Wide Approaches*. Africa Region Human Development Series. World Bank, Washington, DC.

39 Ouattara B (2007). Foreign aid, public savings displacement and aid dependency in Cote d'Ivoire: an aid disaggregation approach. *Oxford Development Studies*, **35**(1), 33–46.

40 IHP (2009). *International Financing Mechanisms to Support Health Systems Strengthening: Multi Donor Trust Funds (MDTFs)*, International Health Partnership, Washington, DC. Available at: www.internationalhealthpartnership.net

41 Carter R, Lister S (2007). Budget support: as good as the strategy it finances. In Pallares L (ed) *Social Watch Report 2007 In dignity and rights*, pp.62–7. Social Watch, Uruguay.

42 Piva P, Dodd R (2009). Where did all the aid go? An in-depth analysis of increased health aid flows over the past 10 years. *Bulletin of the World Health Organization*, **87**(12), 930–9.

43 IHP (2009). *International Financing Mechanisms to Support Health Systems Strengthening. European Commission: MDG Contracts and General Budget Support*. International Health Partnership, Washington, DC. www.internationalhealthpartnership.net

Chapter 10

The health system and wider social determinants of health

Rene Loewenson and Lucy Gilson

10.1 Introduction

Health is an outcome of the circumstances of people's lives, the communities and environments in which people live and work, the nature of the social relationships, goods and services people encounter, and the choices people make around these conditions [1].

In this chapter we identify these influences over the distribution of health and well-being across population groups, countries, and regions. We outline models used to summarize and explain the social determinants of health. Further, we consider the types of interventions and actions that must be taken outside the health sector to improve the distribution of health and well-being, and what that implies for the role of the health sector within the wider health system. In some aspects, the chapter draws on the learning from the work in the World Health Organization (WHO) Commission of the Social Determinants of Health (CSDH), and particularly the Health Systems Knowledge network of the CSDH [2], and the learning and analysis from work in the Regional Network for Equity in Health in East and Southern Africa (EQUINET) [3].

10.2 Understanding the distribution and determinants of health

The variations in the conditions in which people grow, live, and work enable some people to lead long and healthy lives, and undermine these chances for others. Table 10.1 illustrates the associations between social determinants health and health equity outcomes.

Populations disadvantaged along one or more of these determinants are often both heavily burdened by disease, whilst also having poor access to health services. There is debate about whether interventions that aim to improve the distribution of household health and well-being should focus on improving the health of the poorest groups in society, should narrow the gap between

Table 10.1 Examples of influences of social determinants on health and health equity

Social determinant	Examples	Source
Social position, gender, ethnicity	Life expectancy at birth is lower for indigenous Australians than for Australians generally	[5–7]
	Social, political, and civil rights in Nordic countries in the 19th century were an important contributor to health improvements across social groups	
	Raising the health status of people lower in the social hierarchy improves overall health	
Occupation and income and working conditions	Maternal mortality, infant mortality, and uptake of health services varies by income group in high- and low-income countries	[2,8]
Education, including early child education and care; literacy	Experiences in early childhood and education affect health throughout the life course. Investments in early child development have the largest effects on the most deprived children	[2,8–10]
	Maternal education is associated with improved health outcomes and health care uptake in women and children	
	Education attainment is associated with adult income, employment and living conditions, and improved health outcomes	
Material circumstances: living conditions, community environments	Underinvestment in rural infrastructure and amenities leads to poverty, poor health outcomes and outmigration into insecure urban environments; informal and concentrated low income urban settlements are associated with a cluster of non communicable disease, violence, and drug use, increasing injury and mortality	[2,11]
	Differences in morbidity and mortality outcomes across countries and social groups are associated with food and employment insecurity; poor access to safe water, sanitation, energy, transport, and shelter.	
Employment and working conditions	Temporary workers on insecure contracts have higher illness and mortality than permanent workers	[12,13]
	Poor working conditions and work related stress associated with increased risk of coronary heart disease; mental ill health, with effects of poor quality work almost as large as loss of work	
Health care and social protection systems	Absolute mortality in disadvantaged people is lower in countries with more generous, universal social protection schemes.	[6,14,15]
	Social protection schemes mitigate globalization-related economic shocks and insecurity limiting negative health outcomes	
	Health systems organized on the basis of universal coverage and primary health care can close inequalities in health, even in the absence of wider economic improvements	

groups, or should aim to close the gradient across social groups [4]. In this chapter we argue for policies that close the gradient, while also paying attention to the specific measures needed to reach disadvantaged groups. This is because programmes targeted directly at poor people can play a constructive role in meeting their greater needs, as long as they do not become the sole form of action, are located within the framework of wider universal social protection, and do not obscure the need to address the wider structural determinants of health and health inequality.

While much epidemiology has been preoccupied with establishing the immediate factors that produce ill health (e.g. water, food, work environments), attention has increasingly turned to the social structures and systems that shape people's chances to be healthy. A number of factors are driving this. Opportunities for health have grown, but so too have inequalities in access to those opportunities and in health outcomes. Knowing the risk factors for ill health in individuals has not been sufficient to understand or change the distribution of health in *populations*. Further, as the burdens of non-communicable disease, the expectations of improved quality of life and the costs of personal medical care have all increased, so too has the demand to understand what helps people stay *healthy,* rather than focussing exclusively on what makes them ill. Moving upstream then, to understand and act on the structural drivers of ill health, is necessary if we are to create the conditions for health. As the report of the Commission on the Social Determinants of Health explains it: 'Poor and unequal living conditions are, in their turn, the consequence of deeper structural conditions that together fashion the way societies are organized – poor social policies and programmes, unfair economic arrangements and bad politics' [2; p.26].

The different conceptual frameworks discussed below demonstrate a progressively deepening understanding of the complexity of pathways between the social determinants of health and health outcomes.

Mackenbach et al. [16] outlined the lifestyle, environmental, and psychosocial stress-related factors that are intermediaries between socioeconomic position and health problems. In an analysis of data from 22 European countries, for example, mortality rates and poorer self-assessments of health were substantially higher in lower socioeconomic groups, and the magnitude of the health inequalities between socioeconomic groups in different countries could be explained by the influence of lifestyle factors of smoking or alcohol use [17]. Such analysis established associations between socioeconomic status, more immediate social determinants, and health outcomes, without seeking to show the network of relationships across different social determinants [18]. The work suggested that although offering important health and other gains in

Europe, the welfare state had not eliminated socioeconomic inequalities, and that these were associated with particular lifestyle and environmental factors that lead to inequalities in health outcomes. This argument that the universal social protection schemes of the welfare state were insufficient to close inequalities was used to motivate specific, targeted actions for disadvantaged groups. The Acheson report [19] added further to this analysis to explore the manner in which genetic, early life and culture factors mediate these relationships across the life course.

The work of Mackenbach and others elucidates the social determinants that lie between socioeconomic position and health outcomes and gives valuable information on immediate determinants for design of health interventions. However, this analysis does not explain the structural determinants of these outcomes. A recent review of evidence from east and southern Africa, for example, looks further upstream to explore whether improved economic growth translates into improved health outcomes [8]. As shown in Figure 10.1, in many countries economic growth translates poorly into improvements in human development (life expectancy, literacy, and income per capita). This weak and often inverse relationship points to the fact that the benefits of growth are not distributed to disadvantaged groups through the usual routes of employment, education, gender equity, food security, access to safe water and to healthcare, and that in each

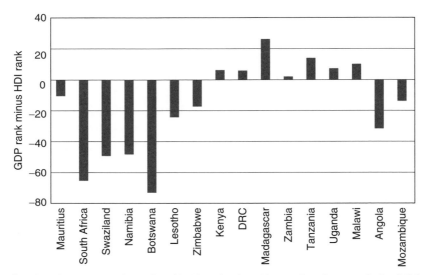

Fig. 10.1 Gross Domestic Product (GDP) rank minus Human Development Index (HDI) rank for ESA countries, 2004 (negative bars signal that countries perform relatively poorly on HDI relative to GDP).
Source: UNDP 2005 data analysed in [8]. Reproduced from EQUINET Steering Committee (2007). Reclaiming the resources for health: A regional analysis of equity in health in east and southern Africa. EQUINET Weaver Press, Harare with permission from EQUINET.

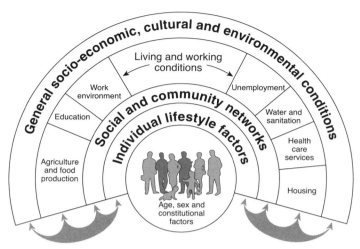

Fig. 10.2 The 'rainbow' model of determinants of health.
Source: Dahlgren and Whitehead, 2007 [21]. Reproduced with permission from
Dahlgren and Whitehead, 1993, easily accessible in Dahlgren and Whitehead, 2007.

country these pathways need to be better understood to explain the deeper structural drivers of differences in health outcomes.

Health outcomes appear to be associated with determinants that go beyond individual socioeconomic characteristics. Studies report, for example, that even after adjusting for individual level factors, including socioeconomic status, the socioeconomic characteristics of the environment people live in (e.g. neighbourhood) can have an independent effect on health [20].

Dahlgren and Whitehead's model [21], shown in Figure 10.2, presents a multi-layered model of determinants that shows the different levels and types of social factors and social processes that interact to influence the social stratification that determines health opportunity. The model draws attention to more distal or upstream determinants of health, and is a useful analysis for health promotion, to point to the changes in the socioeconomic environment needed to enable people to make healthy choices. Similar models across levels and factors have been applied to understand the relationships between national policies, food security, and nutrition outcomes, to identify the spectrum of policy and programme interventions to improve child nutrition, for example [22], or to understand the determinants of HIV to inform the behavioural and biomedical interventions that reduce susceptibility to HIV infection and the changes to risk environments that are needed to support them [23,24].

The ways in which health can be protected through action across sectors and levels of determinants even in times of economic crisis, is shown by experience from Thailand. In the economic crisis of 1997 onwards, policy responses were applied at national, sectoral, and household level, within and beyond the health sector. Government health and education expenditure held steady and spending on social safety nets was increased. The low income Health Card Scheme that gave free access to health services was extended to the newly unemployed, and government subsidies for the Voluntary Health Card Scheme were increased. Scholarships were introduced for children who dropped out of school, vouchers were issued to children in private schools to keep them enrolled and the education loan program was expanded for the children of the unemployed [25]. Despite the economic shocks, therefore, the Thai under five mortality rate *fell* by 44% among the poorest income groups over the 1990s and by 13% among the richest [26]. At the same time, the actions taken maintained effective control of the AIDS epidemic, even in an economically difficult period [25].

The WHO CSDH conceptual framework, the most recent synthesis of this hierarchy of 'causes of causes', makes connections between global and national 'drivers' and the immediate circumstances of daily life that affect health (Figure 10.3). The model includes the structural and intermediate determinants that reflect, or generate social *stratification* (e.g. income, education, gender, ethnicity). It integrates differences in exposure and vulnerability to conditions that boost or compromise health (e.g. social cohesion, material

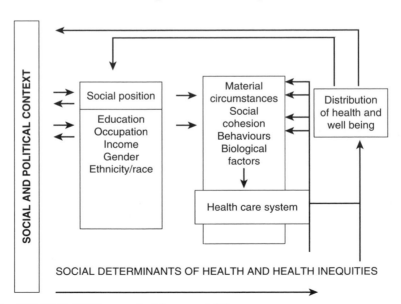

Fig. 10.3 WHO CSDH conceptual framework [2].
Source: Reproduced from [2] with permission of the World Health Organization.

circumstances). It is concerned not just with determinants of health, but of health *equity,* including the health sector. The latter, encompassing the organizations, people, and actions whose primary intent is to promote, restore, or maintain health [27], is an intermediate determinant of health itself, affected by other determinants, as discussed in more detail later. The CSDH framework attempts to go beyond the circumstances of daily life to explore the pathways that link these to the structural drivers of the social stratification associated with health outcomes, including social norms, global policies, and the distribution of power and governance processes from local to global level.

This is important as globalization has had increasing effect on other social determinants, through effects on power, resources, labour markets, policy space, trade, financial flows, and access to essential services and inputs for health (as outlined in other chapters in this volume). By incorporating the pathways linking globalization to health outcomes, the CSDH model widens our understanding of the social determinants of health [14].

The CSDH points to the social processes and power differentials that make a difference to health outcomes [2]. Studies suggest, for example, that social support and power differentials within communities are an important determinant of how and whether available resources are allocated to and reach households and individuals affected by AIDS [23,24]. In southern Africa, where AIDS has dominated the health profile in the past two decades, HIV infection spreads from more socially and economically powerful adult males to poor and economically insecure females, particularly female adolescents [28,29]. The HIV prevalence in young women aged 15–24 years is currently more than twice that of their male counterparts throughout the region [30]. At the same time studies have found, under the generic term 'social cohesion', a range of 'protective' characteristics of communities that have been associated with lower susceptibility to HIV and vulnerability to AIDS [23,24,31].

The relationships between social determinants and health are thus not fixed across time or place, but are shaped, and confronted, by societal and political processes. This includes the extent to which there is procedural justice, so that decisions over resources are made through processes that are transparent, accessible to and inclusive of the input of those affected by them [32].

There is just critique that analytic models and health research have yet to adequately and explicitly capture and portray issues of individual and collective power as a social determinant of health [33]. Nonetheless, as we discuss later in this chapter, work in this area is expanding, and attention is being given to understanding and implementing measures that build the power and ability people (and social groups) have to make choices over health inputs and to use these choices towards health, such as through rights frameworks [8,34].

In sum, this section highlights the range of social determinants that influence household health and well-being, indicating examples of social position, gender, ethnicity; occupation and income; education, material circumstances, employment, healthcare, and social protection systems. The conceptual models show how these arise at different levels, through pathways that become more complex the more upstream, or structural the determinant. Later in this chapter we discuss how health sectors, both as a determinant themselves, and through their organization, functioning and leadership, can engage with these wider determinants of health, and how they can create conditions for people to be empowered in the way they do this.

10.3 Health in all policies: actions outside the health sector to improve equity in health

The social determinants highlighted in the previous section, and the persistence of a 'vicious circle' between poverty and poor health, demonstrates the importance of linking the activities of the health sector with those of other sectors such as education, housing, water and sanitation, labour, public works, transportation, agriculture, environment, and industry.

Whether individually, or through collaborative intersectoral action between different departments and bodies within government, sectors such as agriculture, culture, education, employment, environment, finance, housing, information and communications, justice, manufacturing and technology, and transport services can have an important positive impact on health (as shown in relation to nutrition, in Box 10.1). Thus, in Sri Lanka, for example, Ministry of Health efforts to control sexually transmitted and vector-borne diseases were supported by actions of the education and public broadcasting sectors (through health education at schools and on radio), the water and sanitation sectors (reducing vector breeding through environmental controls), the tourism sector (through health education to tourists and workers in industry) and the transport sector (through providing an extensive road network and cheap public transport to ensure access to health services) [35].

The integration of health across sectors is not only an issue for low income countries. In high income countries promotion of sustainable production, marketing and distribution of health foods promotes healthy nutrition in all age groups. As an example, the local Public Health institute, the Centre for Health and Development, in Pomurje region in Slovenia, one of the most deprived regions in Slovenia, worked with farmers to support organic farming, negotiated amendments to procurement practices of public institutions to support demand for locally produced foods, integrated demand for organic

Box 10.1 Inter-sectoral action for food security and nutrition

Food availability, access, intake, and dietary choices and patterns affect health outcomes. These determinants have been increasingly affected by markets and the actions of large corporates involved in the manufacture and marketing of food. For east and southern Africa, where levels of underweight children are commonly above 20%, the agricultural and trade policies have a significant bearing on health, especially for the lowest income groups who have up to 2.6 times higher levels of chronic undernutrition than those with the highest incomes [36], and in a context of worsening household food security [37].

It is argued that nutrition would be improved by prioritizing food production for domestic and local markets, promoting women's role in food production and supporting equitable access to productive resources [38]. Women, although responsible for 80% of food production in Africa, own less than 1% of land and access less than 10% of credit provided to small farmers. Health surveys have found improvements in women's productivity to be associated with improved childhood nutritional status [37].

By 2004, the scale of food insecurity and malnutrition led the Ministers of Agriculture in the Southern African Development Community (SADC) to propose policies for improved nutrition through measures in their sectors that support to household production and local marketing, including: promoting equal access for men and women, as well as child-headed households, to land, credit, technology, and other key agricultural inputs and supporting empowerment of women [39]. Added to this, the regulation, labelling and marketing of food has been noted to affect dietary patterns, while involvement of community networks and community level services enhance the likelihood that support for food production, home gardens and relief reach the families that most need them [40,41].

foods in the tourism sector and carried out extensive promotion of healthy nutrition. The intervention was associated with significant improvements in food preparation and dietary patterns and a reduction in ischaemic heart disease in the region compared to the rest of the country [42].

The action of different sectors in health not only brings material resources and services to communities in disadvantaged areas, it also has the potential to intervene in the asymmetries of power related to gender, wealth, and social status that influence health outcomes, discussed earlier. For example, a series of six field studies in Asia, Africa, and South America found that the gender related determinants of susceptibility to HIV could be addressed by open dialogue between individuals and their parents and partners, shared decision-making between partners, young women's access to training, job opportunities, employment, and decent work reduced susceptibility [24,43]. Interventions that promote these outcomes have been campaigned for by social movements of people living with HIV (PLWHA), with some degree of success at national and global level, and are recognized in UNAIDS' 'combination prevention' approach [24,44].

The range of intersectoral actions identified by the CSDH as necessary to promote health equity includes action on the physical, social, emotional and cognitive nourishment of children in early life, shown to have positive impact throughout the life course; quality housing, clean water and sanitation in cohesive community environments, particularly in growing urban populations; secure employment in decent working conditions; and redistributive welfare and health systems [2]. But what forms might such integrated and co-ordinated action across sectors take and how can it be leveraged?

Table 10.2 summarizes the four main approaches to intersectoral action identified from experience, also providing brief comments on the key challenges, and some specific examples, of each. These approaches may reflect different levels of intersectoral action, from information sharing, to coordination and cooperation across sectors, to integration of health goals within the policies and actions of other sectors. Coordinated action across sectors becomes more complex and harder to achieve at higher levels of government, given territorial competitiveness and the growing numbers of actors involved [45]. More focused institutional entry points, such as in the healthy schools programme, provide opportunities for managing this complexity in different settings. More commonly, success stories of IAH tend to be documented at the local level, where the smaller, more human scale allows for closer ties among participants in local projects; policy-makers live where they work so they are more accountable for their decisions; and bureaucratic structures are smaller and relatively more accessible. However, successful local action can also promote effective higher-level action with wider and longer-term impacts on population health by addressing the structural causes of ill health—such as through fiscal interventions like tobacco and alcohol taxation. Commitments made to international conventions, such as those on the WHO Framework Convention on Tobacco Control, have also been useful to encourage collaborative alliances and actions around priority areas within and across countries.

The available experience of IAH also suggests that there is often a central role for Ministries of Health in at least initiating and monitoring, if not also

Table 10.2 Approaches to intersectoral action for heath (IAH)

IAH Approach	Examples
Targeted approaches focusing on a specific population or issue, given resource constraints and a desire for visible or timely results. But danger of taking a narrow focus on downstream issues, with potential to duplicate efforts	Programmes for indigenous peoples or for out of school youth National tobacco strategies or campaigns on breast milk substitutes
Place-based approaches at local level, facilitating horizontal engagement and offering tangible results. But can be complex and may require sustained support by wide range of actors.	WHO Healthy Communities/Healthy Cities initiative; UK's Health Action Zones. Informal settlement programmes Healthy schools programme
Incremental approaches on a large scale, based on review of evidence on sectoral policies and choices. But longer timescale makes them vulnerable to vagaries of political support.	Water, Sanitation and Health Protection within the Human Environment initiative
Broad policy frameworks that can be adopted by governments as a whole to guide policy-making within and across sectors, towards shared goals. But demand considerable time and resource investment and vulnerable to political reversal	Europe's National Environment and Health Action Plan. Sweden's Public Health Strategy.

managing policies, programmes, and collaboration across sectors [45]. Concern for, and evidence on, population health, together with analysis of the multi-factoral determinants of ill-health, gives the health sector a clear mandate and the necessary skills to participate in IAH. The responsibilities of Ministers of Health in this regard become particularly important when their Cabinet's support for IAH is limited. Engaging in this pivotal role involves making the public case for IAH, building a shared vision of the importance of health equity and IAH, such as through strategic use of evidence, and working strategically to secure the support of other sectors for it [15]. For example, Sweden's National Public Health Strategy in 2003 was underpinned by 19 background papers, commissioned from expert groups, which provided credibility for an IAH-centred strategy. It mobilized a multi-disciplinary research approach to health determinants involving the research community from different disciplines [46]. In Chile, epidemiological information profiled the social determinants of health, thereby encouraging intersectoral solutions to health problems (around family violence and housing for poor families, for example) as well as strengthening support for the PHC approach. In Europe,

Health Impact Assessments and performance reviews of sectoral policies are becoming more commonplace, raising awareness of the social determinants of health [45]. Such periodic assessments, complemented by information from public health surveillance systems, are vital to resource allocation and planning of health sector interventions, but also to engage and monitor interventions in other sectors, and to build and sustain political commitment and alliances.

Health sector personnel often have a catalytic, rather than an, implementing role in these processes. This calls for strategic skills; to identify opportunities and threats and integrate health goals within wider social and economic policies, to manage competition and build mutual trust between government departments; to organize support from the finance sector, to build connections between sectors and different levels of government and to bring in relevant actors at appropriate points in the process [15]. Successfully done, as shown in Sweden in the 1990s [46], this can build momentum for and institutionalize IAH, particularly if it garners support from political leaders, the media and community.

Initiatives that cross sectors or that integrate measures for health in policies and budgets of other sectors are reported to be more likely to be sustained over time when: goals are clear and shared, mutual benefits are perceived, capacities exist to implement and assess initiatives and to manage complex communication and negotiation processes, and where decision-making authority rests with those responsible for implementing such action [45]. In addition the longer term stability of integrated action appears to be more likely where:

- Health impact assessment and integration moves from a voluntary to a mandatory requirement (such as through legislation).
- Arrangements and responsibilities to facilitate ongoing dialogue across sectors are institutionalized (such as through boards and sectoral clusters).
- Financial provisions, budgets and accountability frameworks are organized to provide performance incentives for integration of health goals in other sectors and for participation in IAH.

The decision to act on unfair differentials in health is finally, primarily sociopolitical, driven by the norms and interests of society and their expression in the state. Influencing the sociopolitical environment through evidence, awareness, debate and alliances may be critical if such policies are to weather political change.

10.4 Health systems that act on the social determinants of health and improve the distribution of household health and well-being

The previous section refers to the leadership role of the health sector in building action across sectors to address the social determinants of health inequity.

However, the health system itself also acts as a social determinant of health and health equity, as portrayed in Figure 10.4. The solid arrows show how health inequity results from a mal-distribution of power, whereas the dotted arrows show how a progressive health system can mitigate these effects [15].

Every health system both reflects existing patterns of social inequality and provides a site from which to contest them [47]. As shown in Figure 10.4, adopting a primary healthcare (PHC) approach within the health system, as an organizational strategy and underlying philosophy, strengthens its positive role as a social determinant [48]. PHC-oriented health systems act first, to promote population health and address differential exposure and vulnerability to ill health through the types of intersectoral action already discussed. Second, health system investments in strategies for social empowerment can have direct influences over social cohesion and social stratification [49]. Third, through their financing and provision arrangements they can both modify the impact of differential exposure and vulnerability on health inequity [50], and tackle differential access, use and experience of healthcare [51,52]. As a major national employer, public health systems also influence their employees' lives, and specifically women [53], through workforce structures and practices. Health systems may even be influential in building and sustaining societal and political support for governments that promote health equity [35,54]. They can thus address the circumstances of disadvantaged populations and generate wider benefits: a sense of life security, well-being, social cohesion, and confident expectation of care in times of illness.

However, health systems often fail to realize this positive potential (e.g. China [55] and the United States [56]) and may perpetuate injustice and social stratification. The layers of sociopolitical forces underpinning these failures start with the norms and practices embedded within health systems, which often work against heath equity. Gender discrimination within the workforce contributes to gender inequities, for example, by: generating gaps in the services needed by women; failing to support the critically important community-based activities undertaken by women; and sustaining interpersonal interactions that challenge patient dignity and autonomy [57].

Health system policies that have increased cost, geographical or technical barriers to care, focused on individual curative care at the expense of the promotion of population health and/or prevention of disease, or that have weak opportunities for engagement with civil society, have heightened access barriers for disadvantaged groups, increasing the impoverishment and social stratification [8,15]. Such policies have, moreover, been entrenched by the macro-economic policies and neo-liberal health sector reforms that have dominated recent health system development in many countries, driven by

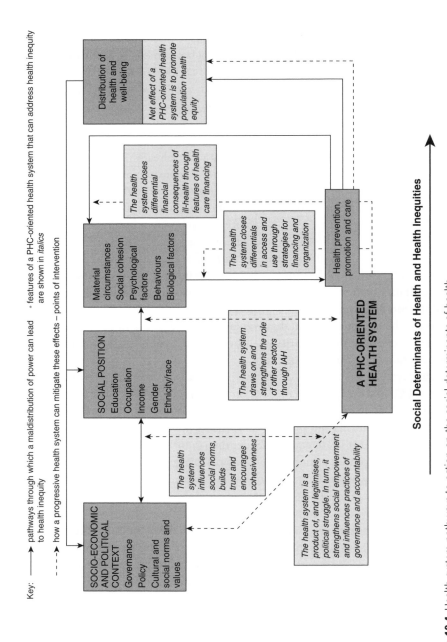

Fig. 10.4 Health system pathways to action on the social determinants of health.
Source: Reproduced from [15] with permission.

international agencies, commercial actors and higher income and medical groups [58]. These are reflected in, for example, fees charged for public health services, and the internal and international migration of scarce human resources from poor to wealthier communities [59].

We argue that for health systems to act as a positive social determinant of health and health equity, four sets of actions are critical:

1 Financing and provision arrangements that recognize the right to health, aim at universal coverage and redistribute resources towards poorer groups with greater health needs.

2 Empowering population groups and involving them and their organizations (particularly those working with socially disadvantaged and marginalized groups) in decisions and actions on health, including those that identify, address and allocate resources to health needs.

3 Building or revitalizing the comprehensive primary healthcare approach as a strategy that reinforces and integrates these and other health equity-promoting features.

4 Ensuring the wider political action needed to introduce and sustain this comprehensive primary healthcare approach.

5 Health for all: the right to health and universal coverage.

Our growing understanding of the social determinants of health encompasses an understanding of the Right to Health as more than just about rights to healthcare, but also as concerning rights to the underlying determinants of health [60] and to sustainable health systems based on equity and social justice [61]. Internationally, the Right to Health imposes four obligations on states: to respect, protect, promote and fulfil the enjoyment of the right to health. The last obligation means taking positive measures to ensure that a right is met, recognizing that the current, limited availability of resources may require the 'progressive realization of the right'. In other words, even if government cannot afford to ensure or provide a level of provisioning for water, food security, shelter or form of healthcare now, it must, over time, take measures to ensure that it will, in future, be able to provide this [34].

This understanding of entitlements to the determinants of health and healthcare implies that health systems should be organized on the basis of universal coverage. In such systems everyone within a country can access the same range of services on the basis of need and pays for these services on the basis of their income. Deliberate efforts are, however, still needed to ensure that socially marginalized groups really do have access to effective health services. These include efforts to widen geographic access, reduce transport cost barriers, and improve referral linkages between primary and secondary levels; as well as making public services more acceptable, particularly for women and marginalized groups. These actions will, in turn, require re-allocation of the available tax funding between populations and areas relative to need. Four other core principles of universal systems are that: public funding plays a central role in their financing, no or very low fees are charged for public services, a comprehensive package of services is provided and policy and regulatory action is taken to ensure that the private sector serves, rather than undermines, redistributive goals [15].

Achieving universal coverage will inevitably be a long-term goal for most countries, and the set of feasible policy actions necessary to move towards it will vary between settings and across time frames. These issues are also considered in greater detail in other chapters of this book. Implementation of the policy actions also depends on how far social and civil society pressure levers and reinforces them.

10.6 Social empowerment within and through the actions of health systems

Social empowerment refers to the ability of people to act collectively on many reciprocal levels in different domains [62]. Not only are disempowerment and social exclusion themselves social determinants of health, but social support and power differentials within communities are also important determinants of how and whether available resources are allocated to and reach households and individuals. The CSDH notes, for example, that one of its three pillars of action is to 'Tackle the inequitable distribution of power, money and resources – the structural drivers of those conditions of daily life- globally, nationally and locally' [2; p.43].

Health systems can, through their processes and organization, reinforce or address the inequitable distribution of power by strengthening or ignoring the collective ability of people to act on health [63]. However, their ability to do this depends on the broader context [64]. Stable, egalitarian sociopolitical contexts, organized and capable civil society, and social networks and social conditions that promote collective claims to social rights have, for example, facilitated social participation [35,54,65]. Approaches for strengthening social empowerment must, thus, be context-specific, taking into account of the nature of the relationships between the state and society and the underpinning values, norms and political culture.

Nonetheless, available experience suggests that health systems interventions have in the past strengthened social empowerment when they have:

◆ Promoted better health through building the collective capability of individuals and social groups to act on the structural determinants of health, or by encouraging greater healthcare use.

- Addressed health inequity by generating preferential gains for socially disadvantaged groups either by impacting on the structural factors that disadvantage these groups (such as women's autonomy) or by strengthening the ability of these groups to claim health resources or implement health actions.
- Enhanced psychological empowerment and autonomy, particularly in disadvantaged groups [64–66].

As a first step towards social empowerment, social mobilization strategies have encompassed activities aimed at increasing social awareness of health and health systems, strengthening health literacy, and enhancing social capacities to take health actions. They include increasing citizen's access to information and resources through community monitoring and information campaigns, involving population groups in priority-setting for planning and involving disadvantaged and, marginalized groups in strengthening specific healthcare programmes [66]. Such strategies can improve the performance of health systems and population health outcomes, especially in relation to health promotion and public health activities [65].

However, acting on social determinants and influencing the distribution of power and resources needs more than social mobilization. It calls for greater autonomy and participation in decision-making, and greater control over the resources for health, particularly by relatively powerless groups who also bear the burden of health problems in every society. To facilitate this deeper level of social empowerment and to promote equity, central and local government structures, including Ministries of Health, must provide opportunities for disadvantaged and marginalized groups to engage in decisions on health and facilitate such input by making health systems more responsive to need. They could achieve this by establishing rights to information for the public and funding mechanisms to enable direct participation in decision-making by population groups. Enhanced relationships and communication between health workers and the population are also important to social empowerment. Civil society organizations, on the other hand, need to facilitate social processes and population-led action, including those which expose and redress power imbalances that harm opportunities for health in disadvantaged groups. This inevitably takes time, resources, leadership, and must be sensitive to local contexts [65]. The processes for empowerment can be supported by tools and methods, but cannot be reduced to these; and any experience or method from elsewhere needs to be 'recreated' in the context of the political values, systems, and institutions within different societies and settings. This makes the exchange of information through learning and mentoring networks more valuable in building social empowerment in health systems than more traditional forms of knowledge transfer [67].

10.7 **Implications for strengthening health systems: building and revitalizing comprehensive primary healthcare-oriented systems**

Primary healthcare was declared the model for global health policy at the 1978 Alma Ata conference and was it was directly linked to action on the wider determinants of health and right to health raised earlier in this chapter [68]. As envisioned at Alma Ata it involved a strategy that would respond equitably, appropriately, and effectively to basic health needs and address the underlying social, economic, and political causes of poor health. It was to be underpinned by universal accessibility and coverage on the basis of need, with emphasis on disease prevention and health promotion, community participation, self-reliance, and inter-sectoral collaboration. Thirty years after Alma Ata, and despite experience of the challenges and obstacles to PHC, there is a widely shared view that revitalizing PHC is critical to address rising inequity in health and the significant burdens to global health generated by their social determinants [48]. Indeed, a review of PHC and health outcomes in low-income and middle-income countries since Alma-Ata found that scale-up of comprehensive primary healthcare, as distinct from a smaller package of selective interventions, was associated with progress in governance and in health and mortality outcomes, despite very low income per person, political instability, and high HIV prevalence in some [69].

Implementation of action in all areas already discussed in this chapter will, therefore, help to build health systems oriented to comprehensive primary healthcare. However, additional actions are also necessary to revitalize the PHC approach within most health systems, and so capture the health and health equity gains that it can deliver. Key amongst these are:

- Strengthening the local level (e.g. the District Health System) as the focal point for wider action to address the social determinants of health inequity as well as the entry point to the health system [70].

- Investing in primary and community level services and interventions, including improved infrastructure (such as health facilities and equipment, roads, water and electricity supplies and telecommunications) and logistical support (such as the supply and distribution of affordable pharmaceuticals based on an Essential Drugs List and transport for outreach services) [71].

- Ensuring adequate numbers of appropriately skilled health workers are available at the local level and tackling skills' imbalances, geographic maldistribution, poor working environments, and weak information on the health workforce [15]. Existing evidence suggests that this calls for improved salaries and payment mechanisms, ensuring availability of supplies to do one's job, and flexibility and autonomy to manage work [72]. East and southern African experience also suggests that non-financial incentives (e.g. training, welfare provision, career paths, support, and supervision) play a significant role in motivating health worker retention, and may have a more sustained effect in situations of high inflation and economic instability [73]. More equitable distribution of the health workforce is, finally, likely to require measures to improve overall human resource availability, as well as differential implementation to address the particular needs of under-served areas and levels of the system.

◆ Strengthening interpersonal relations between providers, patients and community groups, and reorienting health worker attitudes towards combining promotion, prevention and curative care, so that health workers feel valued and respected and provide client-centred, relevant and better quality services [74]. Improved provider–patient–community relationships may be reinforced by codes of conduct for health workers; basic amenities such as privacy during consultation; supervision (with quality improvements); and team-based interventions that allow health workers to innovate [72].

◆ Supporting local public sector health managers to play key roles in taking action on the social determinants of health inequity [75]. Low-cost investments in strengthening local level management and supervision can also improve the performance of a much larger number of staff. However, to perform their roles, managers, like other staff, need relevant skills, as well as incentives to sustain their motivation; and they need information to take informed decisions.

10.8 Strengthening political action on the social determinants of health

After three years of work the Commissioners and contributors to the CSDH observed in their final report that: 'Changing the social determinants of health and health equity is a long-term agenda requiring sustained support and investment', recognizing that 'At the centre of this action should be the empowerment of people, communities and countries that do not have their fair share' [2; pp.27–28]. The possibilities for addressing the social determinants of health, and strengthening health systems, have never been greater: the knowledge, awareness, capabilities, demand, and experience exist to inform effective action.

Yet policy choices are always subject to challenge, particularly from those with competing agendas who fear a loss of power, status or income. Reforming health systems involves battles between opposing groups holding different values bases, and even within supportive national contexts, good intentions and policies may face obstacles for their translation into systems and practice [76].

Progressive policy actors must, therefore, think strategically about the processes of policy development and implementation needed to sustain the health system and wider actions discussed in this chapter as necessary to address the social determinants of health [15,48]. This includes thinking about how to build coalitions that engage other potentially powerful actors who have their own circles of influence, as well as what actions can offset policy opposition. Careful thought is also required about how to sustain implementation of critical policies. In strengthening health systems to address the social determinants of health it is vital to: secure the legislative and funding base of new health policies, through constitutional rights to health or healthcare as well as specific legislation; establish policy frameworks that enable a balance of local autonomy and central direction in particular areas of health system decision-making; and engage with actors outside government structures in monitoring and evaluating their implementation. At the same time, civil society organizations and parliamentarians must initiate the wider social processes that support health system leaders and managers in these actions and hold them accountable to the principle of health equity.

References

1 Tarlov A (1996). Social determinants of health: the sociobiological translation. In Blane D, Brunner E, Wilkinson R (eds) *Health and social organization*, pp.71–93. Routledge, London.

2 WHO Commission on the Social Determinants of Health (2008). *Closing the gap in generation* Final report of the WHO CSDH. WHO, Geneva. Available at: http://www.who.int/social_determinants/en/.

3 Regional Network for Equity in Health in East and Southern Africa (EQUINET). Available at: www.equinetafrica.org.

4 Graham H, Kelly M (2004). *Health inequalities: concepts, frameworks and policy* (Briefing paper). NHS Health Development Agency, London.

5 Aboriginal and Torres Islander Social Justice Commissioner (2005). *Social justice report*. Human Rights & Equal Opportunity Commission, Sydney. Available at: http://www.hreoc.gov.au/social_justice/sj_report/sjreport05/pdf/SocialJustice2005.pdf (accessed February 2008).

6 Lundberg O, Åberg Yngwe M, Stjärne M, Kölegård, Björk L, Fritzell J (2008). *The Nordic experience: welfare states and public health (NEWS)*. Health Equity Series no. 12 Centre for Health Equity Studies (CHESS). University/Karolinska Institutet, Stockholm.

7 Mackenbach JP, Meerding WJ, Kunst AE (2007). *Economic implications of socio-economic inequalities in health in the European Union. Luxembourg: European Commission. Measurement and Evidence Knowledge Network of the Commission on Social Determinants of Health*. World Health Organization. Geneva.

8 EQUINET Steering Committee (2007). *Reclaiming the resources for health: A regional analysis of equity in health in east and southern Africa*. EQUINET Weaver Press, Harare.

9 ECDKN (2007). *Early child development: a powerful equalizer.* Final report of the Early Child Development Knowledge Network of the WHO Commission on Social Determinants of Health. WHO, Geneva.

10 Bloom DE (2007). *Education, health, and development.* American Academy of Arts and Sciences, Cambridge, MA. Available at: http://www.amacad.org/publications/ubase_eduhealth_dev.pdf, cited in WHO CSDH (2008).

11 WHO Afro (2006). *The African Regional Health Report 2006.* WHO-Afro Region: Brazzaville, Available at: http://www.afro.who.int/regionaldirector/african_regional_health_report2006.pdf.

12 Kim IH, Muntaner C, Khang YH, Paek D, Cho SI (2006). The relationship between nonstandard working and mental health in a representative sample of the South Korean population. *Social Science and Medicine*, **63**, 566–74.

13 EMCONET (2007). *Employment conditions and health inequalities* (Final report of the Employment Conditions Knowledge Network of the WHO Commission on Social Determinants of Health). WHO, Geneva.

14 Labonte R, Shrecker T (2008). *Towards Health-Equitable Globalisation: Rights, Regulation and Redistribution* (Final Report to the Commission on Social Determinants of Health of the Globalisation Knowledge Network). University of Ottawa Institute of Population Health, Ottawa.

15 Gilson L, Doherty J, Loewenson R, Francis V (2008). *Challenging inequity through health systems* (Final report of the Knowledge Network on Health Systems, WHO Commission on the Social Determinants of Health). Johannesburg: Centre for Health Policy, EQUINET, London School of Hygiene and Tropical Medicine, London.

16 Mackenbach JP, Van de Mheen, Stronks (1994). A Prospective cohort study investigating the explanation of socioeconomic inequalities in health in the Netherlands. *Social Science and Medicine*, **38**, 299–308.

17 Mackenbach JP, Stirbu I, Roskam A, *et al.* (2008). Socioeconomic Inequalities in Health in 22 European Countries *New England Journal of Medicine*, **359**(12), 2468–81.

18 Mackenbach JP, Bakker M (2002). *Reducing inequalities in health: a European perspective.* Routledge, London.

19 Acheson D (1998). *Inequalities in health: report of an independent inquiry.* HMSO, London.

20 Government of Northern Ireland (2004). *Equalities and inequalities in health and social care in Northern Ireland.* Available at: http://www.dhsspsni.gov.uk/equality_inequalities2.pdf.

21 Dahlgren G, Whitehead M (2007). *European strategies for tackling social inequities in health: Levelling Up Part 2.* European Region of the World Health Organization, Copenhagen. Available at: http://www.euro.who.int/__data/assets/pdf_file/0018/103824/E89384.pdf.

22 Jonsson U (1996). *An Approach To Assess And Analyse The Health And Nutrition Situation Of Children In The Perspective Of The Convention Of The Rights Of The Child.* WABA Forum, 2–6 December 1996, Bangkok.

23 Barnett T, Whiteside A (2002). *AIDS in the twenty-first century: Disease and globalisation.* Palgrave McMillan, Basingstoke.

24 Loewenson R (2007). Learning from diverse contexts: Equity and inclusion in the responses to AIDS. *AIDS Care*, **19**,(1), 83–90.

25 Ainsworth M. (1999). AIDS, development and the East Africa crisis. Plenary address to the 5th International Conference on AIDS in Asia and the Pacific. Kuala Lumpur, Malaysia, October 25.

26 Vapattanawong P, Hogan MC, Hanvoravongchai P, *et al.* (2007). Reductions in child mortality levels and inequalities in Thailand, analysis of two censuses. *Lancet*, **369**, 850–55

27 World Health Organization (2000). *World Health Report: Health Systems Improving Performance*. WHO, Geneva.

28 Gillies P, Tolley K, Wolstenholme J (1996). Is AIDS a disease of poverty? *AIDS Care*, **8**(3), 351–64.

29 International Labour Organization (ILO) (1995). *The Impact of HIV/AIDS on the productive labour force in Africa. EAMAT Working Paper 1*. ILO. Addis Ababa.

30 Southern African Development Community (SADC) (2003). *SADC HIV/AIDS framework and strategic programme of action 2003–2007*. SADC, Gabarone.

31 Decosas J (2002). *The social ecology of AIDS in Africa*. Paper prepared for the UNRISD project on HIV and Development, March 2002. UNRISD, Mimeo, Geneva

32 Gilson L (1998). In defence and pursuit of equity. *Social Science and Medicine*, **47**(12), 1891–96.

33 Kreiger N (2008). Ladders, pyramids and champagne: the iconography of health inequities. *J Epidemiol Community Health*, **62**, 1098–104.

34 London L (2003). *Can human rights serve as a tool for equity?* EQUINET Policy Paper 14. South Africa, Ideas studio. Available at: http://www.equinetafrica.org/bibl/docs/POL14rights.pdf (accessed 07 November 2006).

35 Perera M (2007). *Intersectoral Action for Health in Sri Lanka*. Paper prepared for the Health Systems Knowledge Network of the World Health Organization's Commission on Social Determinants of Health, Geneva.

36 United Nations Development Programme (UNDP) (2005). Human development report 2005–International co-operation at a crossroads: Aid, trade and security in an unequal world, OUP, New York. Available at: http://hdr.undp.org/reports/view_reports.cfm?type= (accessed 1 June 2007).

37 Chopra M (2004*). Food security, rural development and health equity in southern Africa'. EQUINET Discussion Paper 22*. EQUINET, Harare.

38 Rosset P (2003). Food sovereignty global rallying cry of farmer movements. *Food first*, **9**(4). Available at: http://www.foodfirst.org/pubs/backgrdrs/2003/f03v9n4.pdf (accessed April 2010).

39 SADC (2004). *Enhancing agriculture and food security for poverty reduction in the SADC region*. Communique of SADC Ministers of Food, Agriculture and Natural Resources, Tanzania. Available at: http://www.waterberg.gov.za/docs/agriculture/food/P792-Statement_20040214.pdf (accessed 14 February 2010).

40 Food and Agricultural Organization (FAO) (2004) *FAOSTAT*. FAO, Rome.

41 Chopra M, Tomlinson M (2007) *Food sovereignty and nutrition in east and southern Africa: A synthesis of case study evidence,' EQUINET discussion paper 47*. EQUINET/MRC, South Africa.

42 Buzeti T, Zakotnik JM (2008). *Investment for health and development in Slovenia: Programme Mura*. Centre for Health and Development, Murska Sobota, Slovenia.

43 Chacham A, Maia M, Greco M, Silva A, Greco D (2007). Autonomy and susceptibility to HIV among young women living in a slum in Belo Horizonte, Brazil. *AIDS Care*, **19**(Suppl 1), S12–S22.

44 UNAIDS (2009). *No single magic bullet For HIV prevention*. UNAIDS Newsletter/09, Geneva. Available at: http://data.unaids.org/pub/Periodical/2009/20090323_unaids_newsletter_issue1_en.pdf (accessed February 2010).

45 Public Health Agency of Canada (PHAC) (2007). *Crossing sectors: experiences in inter-sectoral action, public policy and health*. Paper prepared for the Health Systems Knowledge Network of the World Health Organization's Commission on Social Determinants of Health, Geneva.

46 Östlin P, Diderichsen F (2001). *Equity-oriented national strategy for public health in Sweden: A case study Policy Learning Curve Series Number 1*, WHO European Centre for Health Policy, Brussels. Available at: http://www.who.dk/Document/E69911.pdf.

47 Mackintosh M (2001). Do health care systems contribute to inequalities? In Leon D, Walt G (eds) *Poverty, inequality and health: An international perspective*, pp.175–93. Oxford University Press, Oxford.

48 WHO (2008). *The World Health Report 2008. Now more than ever: Primary Health Care*. WHO, Geneva.

49 De Maeseneer J, Willems S, De Sutter A, Van de Geuchte I, Billings M (2007). *Primary health care as a strategy for achieving equitable care*. Paper prepared for the Health Systems Knowledge Network of the World Health Organization's Commission on Social Determinants of Health, Geneva.

50 Starfield B, Shi L, Macinko J. (2005). Contribution of primary care to health systems and health. *Milbank Quarterly*, **83**(3), 457–502.

51 Gilson L (2007). *Acceptability, Trust and Equity*. In Mooney G, McIntyre D (eds) *The economics of health equity*. Cambridge University Press, Cambridge.

52 McIntyre D, Thiede M, Dahlgren G, Whitehead M (2006). What are the economic consequences for households of illness and of paying for health care in low- and middle-income country contexts? *Social Science and Medicine*, **62**(4), 858–65.

53 George A (2007). *Human resources for health: A gender analysis*. Paper prepared for the Women and Gender Equity Knowledge Network of the WHO Commission on Social Determinants of Health, Geneva.

54 Laurell A (2007). *Granting universal access to health care: The experience of the Mexico City Government*. Paper prepared for the Health Systems Knowledge Network of the World Health Organization's Commission on Social Determinants of Health. Available at: (http://web.wits.ac.za/Academic/Centres/CHP/Collaboration/HSKN.htm (accessed April 2010).

55 Meng Q (2007). *Developing and implementing equity-promoting health care policies in China*. Paper prepared for the Health Systems Knowledge Network of the World Health Organization's Commission on Social Determinants of Health, Geneva.

56 Dubowitz T, Anthony R, Bird C., Cohen D, Lurie N. (2007). *The experience of the USA: health inequity within a high-income setting*. Paper prepared for the Health Systems Knowledge Network of the WHO Commission on Social Determinants of Health. WHO, Geneva.

57 Govender V, Penn-Kekana L (2008). Gender Biases and Discrimination: a review of health care interpersonal interactions. *Global Public Health*, **3**(S1), 90–103.

58 Homedes N, Ugalde A (2005). Why neoliberal health reforms have failed in Latin America. *Health Policy*, 71(1), 83–96.

59 Mackintosh M, Koivusalo M (2005). *The commercialisation of health care: global and local dynamics and policy responses.* Palgrave Macmillan, Basingstoke

60 Committee on Economic, Social and Cultural Rights (CESCR) (2000). *General Comment No. 14, The Right to the Highest Attainable Standard of Health*, UN Doc. E/C. 12/2000/4 (2000). Available at http://cesr.org/generalcomment

61 Hunt R, Backman G (2008). Health systems and the right to the highest attainable standard of health. *Health and Human Rights*, 10, 81–92.

62 Wallerstein N (1992). Powerlessness, empowerment, and health: implications for health promotion programs. *American Journal of Health Promotion*, 6(3), 197–205.

63 Marmot M (2006). Harveian Oration. Health in an unequal world. *Lancet*, 368, 2081–94.

64 Wallerstein N (2006). What is the evidence on effectiveness of empowerment to improve health? WHO Regional Office for Europe (Health Evidence Network), Copenhagen.

65 Loewenson R (2003). *Civil Society–State interactions in national health systems.* Annotated Bibliography on Civil Society and Health. WHO/TARSC. Available at: http://www.tarsc.org/WHOCSI/ (accessed 26 June 2007).

66 Goetz A, Gaventa J (2001). *Bringing citizen voice and client focus into service delivery.* IDS Working Papers - 138. Institute of Development Studies. UK. Available at: http://www. ids.ac.uk/ids/bookshop/wp/wp138.pdf (accessed 27 June 2007).

67 Loewenson R (2008). *Neglected Health Systems Research: Governance and Accountability.* Alliance for Health Policy and Systems Research: Research Issues 3, AHPSR, Geneva.

68 WHO (1978). Declaration of Alma Ata: International Conference on Primary Health Care, Alma Ata, USSR, 6–12 September 1978. Available at: www.who.int/hpr/NPH/ docs/declaration_almaata.pdf (accessed 18 February 2004).

69 Rohde J, Cousens S, Chopra M, *et al.* (2008). 30 years after Alma-Ata: has primary health care worked in countries? *Lancet*, 372, 950–61.

70 Baez C, Barron P (2006). *Community voice and role in district health systems in east and southern Africa: A literature review* (Discussion paper 39). In Regional Network for Equity in Health in East and Southern Africa (EQUINET), Harare.

71 Mills A, Rasheed F, Tollman S (2006). Strengthening health systems. In Jamison D, Breman J, Measham A, *et al.* (eds). *Disease Control Priorities in Developing Countries*, pp.87–102. Oxford University Press and the World Bank, Washington.

72 WHO (2006). *World Health Report 2006. Working together for health.* WHO, Geneva

73 Iipinge S, Dambisya YM, Loewenson R, *et al.* (2009) Policies and incentives for health worker retention in east and southern Africa: Learning from country research. EQUINET, ECSA-HC, *EQUINET Discussion Paper 78.* EQUINET, Harare.

74 Macinko J, Guanais FC, de Fatima M, de Souza M (2006). Evaluation of the impact of the Family Health Program on infant mortality in Brazil, 1990–2002. *Journal of Epidemiology and Community Health*, 60(1), 13–19.

75 De Savigny D, Kasale H, Mbuya C, Reid G (2004). *Fixing Health Systems.* International Development Research Centre, Ottawa.

76 Chetty K (2007). *Equity promoting health care policies in South Africa.* Paper prepared for the Health Systems Knowledge Network of the World Health Organization's Commission on the Social Determinants of Health, WHO, Geneva.

Chapter 11

The health system and global changes

Richard D. Smith

11.1 Introduction

There is growing recognition that many of the greatest challenges facing population health this century will be from areas not traditionally seen as within the remit of the domestic health sector. As Chapter 10 presented, there is renewed interest in the 'social determinants of health', such as income, education, and the environment, especially given the recent report of the World Health Organization's (WHO's) Commission on Social Determinants of Health [1]. However, work in this area often remains focused upon the specific national context, and has little concern with the changes happening on a global level that are less within the direct control of nation states. For example, the recent crisis of food prices, generated by commodity markets and demand for bio-fuels, has generated concerns for food security; the expansion in movement of people, animals, and animal products has been linked with infectious disease transmission; and demographic changes associated with population growth and profile have already generated stresses upon fragile health systems.

Yet, the pace of global change in many areas relevant to health sectors and systems is accelerating, presenting significant challenges, and perhaps opportunities, for health. Many factors, such as those outlined, are increasing the demands placed upon health sectors by their populations (e.g. from changing demographics, economic prosperity, changing disease burdens), but are also influencing the ways and means by which health sectors are financed and provide services (e.g. public financing of health systems, provision of new technologies). Further, changes within wider realms of national, international and global governance structures are imposing changing structures within which health sector sovereignty may operate. This chapter therefore builds on Chapter 10 by adopting a broad perspective to consider how a nation's health system may be impacted upon by changes at the global level.

Clearly, there is a complex and interwoven spectrum of many possible global influences upon the health sector and system. This chapter therefore begins with delineating the boundaries for an analysis of the effects of global changes. It then proceeds to provide an overview of the main global influences that may impact on both health system demand and supply sides, discussing how health systems have, or may, respond to these at the domestic and global level. Section 11.4 then concludes.

11.2 Defining global change

There are extensive theoretical and empirical analyses of the distinct characteristics of that which is 'global' [2]. In international relations, for example, there is a distinction that 'international' exchanges occur between country units, while 'global' transactions occur within a planetary unit [3]. Whereas international relations are *inter*-territorial relations, global relations are *trans*- and sometimes *supra*-territorial relations. In economics, global refers to 'the state of development where geographical location no longer matters' such as in trade and finance. In public health, the failure to similarly engage with theorizing about what is *global* about *global health* is due, perhaps, to a desire to avoid the 'danger of succumbing to pedantic word games while the world succumbs to deadly pandemics, irreversible environmental degradation and deteriorating health systems' [4]. Nevertheless, eschewing theory and definition results in a lack of analytical boundaries and, in turn, practical focus, so it is worth briefly outlining how global (change) is to be interpreted in this chapter.

Certainly global could easily refer to transnational issues on a geographical basis. However, this may be limited in a similar manner to 'global public goods', in that there are very few issues that will be truly global in the sense of affecting all nations and peoples (and, as often has been added in the case of global public goods, generations) [5]. Broad environmental changes, such as climate change, are perhaps the only truly global issue in this respect. However, one could take global to encompass a more normative, choice-related, definition of aspects of change within certain areas that are of interest globally if not necessarily of effect globally from a geographical perspective. For instance, the exploration and exploitation of space may be of interest to most, if not all, nations, yet only affect directly very few nations. Similarly, global could be taken to refer to those aspects of change that will affect institutions other than just nation states. For the purposes of this chapter 'global' is taken to refer to a loose geographical definition of affecting a considerable number of countries across a number of regions, although not necessarily affecting literally all countries. This will then differentiate global issues from regional or local issues, but will not be unnecessarily restrictive.

Change is perhaps a somewhat easier concept to define, referring to 'difference over time'. Global change must identify what differences are expected to occur between now and some point in the future, raising the issue of how far to go in to the future to assess and predict this change. In some areas changes may be very slow to operate, such as environmental, whereas in others the velocity of change may be considerably higher, such as technology. There is also a link with the definition of global as above. For instance, must global change refer to a change that is simultaneously occurring everywhere? Might changes be occurring at different rates in different areas, or would this not be considered global? Must it refer to change that resonates with all global players? How would regional change, which may impact subsequently on others (e.g. through externality effects) be considered? For the purposes of this chapter, change is considered to be related to the above definition of global—occurring in many places simultaneously, but not necessarily equally, and across a time frame of a few decades, to allow for slower as well as quicker aspects of global change to be considered.

Finally, in setting the boundaries, one needs to remember that the specific interest here is with the likely implication that global changes will have for health systems. In this respect, the areas identified will be expected to present challenges or opportunities for domestic health systems from two perspectives; of the demands placed upon health systems and of the ability of health sectors to supply health services. In the analysis presented below, each area of global change is therefore analysed from these two perspectives.

11.3 Mapping areas of global change important for health systems

The implications of various global changes for health systems are many and manifest. For instance, the demands placed on health systems may increase with climate-related impacts, such as increased extreme weather events, or as a result of changes in food security resulting from changing agricultural production. Similarly, increased migration may increase demands through movement of communicable disease, but also change the profile of demands through changes in the age structure of the population, genetic changes in future generations and factors associated with culture changes (e.g. diet and exercise). Changes in the global economic and financial system may impact upon how health systems are funded, such as changes in the forms of taxation for public services, and changes in technology may generate changes in the way in which health services are delivered, such as through the use of bio- and nanotechnology. There are also very direct influences through changes in the way in which health-related goods and services themselves are traded on the global market, as discussed in detail in Chapter 12.

Given the immense breadth of possible connections between events at the global level and the domestic, it is perhaps unsurprising that there has been no attempt to comprehensively catalogue the full range of possible impacts of global changes from a health perspective. There have been various 'foresight' initiatives, many of which have included health specifically, or have highlighted the health effects of other areas, in their analysis of the likely key areas of future global change. Taking various reports and analyses such as these, together with expert opinion and workshop discussions, a report commissioned for WHO in 2008 sought to provide a consensus on the most pressing aspects of global change from a health perspective [6]. These are summarized in Table 11.1, where the left column outlines the 'top five' areas of global change that potentially influence health (alphabetically listed), and the right column shows the main issues within these areas that will affect health.

One can see from Table 11.1 that a number of the issues relevant to these areas of global change will be likely to impact upon the demands made of health systems by the population covered. These are principally those changes that will influence levels of ill-health within populations and/or change population behaviour with respect to health. Similarly, several are likely to impact upon health sectors from the supply side, influencing the ability to finance, provide, and organize health service delivery. In this section, the core areas identified above, reflecting the typology provided in Table 11.1, are considered as they relate to both these demand and supply sides.

11.3.1 Global agricultural changes and health systems

Agriculture, which provides for the most basic of human needs—food—has and will continue to undergo substantial changes in the 21st century. Increasing production of cash crops, trade in agricultural products, concerns for food-borne disease and quality standards, responding to climate change, changes in tastes and preferences in the developing world, increased demand for bio-fuels, and many other changes all provide a challenge for human health. From a health system perspective, the most critical will be those which generate increased demand upon the health sector due to exacerbation of ill-health through non-optimal food consumption and exposure to food-borne disease transmission.

11.3.1.1 Non-optimal food consumption

Health systems in all countries face demand related to the health effects of non-optimal consumption of food, which is influenced primarily by food

Table 11.1 Summary of issues that will influence health

Area	Issue
Agriculture	1. Food security:
	Food prices
	Impact of trans-national companies
	2. Disease transmission:
	Communicable disease
	Non-communicable disease
Demography	1. Population growth
	2. Migration:
	General
	Healthcare workers
Economics and governance	1. Development
	2. Trade:
	Hazardous/harmful products
	Intellectual property
	3. Finance:
	Economic insecurity
	Change in global structure
	4. Change in power, regulation and governance
Environment	1. Climate change:
	Fatalities
	Communicable diseases
	Water supplies
	2. Energy
	3. Water/sanitation
Technology	1. Information and communication technology:
	Satellite technology
	Diagnostics
	2. Biotechnology
	3. Nanotechnology

prices and availability, increasingly subject to the control of trans-national corporations (TNCs) [7]. For most low- and middle-income countries the concern is primarily with food security, referring to 'access by all people, at all times, to sufficient, affordable, safe and nutritious food, necessary and appropriate for a healthy life, and the security of knowing such access is sustainable in the future' [8]. The principal result of a lack of food security is under- and malnutrition, which affects some 820 million people and an estimated two billion experience diet-related ill-health [9]. Although childhood undernutrition declined worldwide between 1980 and 2005, approximately 25% of all children in the developing world are still estimated to be underweight (137.95 million children in 2005). In Africa, the proportion and number of underweight children actually *increased* between 1980 and 2005. Micronutrient deficiencies are even more widespread, particularly of vitamin A, iron, zinc, and iodine, and disproportionately affect women and children [10].

Inadequate diet is implicated in increased risk of infectious diseases, particularly in children, along with the effects of over-crowding, poor sanitation, and contaminated water supplies [11–13]. Nearly 13 million children aged five and under die annually, and malnutrition is associated with, or contributes to, at least 25% of these premature deaths. Malnourished children and adults have higher rates of morbidity; decreased cellular immunity, increased incidence and/or duration of illness, and experience higher mortality. On the positive side, a good diet can also protect against some infectious diseases and thus contribute to improving the length and quality of life [14].

In addition to food security, there is concern about the change in consumption patterns associated with decreased poverty; that an increase in unhealthy eating, promoted by a surge in TNCs, will result in 'overnutrition' resulting in higher levels of non-communicable diseases [15,16]. According to WHO, diet-related chronic diseases (DRCD) are the largest cause of death globally, led by cardiovascular disease (17 million deaths in 2002) and followed by cancer (7 million deaths), chronic lung diseases (4 million), and diabetes mellitus (almost 1 million) [17]. Although chronic diseases have been the leading cause of death in developed countries for decades, they now represent the leading cause of death in developing countries [18]. The global prevalence of DRCD is projected to increase substantially over the next two decades. For example, the number of individuals with diabetes is estimated to rise from 171 million in 2000 to 366 million in 2030, 298 million of who will live in developing countries [19]. In India, for instance, the incidence of diabetes climbed from 15 million cases in 1990 to 35 million by 2000, concentrated among urban populations adopting developed country lifestyles (increased consumption of meat and dairy fats, salt and sugary foods and drinks, fewer cereals and legumes, and a reduction in physical activity). Evidence shows that diets high in fats, especially saturated fats and *trans*-fatty acids, free sugars, and salt and low in fruits, vegetables, pulses (legumes), whole grains, and nuts pose significant risks for chronic diseases [20]. In what is termed the 'nutrition transition', populations in developing countries are shifting away from diets high in cereals and complex carbohydrates, to high-calorie, nutrient-poor diets high in fats, sweeteners, and processed foods [21,22]. This is leading to concerns that DRCDs will become an even more significant burden in developing countries. For instance, between 1997 and 2002, average annual sales growth of carbonated soft drinks was 1.4% in the United States, compared with 8.8% in China, 7.9% in India, 7.8% in Indonesia, and 6.2% in South Africa [23]. Developing countries are expected to account for most of the future increases in sales—and therefore consumption—of processed foods [23]. Thus, as countries experience rising incomes, they may experience changes in the burden of diseases that present to health sectors, necessitating a shift in the balance of services provided.

Changes in food production processes through trade liberalization and the rise of TNCs present challenge to health sectors; which will face higher demands to deal with the consequences of these health effects. For instance, in the provision of maternal and child care for those experiencing undernutrition, and treatment for heart disease and diabetes where there is overnutrition. However, there is also a challenge for health sectors to be actively lobbying for agricultural reforms and policies to target agricultural commodity and food retail prices and other influences over food security, such as food safety, security within the food supply chain, and the balance in the use of agricultural land for bio-fuels and other 'cash crops' versus nutritional foodstuffs [24]. For instance, the 'hypermarket revolution' entails a restructuring that drives out smaller shops which are more accessible to the less mobile; thus provision for the affluent consumer excludes the poor [25–27]. Furthermore, those shops that tend to remain where poorer people live tend to charge higher prices for the same basic basket of goods, because of economies of scale and wholesale market access. There may therefore be a case for health sector involvement to influence policy over advertising and other food marketing techniques, especially those targeted at children [28-32]. This creates a very different role for the health sector, as discussed further in Chapter 12.

11.3.1.2 Disease transmission

Food-borne disease is a leading global public health concern, affecting millions of adults and children every year, especially in developing countries [33]. The core cause of food-borne diseases is unsafe food contaminated with microbiological or chemical hazards, or unconventional agents. Microbiological contaminants include bacteria (e.g. *Escherichia coli, Listeria, Salmonella, Campylobacter*), viruses (e.g. calcivirus), and parasites (e.g. trematodes) while chemical contaminants include natural toxicants such as mycotoxins, environmental hazards such as mercury, and persistent organic pollutants such as dioxins. Ingestion of chemicals introduced during food production, such as pesticides, antibiotics, and growth promoters, can also pose health risks. For example, the leading cause of sickness and death among children under five in developing countries are diarrhoeal diseases which are often transmitted by unsafe food.

During the last decade there has been a massive growth in meat product consumption and livestock production. As indicated above, increased income tends to move diets to more animal-based products and on to more processed animal products. It is therefore vital to ensure the safety of livestock rearing and food processing. Increased trade in food and agricultural products, such as feedstuffs, also increases the potential for the transmission of communicable disease. However, there is little evidence that at present this potential risk has been translated into disease [34]. Border control and other procedures play an important role in reducing food safety risks, and of the estimated 1%, or US$3.8 billion worth, of all agro-food trade rejected for safety reasons, some US$1.8m were rejected by developing countries, although process of control and standards still tend to focus on foods exported to developed countries [35]. It is also the case that increased control may have perverse effects on food security. For example, when substandard foods have been found in internationally marketed foods, this has led to curtailment of trade, creating insecurity for the livelihoods of food producers in developing countries.

Another major factor of concern in the role of agriculture in the development and transmission of diseases is the role of zoonoses, and especially the changes in global conditions that may increase the development and transmission of these [36]. Of 1415 known human pathogens, 62% are zoonotic, and 75% of all emerging diseases that have affected humans over the last two decades have resulted from an animal pathogen moving into the human host from animals or animal products. In addition to the public health concerns of this specific group of diseases, many of the major zoonoses also prevent the efficient production of food of animal origin and create obstacles to international trade in animal products.

Given the history of zoonoses development and the dynamics of host, pathogen, and environment interaction (disease ecology), it is difficult to predict what zoonosis is likely to emerge next. However, the exponential growth of the human population, ecological, climatic, and agricultural practice changes, lifestyles, modernization and globalization, international trade and travel, the emergence of chronic and immunosuppressive diseases, the growing number of ageing and adolescent members of society, the development of antimicrobial resistance, and increased contact with wildlife species have all come together to create a novel environment for the emergence of disease. Establishing causal linkages is very difficult, but there is widespread consensus that trade and travel, geography, economic and biotechnological developments, urbanization, land use, climate change, and the 'livestock revolution' form causal links with the reported increases in the spread of trans-boundary animal diseases, food safety hazards and other veterinary public health risks.

The enormous potential for increases in zoonotic outbreaks, as recent cases of variant Creutzfeldt–Jakob disease (vCJD), severe acute respiratory syndrome (SARS), avian and swine flu have demonstrated, should concern health systems worldwide. There is a need for health sectors to have adequate facilities to treat cases of newly and re-emerging zoonotic illness, have preparedness plans for possible outbreaks, and consider how the system will respond in the event of a significant influx of those affected, as well as maintain its own workforce. The global linkages and dimension within this aspect of disease transmission again necessitate the health sector to be involved in global level activities, as discussed in Chapter 12.

11.3.2 Global demographic changes and health systems

Health systems cover a specified population. Changes in global demography—the growth and movement of populations—will affect the size, composition, and characteristics of the populations that health systems cover. These will affect the profile of demands made upon the health sector (and, with respect to health worker migration, the ability of the health system to respond; as covered in Chapter 12).

11.3.2.1 Population growth

The coming decades will see an immense and challenging increase in population. Demographers project the world population to grow from some 6 billion people to over 9 billion by 2050. All of the additional 3 billion are predicted to be living in LIMCs. Ironically, there are concerns that if this population growth coincides with reductions in poverty, then the pressures placed on agriculture and the environment will be even more severe than if that population remains impoverished [37].

Population growth in itself would not be a significant issue. However, its potential to aggravate all the other challenges of global change makes it essential to tackle it. In terms of health systems, the key implications of increases in population and, for developed countries especially, a change in demographic pattern to those of an older age, are fourfold. First, there will be increased pressure on resources, especially water and food, which, in turn, may exacerbate food and water shortages and quality [38]. However, there will also be great pressure on resources for power and transportation, shortages of which could again impact directly upon health. Second, there are direct health repercussions for women and babies of changes in reproduction—having children at later age, having fewer children or having no children, increases the risk of specific forms of illness. Third, changes in the balance of the world's population from developed to developing nations will influence the pattern of global disease burden, as well as link to migration patterns as discussed below. Finally, there will be implications for the affordability of health and social care (for countries with aging populations, increased pressure on working population and higher taxes, reduced benefits for elderly or later retirement) and increased demand and utilization of medical services.

11.3.2.2 Migration and mobility

In addition to global population growth, there are also concerns related to the movement of people on an unprecedented scale through population mobility (the process common to evolving patterns of human movement across borders) and migration (the legal and administrative aspects of the movement of individuals and groups). Population mobility and migration patterns are changing. Migration and mobility used to be a relatively slow and unidirectional process, involving the permanent resettlement of individuals. Now, and increasingly in the future, migration is multidirectional—people move through a succession of countries, including their country of origin—and on a temporary as well as permanent basis. There is a significant proportion of mobility that is not migration—that is, outside of legal and administrative structures. Movement may be for economic, education, humanitarian or other reasons (including those who are trafficked). Modern migration and mobility is fuelled by the traditional push (what prompts people to leave a country) and pull (what attracts them to a specific country) factors, as well as developments in other areas. For instance contextual factors that play a role in decisions, such as similarity of language/culture between source and destination (hence cyclical pattern between Australia, Canada, Ireland, United Kingdom and United States) and historic (colonial) ties (e.g. India to United Kingdom, North Africa to France, and Mozambique to Portugal) are becoming less important with globalization. Similarly, developments in transportation have escalated this movement, as well as the development of regional blocs that facilitate migration through easing legal and administrative processes. This has been well demonstrated in the accession of former Soviet-bloc countries to the European Union. The new volume, pattern, and diversity of population mobility and migration represent a challenge for health as well as foreign policy, trade and security.

In terms of health sectors and systems, migration and mobility raise challenges in the delivery of services in four ways.[1] First, changes in population

---

[1] Note, the interest here is with global change, but health systems will also be affected by internal migration, especially the increasing rates of urbanization seen across the

demographics (age, gender, fecundity) will alter the pattern of disease (e.g. movement of people into indigenous areas and mixing of indigenous with non-indigenous could alter patterns of mortality and morbidity), and consequently the pattern of demand for services. Second, such movements could influence economic and social factors that are key determinants of disease. Third, there will be changes in health service needs to be culturally and linguistically appropriate. Finally, the health of migrants is transferred with them, and may be spread in receiving populations—the traditional communicable disease concern, but also aspects of genetics, exposure and behaviour. International mobility is central to the globalization of both communicable and non-communicable disease. This is recognized in various aspects of international legislation, such as GATS (General Agreement on Trade in Services) and IHR (International Health Regulations 2005), for example, although focused predominantly on infectious disease. Certainly recent outbreaks, such as SARS and swine and avian influenza, have further fuelled public, political, and economic pressure for global surveillance and other management measures for infectious disease. Again, activities in these realms require health to engage in international negotiations, as outlined in Chapter 12.

11.3.3 Global economic and governance changes and health systems

It is well recognized that health and wealth are interconnected. To the extent that economic development, changes in trade, or other economic aspects may impact on health, this will be translated in to changes in the demands placed upon health systems (more, less or different patterns of demand). However, perhaps as importantly, global economic factors are increasingly important for the ability of health sectors to finance and provide services.

11.3.3.1 Economic development

Macro-economic policy is concerned with gross domestic product (GDP), which represents national income, or wealth, and the rate of increase in GDP represents economic growth. The basis of macro-economic policy is that higher GDP will lead to greater consumption that, in the specific context here, will result in better health. In general, analyses suggest that 'wealthier countries are healthier countries'. The relevant factors in this relationship are generally

---

world. According to the United Nations Population Fund, in 2008 3.3 billion people live in cities (over 50% of the world's population), whereas by the year 2030, this number will amount to 4.9 billion [39]. Urbanization will have great impacts on health as there will be more crowding and fewer resources, such as water and food. Furthermore, if people are leaving the countryside, there will be fewer farmers, which may decrease the amount of food produced.

improved nutrition, sanitation, water, and education. Clearly the direction of causation is also subject to some debate, although received wisdom is that a 'virtuous circle' is engendered.

However, as indicated elsewhere, increased wealth can lead to challenges in other areas that affect health, such as strains on food production, water, and other natural resources, as well as impacts on migration and demographic factors and demands on health systems. Increased wealth also leads to an expansion not just in consumption that improves health, such as clean water, safe food and education, but also that which may be harmful or hazardous to health. Increased trade liberalization, through expansion of World Trade Organization (WTO) membership and numerous regional and bi-lateral trade agreements, will reduce the price of imported 'bads', through reduced tariff and non-tariff barriers, and increase the marketing of 'bads', such as tobacco, alcohol and 'fast food'. Further, increased trade in, and therefore consumption of, technology, such as mobile phones and computers, leads to increased 'trade' in toxic products and waste. This may result in direct health impacts to those who may recycle or otherwise dispose of such products and waste, and consequent environmental degradation may also lead to indirect health impacts.

The form of economic development also affects government income and hence the ability to finance and/or provide public services, including those that are health-related. For instance, although economic growth may appear to offer greater ability to finance healthcare, the drivers of this growth may negate this, such as through changes to the tax revenue structure. Although theoretically governments should be able to shift tax bases from, say, tariffs to domestic taxes, such as sales or income taxes, in practice developing countries, especially low income countries, find this difficult, especially because of the informal nature of their economies with large subsistence sectors. For instance, high income countries are usually able to recover 100% of the lost tariff revenues, middle-income countries recover around 40–60%, but low-income countries only around 30%. The extent to which limitations on raising the domestic share of total revenue impact on the health sector were considered in Chapter 4.

The stability of such development and growth is also critical. Economic instability results in volatile markets, increased frequency of external shocks, and increased impact of such shocks. These include, especially, financial crises, currency devaluation, and rapid changes in employment. These translate into economic insecurity for an individual, which is closely linked to increased stress-related illness. It will also affect the adequacy of financial planning for ill-health by the household and the (public and private) health sector, and generate investor reluctance (including within the health sector itself).

The dynamic nature of economic insecurity and poverty also means that non-poor households may become poor, affecting material conditions, such as housing, nutrition, etc., in addition to the psychological burden of distress.

The Asian crisis of the 1990s is the most quoted example of this impact of economic instability on health. However, in 2007 the 'credit crunch' for millions of homeowners in the United States (rising mortgage interest rates and falling housing values) led to a sharp rise in foreclosures. Within weeks the impact of this spread to other advanced economies as businesses and individuals found that loans were harder to obtain and were unexpectedly expensive and the solvency of major banks and other financial institutions was being questioned (and in the United Kingdom led to the nationalization of one bank). What began as a banking crisis spilled over into equity markets, destabilizing stock markets in industrial countries and rising fears that emerging markets could also be at risk.

11.3.3.2 Changing global governance environment

There will be important changes in the global economy within the 21st century for national and international health governance. First, the transformation of global regulation. The state-centred model, where governments regulate within their borders with some crosscutting commitments to other governments, as entrenched in treaties, has withered. Today, communications technology, non-governmental organizations (and quasi-governmental organizations, such as sovereign wealth funds), and organized and motivated consumer groups provide a more informal governance landscape, not enforced by formal sanctions. Rather, it relies on trans-national advocacy groups, third-party monitors and pressures on companies from shareholders, auditors, insurers, and clients.

Second, the development of a global convergence of governance—rules and norms—through the increased interconnectivity of those involved in the global economy and its regulation. A possible implication of this is that this will simply reinforce common interests and forge informal agreements—principally among the powerful. In the global economy, the G8 is an interesting case study in this respect. The G8 represent around 15% of the world population, but 65% of the world's economic output (GDP) and 70% of the world's total military expenditures, including 99% of the world's nuclear weapons. Initially, the group's focus was on macro-economic policy coordination, but the range of topics now covered in the annual meetings include health, law enforcement, labour, economic and social development, energy, environment, foreign affairs, justice, terrorism, and trade. The G8 has no formal authority, rules of operation, or official governance responsibilities. However, it has served as a network within which its members coordinate their policies with palpable benefits. By virtue of its combined economic, military and diplomatic power, the G8 exercises tremendous influence over the multilateral institutions of global governance—the United Nations Security Council, WTO, International Monetary Fund, World Bank, and Organisation for Economic Co-operation and Development (OECD). Although these institutions have formal structures, institutions, responsibilities, etc., this means that they are, in effect, controlled by a group who has no permanent staff, no headquarters, no set of rules governing its operations, and no formal or legal powers.

All of these will affect the policy space within which domestic health systems are (able to be) governed; even apparently benign global initiatives, such as the Millennium Development Goals, generate domestic political repercussions for health systems. It is therefore critical that health becomes skilled in aspects related to global governance contexts and the ability to engage in negotiation at this level to secure the best advantage for population health, as discussed in Chapter 12.

11.3.4 Global environmental changes and health systems

Clearly there are a whole host of environmental issues and concerns, many of which directly affect health and the remainder arguably affecting health eventually as the environment covers the entire ecosystem within which we live. However, in order to make this issue tractable, the most direct impacts arguably derive from climate change.

Climate change is probably the most high profile of all global changes [40]. According to the Intergovernmental panel on Climate Change (IPCC), the last 50 years of the 20th century were likely the warmest of the last 1300 years in the northern hemisphere [41], and the surface of the earth appears to have increased by some 0.6°C in the 20th century. Various climate change models predict that this increase in temperature will continue by another 1.4–5.8°C during the current century [41]. Climate change has been argued to have already caused an increase in the frequency of extreme weather conditions, including droughts, floods, and storms [40]. Climate change threatens health directly, but also indirectly through food and water resources [42,43]. For instance, regional predictions indicate that by 2020 75–250 million people in Africa will be under increased water stress due to climate change, and in some African countries agricultural yields will drop by up to 50%. In Asia, heavily populated coastal areas and mega deltas will be at greatest risk from flooding, which may lead to mass migration of people [41].

The possible health effects of climate change are numerous and diverse [44–46]. Briefly, the associated health effects are of: 1) (change in pattern of) fatalities from natural disasters, such as heatwaves, floods, and droughts; 2) shifts in infectious disease dynamics—many important diseases are highly sensitive to changing temperatures and precipitation (common vector-borne diseases such as malaria and dengue; as well as other major killers such as malnutrition and diarrhoea); 3) lower agricultural yields, which will cause a decrease in cereal production and ocean acidification that will threaten fisheries; and 4) impacts on fresh water supplies—water scarcity, changes in hydrological systems, and the supplies of freshwater [40,43,47–49].

Clearly these possible events pose major challenges to health sector and system development. Indeed, the 61st World Health Assembly, 2008, mandated WHO to engage more actively in the international multi-agency effort to respond to global climate change, and underscored the urgency of adapting health sectors to deal with the health risks of climate change. In this respect, adaptation should be relatively feasible, as climate change does not present wholly new health risks, but rather exacerbates existing ones. In this sense, the health sector is dealing with a known problem, the effects of which will just increase its magnitude. From a policy perspective, it is important for the health sector to engage in both anticipatory and reactive measures, to reduce vulnerability before the impacts of climate change are felt and respond directly when repercussion of climate change are felt [47]. Critical to these will be public health measures to control vector-borne and water-related diseases, and the maintenance of public health infrastructure, including monitoring and surveillance for new and re-emerging diseases [47]. However, also critical will be engagement with the environmental and climate policy processes to ensure that health co-benefits of control are emphasized [50].

11.3.5 Global technological changes and health systems

Technology covers a huge range of developments in the natural sciences, clinical sciences, communication, engineering, etc. Issues emerging from this cover ground from the generation of electricity, through toxic waste to nanotechnology, and personalized medicine, and even the 'space economy'. However, the most critical developments with respect to health are those that affect personalized medicine: information and communication technology, and biotechnology and nanotechnology.

11.3.5.1 Information and communication technology[2]

Here, one of the most interesting developments concerns satellites. In recent years satellite images of disaster zones, such as earthquakes or flooding, have become a key weapon in the arsenal for those fighting humanitarian

---

[2] One of the most obvious global changes that will affect health sectors is the advances in information and communication technology that will support developments in 'e-commerce'; this is covered in Chapter 8.

emergencies, based on the work of agencies such as Télécoms Sans Frontières. Such images compare the terrain before and after a disaster, and pinpoint the location and impact of effects, such as landslides. In this respect, the International Charter 'Space and Major Disasters', is a key commitment by ten space agencies to provide satellite-based data to countries affected by disaster [51].

However, there are other uses of satellites that may have an impact on health sector developments. For example, as a way to predict and monitor the spread of communicable diseases, as a simple means of communication when land-based systems have failed, and as location and navigation aids when global positioning system (GPS) units locate and track public health information. In the outbreak of Rift Valley fever in Kenya (2006–7), for example, GPS units were used to link surveys to a specific place.

More directly, the European Space Agency (ESA) is collaborating with WHO to establish a European user-driven 'Telemedicine via Satellite' programme. Telemedicine is the use of information technology to deliver medical services or information from one location to another, which may generate substantial benefits for rural locations, and engender significant changes in the way in which many health sectors and systems are structured (considered in more detail in Chapter 8). Other direct applications of technological change concern diagnostics and treatment involved in 'personalized medicine', the use of technology to reconstruct body parts, and so forth. What will be implication of technological change for how healthcare is practiced and delivered, and what is demanded and how supplied? For instance, it could mean that technology for diagnosis and treatment will result in a reduced ability for surveillance, resulting in a lack of information on what people have, how it is treated, and, crucially, how they respond to treatment. This would make epidemiology, public health, and infectious disease control more difficult.

11.3.5.2 Biotechnology and nanotechnology

Biotechnology refers to any technological application that uses biological systems, living organisms, or derivatives thereof, to make or modify products or processes for specific use. Nanotechnology refers broadly to a field of applied science and technology whose unifying theme is the control of matter on the atomic and molecular scale, normally 1–100 nanometres, and the fabrication of devices with critical dimensions that lie within that size range. Both of these technologies are at the cutting edge of various scientific disciplines and may herald significant challenges and opportunities for health sectors in the services provided and the way in which they are provided [52].

For example, modern biotechnology finds promising applications in such areas as pharmacogenomics, drug production, genetic testing, and gene therapy. For example, pharmacogenomics is heralded as yielding: 1) the development of tailor-made medicines; 2) more accurate methods of determining appropriate drug dosages; 3) improvements in the drug discovery and approval process; and 4) better vaccines. Genetic testing is now used for: 1) determining gender; 2) carrier screening, or the identification of unaffected individuals who carry one copy of a gene for a disease that requires two copies for the disease to manifest; 3) prenatal diagnostic screening; 4) newborn screening; 5) pre-symptomatic testing for predicting adult-onset disorders; 6) pre-symptomatic testing for estimating the risk of developing adult-onset cancers; 7) confirmational diagnosis of symptomatic individuals; and 8) forensic/ identity testing. Gene therapy is perhaps the most anticipated development which may be used for treating, or even curing, genetic and acquired diseases like cancer and AIDS by using normal genes to replace defective genes or to bolster a normal function such as immunity.

Nanotechnology uses two main approaches: 1) bottom-up, where materials and devices are built from molecular components which assemble themselves chemically by principles of molecular recognition; or 2) top-down, where nano-objects are constructed from larger entities without atomic-level control. In health terms one of the anticipated developments is quantum dots (nanoparticles with quantum confinement properties, such as size-tunable light emission) which, when used in conjunction with MRI (magnetic resonance imaging), can produce exceptional images of tumour sites. These nanoparticles are much brighter than organic dyes and only need one light source for excitation. This means that the use of fluorescent quantum dots could produce a higher contrast image and at a lower cost than today's organic dyes. Another nanoproperty, high surface area to volume ratio, allows many functional groups to be attached to a nanoparticle, which can seek out and bind to certain tumour cells. Additionally, the small size of nanoparticles (10–100 nanometres), allows them to preferentially accumulate at tumour sites (because tumours lack an effective lymphatic drainage system).

Such potential technological developments will undoubtedly be within high-income countries. However, there is potential for 'technology leaps' to be made (as, for instance, with telecommunication, where many countries leaped over the land-line technology and moved straight into mobile technology). One may therefore find health sector planning considering different paths of developments according to the levels of technological availability and foresight.

11.4 **Conclusion**

This chapter has outlined the 'top five' challenges to health that lie outside the traditional health sector remit and control; these concerned aspects related to agriculture, demography, economics and governance, the environment, and technological change. Within each the primary impacts upon health system demand and health sector supply, the major interdependencies, and interconnectedness between these issues were outlined. These problems and the challenges facing health in the 21st century clearly require far more coordination than is possible within the current fragmented, United States/Europe-dominated, system of global governance. Each of these challenges, even if addressed locally or nationally, has the potential to affect the lives of people everywhere. This requires health systems identifying, monitoring, understanding, and acting on such issues of global concern, moving well beyond the health sector. In this respect, the central issue is to identify those areas where there are critical interdependencies between those affected and the issues themselves, where actions relating to an issue are dependent on the actions others.

A significant limitation on health system development with respect to these wider issues of global change is the lack of monitoring of the effect of these issues on health over time. There are several organizations in place that are already monitoring many of the key issues raised, but not with respect to their relationship to population health. For instance, AQUASTAT[3] is the water and agriculture global information system of the Food and Agriculture Organization (FAO),[4] but does not make any links between water and health. Neither does UN-Water.[5] Although the Food Insecurity and Vulnerability Information and Mapping Systems (FIVIMS)[6] uses three indicators to assess the food situation in the world (*Food insecurity*, food *vulnerability*, and *hunger*)[7], it does not monitor the risk of overnutrition. The same is true for bodies that monitor energy, climate change, and population growth.

A primary issue facing the policy and research communities is therefore which institutions or agencies should be in charge of monitoring each of the key five issues identified as they relate to population health. This would involve choosing between persuading the agencies that are currently monitoring the issues to add a health component to their statistical analysis, finding a new agency to monitor the issues with respect to health, or selecting an institution

---

[3] http://www.fao.org/nr/water/aquastat/main/index.stm

[4] http://www.fao.org/

[5] http://www.unwater.org/

[6] http://www.fivims.net/

[7] http://www.fivims.net/

to produce periodic reports on the state of the five issues and their impact on health. Within this there is a clear need to estimate the direction of the causality between the five issues themselves, and then with health. For example, some will predominantly have impacts *on* health, such as water, whereas others may predominantly be influenced *by* health, like demographics. It would also be useful, at the global and national levels to map the five key issues outlined against current activities, in order to identify overlaps and areas for opportunities.

Of course, the aim of anticipating global challenges to health is so health systems may undertake measures to prevent them from happening, alleviate their effects, or generate positive outcomes. The global nature of the issues highlighted in this chapter requires collective action by people from different regions and across different fields of expertise. The policy implications of this include the need for authorities and international health agencies at all levels, from local to global, to engage in a broader approach to improve health. How this may be achieved is discussed in detail in Chapter 12.

References

1 World Health Organization (2008). *Commission on Social Determinants of Health. Closing the gap in a generation: health equity through action on the social determinants of health*. WHO, Geneva. Available at: http://www.who.int/social_determinants/final_report/en/index.html.

2 Loungani P (2005). In defense of globalization. *Journal of International Economics*, **66**, 544–8.

3 Scholte JA (2005). *Globalization: A Critical Introduction*, 2nd edn. Palgrave Macmillan, Basingstoke.

4 Lee K (2003). *Globalisation and health: an introduction*. Palgrave Macmillan, London.

5 Smith RD, Beaglehole R, Woodward D, Drager N (eds) (2003). *Global Public Goods for Health: a health economic and public health perspective*. Oxford University Press, Oxford.

6 Smith RD (2008). *Global change and health: mapping the challenges of global non-healthcare influences on health* (Trade, Foreign Policy, Diplomacy and Health Draft Working Paper Series). World Health Organization, Geneva.

7 Vorley B (2003). *Food, Inc. Corporate Concentration from Farm to Consumer*. IIED, London.

8 FAO (2003). *Trade Reforms and Food Security*. FAO, Rome.

9 FAO (2006). *The State of Food Insecurity in the World*. FAO, Rome.

10 FAO (2006). *Trade Reforms and Food Security: Country Case Studies and Synthesis*. FAO, Rome.

11 Alberini A, Eskeland GS, Krupnick A, McGranahan G (1996). Determinants of diarrhoeal disease in Jakarta. *Water Resources Research*, **32**, 2259–69.

12 Bozkurt AI, Özgür S, Özcirpici B (2003). Association between household conditions and diarrhoeal diseases among children in Turkey: A cohort study. *Paediatrics International*, **45**, 443–51.

13 Dasgupta P (2004). Valuing health damages from water pollution in urban Delhi, India: A health production function approach. *Environment and Development Economics*, **9**, 83–106.

14 WHO (2004). *Water Related Diseases*. WHO, Geneva. Available at: www.who.int/water_ sanitation_heatlh/diseases.

15 Lang T (1997). *The public health impact of globalisation of food trade*. John Wiley & Sons, Chichester.

16 Hawkes C (2006). Uneven dietary development: linking the policies and processes of globalization with the nutrition transition, obesity and diet-related chronic diseases. *Globalization and Health*, 2(1), 4. Available at: http://www.globalizationandhealth.com/ content/2/1/4.

17 Yach D, Hawkes C, Gould CL, Hofman KJ (2004). The global burden of chronic diseases: overcoming impediments to prevention and control. *Journal of the American Medical Association*, **291**, 2616–22.

18 World Health Organization (2005). *Preventing chronic diseases a vital investment*. WHO, Geneva.

19 Wild S, Roglic G, Green A, Sicree R, King H (2004). Global prevalence of diabetes: estimates for 2000 and projections for 2030. *Diabetes Care*, **27**, 1047–53.

20 WHO/FAO Joint WHO/FAO (2003). *Expert Consultation on Diet, Nutrition and the Prevention of Chronic Diseases*. WHO, Geneva.

21 Popkin BM (1998). The nutrition transition and its health implications in lower income countries. *Public Health Nutrition*, **1**, 5–21.

22 Popkin BM (2006). Technology, transport, globalization and the nutrition transition food policy. *Food Policy*, **31**, 569.

23 Gehlhar M, Regmi A (2005). Factors shaping global food markets. In Regmi A, Gehlhar M (eds) *New Directions in Global Food Markets* (Agriculture Information Bulletin Number 294). United States Department of Agriculture, Washington DC.

24 *The Lancet* (2008). Finding long-term solutions to the world food crisis. *Lancet*, **371**, 1389.

25 Bolling C, Somwaru A (2001).US food companies access foreign markets though direct investment. *Food Review*, **24**, 23–8.

26 Hu D, Reardon T, Rozelle S, Timmer P, Wang HL (2004). The emergence of supermar- kets with Chinese characteristics: challenges and opportunities for China's agricultural development. *Development Policy Review*, **22**(5), 557–86.

27 Hawkes C (2005). The role of foreign direct investment in the nutrition transition. *Public Health Nutrition*, **8**(4), 357–65.

28 Escalante de Cruz A (2004). *The Junk Food Generation: A Multi-Country Survey of the Influence of Television Advertisements on Children*. Consumers International, Asia Pacific Office, Kuala Lumpur.

29 Hastings G, Stead M, McDermott L, *et al.* (2003).*Review of Research on the Effects of Food Promotion to Children*. Food Standards Agency, London.

30 Hastings G, McDermott L, Angus K, Stead M, Thomson S (2007). *The Extent, Nature and Effects of Food Promotion to Children: A Review of the Evidence*. WHO, Geneva.

31 Hawkes C (2002). *Marketing activities of global soft drink and fast food companies in emerging markets: a review. Globalization, Diets and Noncommunicable Diseases*. WHO, Geneva. Available at: whqlibdoc.who.int/publications/9241590416.pdf.

32 McGinnis JM, Gootman JA, Kraak VI (2006). *Food Marketing to Children and Youth: Threat or Opportunity?* National Academies Press, Washington, DC.

33 Kaferstein FK (2003). Food safety as a public health issue for developing countries. In Unnevehr L (ed). *Food Safety in Food Security and Food Trade* (2020 Vision Focus 10; Brief 2). IFPRI, Washington, DC.

34 Buzby JC, Unnevehr L (2004). Food safety and international trade. **In** *Food Safety and International Trade - Research Briefs* (Agriculture Information Bulletin No. AIB789). USDA, Washington DC. Available at: http://www.ers.usda.gov/Publications/ aib789/;2004.

35 Josling T, Roberts D, Orden D (2004). *Food Regulation and Trade*. Institute for International Economics, Washington DC.

36 Ataman Aksoy M. (2005). The evolution of agricultural trade flows. In Ataman Aksoy M, and Beghin J C (eds) *Global Agricultural Trade and Developing Countries* pp.17–35 World Bank, Washington, DC.

37 Eastwood R, Lipton M (2001). Demographic transition and poverty: Effects via economic growth, distribution and conversion. In Birdsall N, Kelley AC, Sinding SW (eds) *Population Matters: Demographic Change, Economic Growth, and Poverty in the Developing World*, pp.213–59. Oxford University Press, Oxford.

38 Pimentel D, Huang X, Cordova A, Pimentel M (1997). Impact of population growth on food supplies and environment. *Population & Environment, 19(1)*, 9–14.

39 UNFPA (2007). *The State of the World 2007: Unleashing the Potential of Urban Growth*. Available at: http://www.unfpa.org/swp/2007/presskit/pdf/sowp2007_eng.pdf.

40 Stern NH, Adger WN (2007). *The Economics of Climate Change: The Stern Review*. Cabinet Office HM-Treasury, Cambridge University Press, Cambridge.

41 Intergovernmental Panel on Climate Change (IPCC) (2007). *Climate Change 2007: Impacts*, Adaptation and Vulnerability. Cambridge University Press, Cambridge.

42 Burke EJ, Brown SJ, Christidis N (2006). Modelling the recent evolution of global drought and projections for the twenty-first century with the Hadley Centre climate model. *Journal of Hydrometeorology, 7*, 1113–25.

43 Cairncross S, Valdmanis V (2006). *Water Supply, Sanitation, and Hygiene Promotion. Disease Control Priorities in Developing Countries (2nd Edn)*, pp.771–792. Oxford University Press, New York.

44 McMichael AJ (1997). Integrated assessment of potential health impact of global environmental change: Prospects and limitations. *Environmental Modeling and Assessment, 2*, 129–37.

45 McMichael AJ, Haines A (1997). Global climate change: The potential effects on health. *British Medical Journal, 315*, 805–9.

46 World Health Organization (2008). *Climate Change and Health* (Sixty-first World Health Assembly). WHO, Geneva. Available at: http://www.who.int/gb/ebwha/pdf_ files/A61/A61_R19-en.pdf.

47 McMichael AJ, Campbell-Lendrum DH, Corvalán CF (2003). *Climate Change and Human Health: Risks and Responses*. World Health Organization, Geneva. Available at: http://www.who.int/globalchange/publications/cchhbook/en/.

48 Checkley W, Epstein LD, Gilman RH, *et al.* (2000).Effect of El Niño and ambient temperature on hospital admissions for diarrhoeal diseases in Peruvian children. *Lancet, 355*, 442–50.

49 Kasisi IE (2001). The Impact of water supply in HIV/AIDS transmission in poor people in Africa: The case of East Africa. International Conference on Freshwater, Bonn. Available at: http://www.water-2001.de/datenbank/756523053.36872.4/hiv%20paper-imani.doc.

50 Haines A, McMichael AJ, Smith KR, *et al.* (2009). Public health benefits of strategies to reduce greenhouse-gas emissions: overview and implications for policy makers. *Lancet*, **374**, 2104–14.

51 Wagstaff J (2008). Space technology: a new frontier for public health. *Bulletin of the World Health Organization*, **86**, 87–8.

52 Dittrich PS, Manz A (2000). Lab-on-a-chip: microfluidics in drug discovery. *Nature Reviews Drug Discovery*, **5**, 210–18.

Section 4

The future of health systems

Chapter 12

Global health diplomacy: the 'missing pillar' of health system strengthening

Richard D. Smith and Kara Hanson

12.1 **Introduction**

A common thread throughout this volume has been that the critical aspect of a health *system*, or even the health sector, is the dynamics of the *linkages* between the various constituent elements, not the elements themselves; that a 'system' implies interconnections and interdependences. For example, the delivery of healthcare is subject to pharmaceutical availability, which depends on local price negotiations, but also international legislation and exchange rates. Similarly, changes in food production processes through trade liberalization will affect health and consequently demands on healthcare. This will require those with a health focus to engage with agricultural reforms and policies to target agricultural commodity and food retail prices and other influences over food security, such as food safety, security within the food supply chain, and the balance in the use of agricultural land for biofuels and other 'cash crops' versus nutritional foodstuffs. Another example is the enormous potential for increases in zoonotic outbreaks, which will require health sector involvement in the development of international rules and legislation concerning movement of people, animals, and food products. The reader themselves can no doubt by now add considerably to this list.

Linkages such as these imply a substantive requirement for those with a health remit to engage in negotiation with those from other sectors and from other geographic locations. Yet, as discussed below, this is a 'missing', or neglected, pillar of 'health system strengthening'. This is perhaps understandable, as concerns beyond health (and especially beyond borders) are recent for most of those involved with health sector development; domestic priorities, and those related specifically to the health sector, such as financing, are more familiar, as indicated by earlier chapters. Yet, the pace of change at the global level creates the imperative to move beyond this form of parochialism, to engage with non-health bodies, especially at global policy levels. This chapter outlines the case for investing in such negotiation and diplomacy skills as an imperative for health system strengthening. Following this introduction, we outline why such skills are vital to health system strengthening. The chapter then moves on to briefly review the concept of 'global health diplomacy', and the developments required to equip those within health to minimize the risks and maximize the opportunities that face health system development in low- and middle-income countries (LMICs) in the 21st century.

12.2 **Why negotiation skills are vital to health system strengthening**

Health, systems that affect health, and even health sectors, cannot be improved through an inward focus on the finance, production, and delivery of health-related services. In the contemporary context, those involved in health policy are required to understand, engage, and negotiate with those outside of the domestic health sector. This raises many issues for those within the health profession. For instance, there are aspects related to the technical aspects of negotiation at different levels and within different fora, challenges presented by interacting with those holding different norms and values, and appreciation of alternative views in the negotiation process needed to identify allies and adversaries. Indeed, there may be opportunities for health to act as a 'broker' between areas, such as environment and agriculture, as it is the body most interested in the links or a more holistic approach, and thus targeting the linkages between health and these other sectors could provide the nexus for health involvement.

It is striking then that this role is seldom emphasized within the literature on health systems strengthening. Rather, the discussion tends to focus upon supporting the technical capacity of health service delivery (e.g. infrastructure, workforce, pharmaceuticals). There is usually mention of governance, but this tends also to be related to the domestic health sector, and is not weighted so heavily in discussion, nor does it feature so predominantly in activities, as these other technical areas. Interestingly, however, governance is generally synonymous with the notion of stewardship, concerning 'the careful and responsible management of the well-being of the population' [1; p.2], which according to the definition of health systems adopted in Chapter 1 would imply greater concern with linkages across other sectors and countries.

As Table 12.1 illustrates, engagement in negotiation to secure collaboration and coalition building, across sectors, in order to influence the determinants of health and health service utilization and connect policy, is seen as a key governance function of the health sector. However, it has yet to be advocated as a

Table 12.1 Leadership and governance sub-functions [1]

Sub-function	Tasks
Policy guidance	• Formulating sector strategies and also specific technical policies
	• Defining goals, directions, and spending priorities across services
	• Identifying the roles of public, private, and voluntary actors and the role of civil society
Intelligence and oversight	Ensuring generation, analysis, and use of intelligence on:
	• Trends and differentials in inputs, service access, coverage, safety
	• Responsiveness, financial protection, and health outcomes, especially for vulnerable groups
	• The effects of policies and reforms
	• The political environment and opportunities for action
	• Policy options
Collaboration and coalition building	Across sectors in government and with actors outside government, including civil society, to
	• Influence action on key determinants of health and access to health services
	• Generate support for public policies; keep the different parts connected—so-called 'joined up government'
Regulation	Designing regulations and incentives and ensuring they are fairly enforced
System design	Ensuring a fit between strategy and structure and reducing duplication and fragmentation
Accountability	Ensuring all health system actors are held publicly accountable. Transparency is required to achieve real accountability

key health sector competency which requires strengthening, as illustrated in Chapter 2.

Yet, the policy space within which this aspect of governance now has to operate has expanded considerably to areas beyond the national context, in to regional and global levels; as indicated in Chapter 11. The pace of change, especially at the global level, has affected the ability of national domestic health sectors to set policy and to engage fully in such activities without wider understanding and capacity in negotiation at the international level. This is colloquially termed 'global health diplomacy' [2].

12.3 What is 'global health diplomacy'?

The manner with which the term 'global health diplomacy' is used exhibits diversity, variously emphasizing the tension between health as an instrument of foreign policy and foreign policy as supporting health goals [2-4]. This makes it hard to understand what the term means and whether people are applying it consistently. Further, while some definitions are descriptive, others are more prescriptive, with strong normative claims about the purpose and impact of global health diplomacy [5].

Historically research interest in diplomacy has been centred in the International Relations field. Here diplomacy is broadly defined as the art or practice of conducting international relations, such as (but not exclusively) in negotiating alliances, treaties, and other agreements. It is ostensibly concerned with dialogue and negotiation designed to identify common interests and areas of conflict between parties, guided by a state's foreign policy and undertaken through professional diplomats from ministries of foreign (external) affairs. More recently the term 'new diplomacy' has been applied to the increasingly globalized context, with its associated diverse array of actors, expanded agenda, and the innovative forms and processes by which diplomacy is conducted. In this respect, the focus of global health diplomacy would be on the specific negotiations which underpin aspects related to health and foreign policy or global health governance.

However, a review of the existing (and limited) GHD literature shows that International Relations scholars have been little involved in the development of GHD [6]. Rather, public health advocates have strongly defined the field, leading to the strong normative basis underpinning its use. GHD has been defined thus far by its expected purposes—namely to further foreign policy goals, advocate for global health goals in non-health settings, or to negotiate health-related agreements—rather than what actually characterizes GHD. Nonetheless, there does appear to be agreement that the core feature of GHD is the process of interaction and negotiation that shapes collective responses by state and non-state actors related to global health, such that GHD may be defined as 'policy-shaping processes through which States, intergovernmental organizations, and non-State actors negotiate responses to health challenges or utilize health concepts or mechanisms in policy-shaping and negotiation strategies to achieve other political, economic, or social objectives'.

This definition reflects three important characteristics of GHD:

1 *Global* refers not only to geographical meaning, but the range of actors involved.

2 *Health* draws attention to problems that involve the protection or promotion of population health, arising either as: (i) a direct threat to human health; (ii) an indirect threat to health; or (iii) unrelated to health but stimulating a health-related response.

3 *Diplomacy* refers to processes in which all actors interact in articulating, advocating for, and defending their interests. Diplomacy is not an end: it is a means to an end.

12.4 Who engages in global health diplomacy?

In recent years the conduct of 'new diplomacy' has been shaped by the greater participation of non-state actors in international relations. While diplomats have traditionally been concerned primarily with interacting with their counterparts, increasingly their constituencies are far more broadly based. In quantitative terms, there are more players, problems, and processes implicated today than in previous eras. This proliferation is part of what makes global health diplomacy difficult to contain descriptively and analytically. In qualitative terms, States increasingly have to deal with non-State actors, and the venues for diplomacy also reveal an unprecedented diversity. The 'pecking order' amongst the traditional actors has therefore been upset and destabilized by the rise of powerful and influential non-State actors, with two important trends.

First, major States, particularly the United States, have re-engaged in global health in significant ways in the post-Cold War period. International health constituted a marginal, neglected area in the foreign policies of major countries during the Cold War era, but, across many agendas and for diverse reasons, these countries have realized the need to focus more on global health concerns. Moreover, the BRIC (Brazil, Russia, India, and China) countries have also developed interests in global health (see Box 12.1). The re-engagement of major States has mixed results for global health diplomacy. On one hand, it raises the political significance of global health problems generally. On the other, they have a degree of independence in their actions that allows them to have significant influence in diplomatic processes [7]. However, it is clear that health policy is increasingly being used as tool of foreign policy and diplomacy by states to further other aspects of their foreign policy agendas. In a sense, this resembles the older imperial motivations of self-interest and humanitarianism that characterized the colonial period, but with a new twist of globalization. Health sectors need to be aware also of this use of the domain of health, and how this may affect their population's health and their abilities in the provision of healthcare to their own or other populations. The current focus on health issues as linked to national security has also raised health from low to high politics, and this has implications for those engaged in the pursuit of health objectives [8,9].

Second, the power now wielded in global health by the Gates Foundation represents an epochal change in terms of the actors in global health. Many

Box 12.1 Global health diplomacy case study: Brazil and the Framework Convention on Tobacco Control

The BRIC countries (Brazil, Russia, India, and China) have been identified as becoming the world's leading economies during the 21st century, expected to overtake the current wealthiest nations as the world's richest by sometime around 2050. As such, they have generated great interest, not just in terms of their economic and military might, but also in the power that emanates from their scale of development, technology, education, and health sector developments; especially in how these are brought to bear on the world stage. Of interest within the context of this chapter is how these countries use their increasing profile to enact what is termed 'soft power'; that which utilizes co-option and attraction rather than coercion and payment ('hard power') [20].

In this sense, Brazil has been an active global citizen in the use of soft power for health concerns, beginning with negotiations on access to medicines for treatment of HIV/AIDS which pitched it against the World Trade Organization and the more developed nations who supported the adoption of the Agreement on Trade-Related Aspects of Intellectual Property Rights (TRIPS). More recently, Brazil used soft power in the negotiation of the Framework Convention on Tobacco Control (FCTC), which has been highlighted as a prototypical example of global health diplomacy [21].

Lee et al. demonstrate through their analysis that Brazil demonstrated consistent commitment to global health diplomacy by serving as an 'exemplar' for domestic tobacco control, engaging in coalition politics, and providing leadership throughout the negotiation process. They chart how the former coordinator of the Brazilian National Tobacco Control Programme led the WHO's Tobacco Free Initiative (TFI), and Brazilian diplomats chaired the Intergovernmental Negotiating Body for the FCTC. On the domestic level, Brazil's National Tobacco Control Programme implemented many innovations in advertising and regulations, which created added gravitas when set in the context of Brazil as one of the biggest producers and exporters of tobacco. The Inter-Ministerial National Commission on the Control of Tobacco Use established in 1999 was backed by nine ministries, including Trade and Development, Agriculture, and Foreign Affairs, which ensured that this issue was seen as more than of just a health system concern. This coalition building was subsequently extended to civil society and non-governmental organizations (NGOs) at domestic, regional, and global levels, and culminated in a broad coalition of developing countries and NGOs to resist efforts by industry and several wealthy countries to oppose the FCTC [22].

Lee et al. conclude that 'a new kind of diplomacy is emerging to achieve collective action on shared challenges such as global health', and that 'Brazil's remarkable example also suggests that engagement in health diplomacy is increasingly seen as a core component of what it means to be a global citizen' [21; p.4].

have raised concerns about the influence the Gates Foundation possesses, influence directly related to the unprecedented funding the Foundation commits to global health endeavours. The non-governmental status of the Gates Foundation, lack of accountability to external bodies, and the scale of the financial resources it has available, gives it the ability to manoeuvre in global health diplomacy largely on its own terms [10]. While governments are tasked with agreeing priorities and negotiating agreements to protect and promote health, as formal representatives of their domestic constituencies, the process and outcomes related to these tasks are influenced by the decisions of non-state actors which are not similarly accountable.

12.5 What does GHD mean for health system development?

The sort of challenges to health systems identified in this volume—direct and indirect—appear across a wide range of political, economic, and social phenomena, and, as a result, intersect with foreign policy and diplomatic activities. This broad scope means that global health diplomacy occurs on many types of problems, involves a diverse collection of actors, takes place in multiple venues, and produces different kinds of collective action outcomes. There is growing interest in the relationship between health and foreign policy and in the dynamics of global health diplomacy at the global level [8,11,12]. However, it is also important that national health actors seize the initiative in the development of capacity in this area [13]. In this respect there are four facets to global health diplomacy of importance: the *topics* to which global health diplomacy is applied, the *actors* involved, the *process*, and the *outcome*.

With respect to the first of these, the principal interest is how health-related problems are identified for diplomatic activities: what is put on the agenda, by whom, how, and why. Countries can be proactive in their pursuit of items on the global agenda, but they also must understand, and hence respond to, those representing the health affairs of other countries or those outside the health fraternity. Here, the health sector needs to undertake surveillance of the frequency of foreign policy, diplomatic, and advocacy activities on health-related problems, providing a sense of the problems that actors prioritize, and comparing these with, for example, evidence about the burdens of disease. For instance, in recent years communicable disease has been considered a global priority in foreign policy, for largely security and trade reasons, but with implications for national health sectors in their involvement in disease surveillance and preparedness plans [14,15]. At various others times, there are concerns and initiatives concerning areas such as tobacco, alcohol, obesity-related diseases, road traffic injuries, and counterfeit pharmaceuticals, as Box 12.1 illustrates. It is highly likely also that the distribution of power in this globalized environment affects the agenda, as does the incidence of the related costs and benefits [16].

With respect to the second facet, once issues are on the agenda the influence and behaviour of different participants in negotiations concerned with global health and other agreements becomes critical to understand; what actors are involved and why they behave as they do illuminates how global health diplomacy occurs. For instance, how different states approach and influence global health diplomacy (e.g. as a donor or recipient country for development assistance) will be important in determining (and reflecting) power relations, forms of power exerted and the success of these, how the non-state actors are aligned and so forth, as Box 12.1 illustrates [16].

In terms of the third facet, the *processes* and the fora (e.g. World Economic Forum) through which foreign policy, diplomatic, and advocacy activities on health occur, understanding them, and their strengths and weaknesses as platforms for health-related diplomacy and collective action, will deepen appreciation and understanding of the complexities of foreign policy, diplomatic, and advocacy activities on health. These processes might include how countries organize themselves to participate in global health diplomacy, on both bilateral and regional bases, and form negotiating 'blocs'. It may also include the relationship between health systems and regional and global bodies, such as those associated with the World Health Organization (WHO). In addition, a range of different forms of collective action for health system development exist, for instance binding treaties (e.g. WHO Framework Convention on Tobacco Control), 'soft law' instruments (e.g. Millennium Development Goals; International Code on Marketing of Breast-Milk Substitutes), new institutions (e.g. Global Fund to Fight AIDS, Tuberculosis, and Malaria), and norms (e.g. authorization for the WHO Director-General to declare the existence of public health emergencies of international concern in the International Health Regulations 2005), as illustrated in Box 12.1.

Finally, it is critical to establish the effectiveness of any engagement with global health diplomacy in terms of securing the desired *outcome:* how well global health diplomacy functions to 'improve the protection and promotion of health'. In this respect, health sectors should generate measures most appropriate to their specific needs and the form of global health diplomacy at hand.

One area of global health diplomacy where the health community, both at WHO level and specific countries, has gained experience in working effectively outside the traditional health sector is in international trade. Box 12.1 discusses this in relation to global tobacco trade, but there are many other examples concerning access to medicines, health worker migration, and medical tourism, where country health systems have directly engaged with those in commerce and foreign affairs. For instance, there have been significant and intense international negotiations concerning a global system for virus sharing and access to resultant vaccines under the auspices of the WHO Intergovernmental Meeting process and discussed at the Sixty-second World Health Assembly, 2009 [17]. The issues raised in this forum clearly affect LMICs in their ability to access essential vaccines, and yet the process has been fraught and separated from the International Health Regulations process. Another health sector issue of high profile has been the WHO Code on the Ethical Recruitment of Health Personnel, the negotiations for which have resulted in a voluntary and very 'soft' statement of desire, which is also of great import to LMICs. Somewhat differently, 2009 also saw the rise on the global health agenda of global rules concerning marketing of food-products to children, following a resolution at the 2007 World Health Assembly (WHA60.23) calling for responsible marketing. The negotiations concerning this issue promise to be as intense, if not more so, than those concerning tobacco in the 1990's. Many of these areas are covered in more detail in Chapter 8, but the diplomatic aspects related to each may provide valuable lessons for health engagement in global health diplomacy more widely. These include the importance of mutual awareness and knowledge between domains, understanding key international regimes, exploiting common principles to achieve coherency (e.g. use of scientific evidence, non-discriminatory measures), investment in interagency or intra-government coordinating mechanisms, and responsiveness to crisis. However, plans for long-term capacity, including significant training and education for health personnel in these issues are rarely institution and/or prioritized.

12.6 **The domestic negotiation context**

Many of the issues raised above concerning the need for the health sector to engage more effectively with other sectors internationally apply equally to the national or domestic level, where opportunities exist to collaborate to address the health impacts of non-health actions, and to use health concepts to shape policies to achieve broader economic and social objectives. These opportunities challenge health sector decision-makers to develop new skills in analysis, advocacy, and negotiation. This can be seen in two examples.

First, as health sectors become increasingly pluralistic, there is a need for governments to strengthen their dialogue with private sector interests in order to assure population health. The scope of interaction may remain within the health sector, include expanding the scope of regulation (a 'stewardship' function) to achieve greater control over private pharmaceutical supply or private healthcare providers; it may include more collaborative interactions such as partnerships in tuberculosis treatment or retail distribution of public health products; or may, indeed, require forging new relationships with private actors outside the health sector, such as with the agriculture (e.g. food policy) or transport (road safety) industries. Relationships with the private health sector have been particularly fraught because of a history of mutual mistrust and perceived lack of shared values and norms. However, developing the skills to negotiate with private sector actors would seem to provide clear benefit to population health.

A second example is the process of negotiating annual budget allocations to the health sector. The challenge that many African countries have faced in securing the Abuja target of 15% of the government budget for health is evidence of the relatively weak position of health ministries in budget negotiations. Ministries of Finance may find themselves constrained overall by macroeconomic conditions and also by the influence of international actors such as the International Monetary Fund; but the analytical and advocacy skills of individual line ministries will influence sectoral allocations. The capacity of planning and budgeting units in health ministries is often limited, particularly with respect to the skills needed to make the *economic* argument for investing in health, accompanied by a persuasive analysis of the costs and consequences (both health and broader non-health) of increased health sector spending [18]. Once armed with evidence, health sector negotiators need to find a common language with which to communicate with finance ministries and identify opportunities to interact with their officials in order to make their case.

12.7 **Conclusion**

The broad nature of the linkages between sectors and countries which constitutes a contemporary, 21st century, 'health system', as defined in Chapter 1, requires collective action by people from different regions and across different fields of expertise. Critically, it requires health professionals to be involved in various degrees and levels of governance, negotiation, and diplomacy [2].

The policy implications of this include the need for local, national, regional, and global authorities and health agencies to engage in a broader approach to improve health. Currently, most efforts to improve health are concentrated on the treatment of, and to a lesser extent prevention of, diseases. Yet even here, as demonstrated in this volume, there are effects on the domestic health sector of the expanding number of actors, requiring a range of new skills and capacities to negotiate. For instance, the regulation of sales of medicines is not just a medical issue but also one of business regulation, yet typical health sector experience and ability to influence regulation and influence this area of business policy making is limited. The limitations of health sectors' skills and influence are even more pronounced once one moves beyond typical health sector concerns, such as to transport and economic growth.

On the international level, global threats to health must also be addressed by international health authorities and agencies, such as WHO. These agencies should focus more on the global-level issues and take a wider approach to improving health. In doing so, they should recognize the global nature of some of the most important determinants of health. They should engage in the necessary activities to ensure that water, food, energy, climate change, and population growth are addressed globally, in order to avoid the potential threats they pose to health worldwide. This will require a diplomatic effort, for which international agencies are best equipped. Indeed, it has been suggested that WHO should develop a 'Committee C'[1] to provide a forum for debate about major health initiatives by WHO Member States and non-WHO organizations, including international agencies, philanthropic organizations, multinational health initiatives, and representatives from major civil-society groups [19]. It would provide an opportunity to address coordination of initiatives and partners, and thus a venue and focal point for global health diplomacy.

Nonetheless, at the local level there is a critical role for national health sectors that goes beyond merely describing how health concerns are global problems; in the world of foreign policy, health's importance is not self-evident or necessarily robust in the face of other priorities. In this respect, negotiation and diplomacy skills are the 'missing pillar' of the health system strengthening discussion. Health actors need new skills, capacities, and insights in this area to be able to operate domestically and internationally if they are to fully protect and promote the health of their populations in the face of the global changes facing the world in the 21st century.

---

[1] Currently the World Health Assembly prepares resolutions and decisions to be taken in two main committees: committee A dealing with programme matters, and committee B with budget and managerial concerns.

References

1 World Health Organization (2000). *The World Health Report 2000. Health systems: improving performance.* WHO, Geneva.

2 Kickbusch I, Silberschmidt G, Buss P (2007). Global health diplomacy: the need for new perspectives, strategic approaches and skills in global health. *Bulletin of the World Health Organization*, **85**, 230–2.

3 Bond K (2008). Commentary: health security or health diplomacy? Moving beyond semantic analysis to strengthen health systems and global cooperation. *Health Policy and Planning*, **23**, 376–8.

4 Adams V, Novotny TE, Leslie H (2008). Global health diplomacy. *Medical Anthropology*, **27**, 315–23.

5 Feldbaum H, Michaud J (2010). Health diplomacy and the enduring relevance of foreign policy interests. *PLoS Medicine* 7(4).

6 Lee K (2009). *Health and International Relations: A review of the literature* (Trade, Foreign Policy, Diplomacy and Health Draft Working Paper Series). World Health Organization, Geneva.

7 Gómez E (2009). The politics of receptivity and resistance: How Brazil, India, China, and Russia strategically used the international health community in response to HIV/AIDS: A theory. *Global Health Governance*, 3(1).

8 Horton R (2007). Health as an instrument of foreign policy. *Lancet* **369**, 806–7.

9 Fidler DP (2005). *Conceptual overview of the relationship between health and foreign policy.* Academy Health in Foreign Policy Forum, Washington DC.

10 McCoy D, Kembhavi G, Patel J, Luintel A (2009). The Bill and Melinda Gates Foundation's grant-making programme for global health. *Lancet*, **373**, 1645–53.

11 Ministers of Foreign Affairs (of Brazil, France, Indonesia, Norway, Senegal, South Africa and Thailand) (2007). Oslo Ministerial Declaration—global health: a pressing foreign policy issue of our time. *Lancet*, **369**, 1373–8.

12 Fidler DP, Drager N (2006). Health and foreign policy. *Bulletin of the World Health Organization*, **84**, 687.

13 Chan M, Støreb JG, Kouchnerc B (2008). Foreign policy and global public health: working together towards common goals. *Bulletin of the World Health Organization*, **86**, 498.

14 Shiffman J (2009). A social explanation for the rise and fall of global health issues. *Bulletin of the World Health Organization*, **87**, 608–13.

15 Shiffman J, Smith S (2007). Generation of political priority for global health initiatives. *Lancet*, **370**, 1370–1379.

16 Smith RD (2010). The role of economic power in influencing the development of global health governance. *Global Health Governance*, III(2). Available at: http://www.ghgj.org.

17 WHO Intergovernmental Meeting process and discussed at the Sixty-second World Health Assembly, 2009 http://apps.who.int/gb/ebwha/pdf_files/A62/A62_5Add1-en.pdf

18 Center for Global Development (2007). *Does the IMF constrain health spending in poor countries? Evidence and an agenda for action. Report of the Working Group on IMF Programs and Health Spending.* Center for Global Development, Washington DC.

19 Silberschmidt G, Matheson D, Kickbusch I (2008). Creating a committee C of the World Health Assembly. *Lancet*, **371**, 1483–6.

20 Nye JS (1990). Soft power. *Foreign Policy*, **80**, 153–71.

21 Lee K, Chagas LC, Novotny TE (2010). Brazil and the Framework Convention on Tobacco Control: Global Health Diplomacy as Soft Power. *PLoS Med* **7**(4), e1000232.

22 Alcazar S (2008). *The WHO Framework Convention on Tobacco Control: A case study of foreign policy and health–A view from Brazil*. Graduate Institute of International and Development Studies, Geneva. Available at: http://graduateinstitute.ch/webdav/site/globalhealth/shared/1894/Working%20Papers_002_Alcazar%20WEB.pdf (accessed 14 December 2009).

Index